THE 20/30
FAT & FIBER
DIET PLAN

The 20/30 Fat & Fiber Diet Plan

By Gabe Mirkin, M.D.
and Barry Fox, Ph.D.

Recipes by Diana Mirkin

A Stonesong Press and LINX Book
HarperCollins*Publishers*

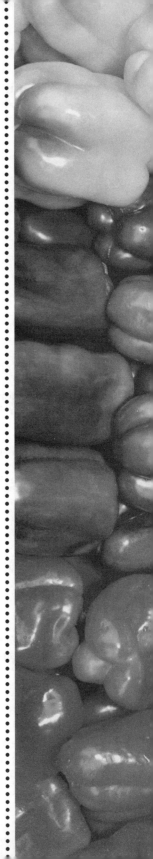

We dedicate this book to Vera Mirkin, who has inspired us with her great spirit and longevity; to Diana's children, Peter, Matthew, Amy, and Chris, and Gabe's children, Gene, Jan, Jill, Geoff, and Kenny.

— **Gabe Mirkin**, M.D.

To Dad, forever young
Thanks to my wife, Nadine, who makes all things possible

— **Barry Fox**, Ph.D.

Copyright © 1998 by The Stonesong Press, Inc. and LINX Corp.
All rights reserved. Published by HarperCollins

No part of this publication may be reproduced in any manner whatsoever without the written permission of the publisher. For information regarding permission, write to HarperCollins Publishers, Inc., 10 East 53rd Street, New York, NY 10022.

Library of Congress Cataloging-in-Publication Data
Mirkin, Gabe.
The 20/30 Fat & Fiber Diet Plan / Gabe Mirkin and Barry Fox.
p.   cm.
ISBN 0-06-270232-7
1. Low-fat diet.   2. High-fiber diet   3. Weight loss.   I. Fox, Barry II. Title
RM237. 7. M549   1999
613.2 63—dc21   98-38136
                                                          CIP

First Edition

10 9 8 7 6 5 4 3 2 1

Designed by Sophia Latto
Photographs Copyright 1998 © PhotoDisc Inc.

Consult your physician before beginning **The 20/30 Fat & Fiber Diet Plan** or any exercise program. Certain medical conditions may be aggravated by diet or exercise, and the material in this book is not intended to replace the advice of a qualified medical professional.

■ TABLE OF CONTENTS

Introduction vii

Chapter One — Counting Your Way to Health 1

Chapter Two — The 20/30 Rationale 9

Chapter Three — Preventing Disease the 20/30 Way 25

Chapter Four — Phytochemicals: The "Medicines" in Foods 41

Chapter Five — Playing For Better Health 47

Chapter Six — High-Fiber, Low-Fat Flavor 63

Chapter Seven — Setting Up For a Slim New You 75

Chapter Eight — The Two-Step Secret To Success 83

Chapter Nine — Low-Fat, High-Fiber Recipes 93

     Recipe Notes 94

     Spices & Special Sauces 98

     Soups 100

     Salads 110

     Entrees 120

     Side Dishes 136

     Snacks 140

     Desserts 145

Chapter Ten — Food Lists 151

     Food List Notes 152

     Beverages 154

     Breakfast Foods & Cereals 160

     Condiments & Sauces 168

     Diary Products 175

     Desserts, Toppings & Baking Ingredients 189

     Fast Foods 198

Fats, Oils & Salad Dressings 211

Fish & Shellfish 214

Fruits 217

Grains & Grain Products 220

Meat & Poultry 232

Prepared Entrees 238

Seasonings 251

Snack Foods 253

Soups 271

Sweetners 276

Vegetables & Beans 278

Notes 285

Index 291

◤ INTRODUCTION

In the midst of an epidemic of obesity and fat-related diseases, *The 20/30 Fat & Fiber Diet Plan* is a hard-hitting, no-nonsense, easy-to-follow solution that has helped thousands lose weight permanently and regain their health.

We can unequivocally tell you that this approach works! It's based on an earlier program Dr. Mirkin presented in his book titled *The 20 Gram Diet*. A best-seller, the book focused on fat consumption, urging people to eat less than 20 fat grams per day. Over forty thousand people following the program have written to tell us how delighted they are. Here are just a few of their comments:

> *"This is the best program I have ever been on (and I've been on them all)."*
> — *CC, Springfield, VA*

> *"It's habit forming and delicious!"*
> — *LB, Oakland, NJ*

> *"I have lost nearly 70 pounds. I feel great and look better than I have in years."*
> — *GV, Bethesda, MD*

> *"It has inspired me to change my eating habits."*
> — *KG, Greensboro, NC*

Now, with research trumpeting the benefits of fiber, we've improved the program by helping you keep track of the fiber you will be eating every day. It's based on the same great diet, backed with the latest scientific information showing that it works and demonstrating that foods you'll be eating are full of the vitamins, minerals, and phytochemicals that help ward off disease and keep you vibrantly healthy.

This is not a theoretical program devised by an ivory-tower scientist who never deals with people. Although it's based on the latest scientific research, the plan has grown out of years of experience with real people facing the same difficulties you are in fighting the "battle of the bulge" and struggling to remain healthy. At last—the safe and sane answer to a hefty problem that has plagued us far too long.

For more information about *The 20/30 Fat & Fiber Diet Plan* visit our Web site at www.2030Plan.com. ∎

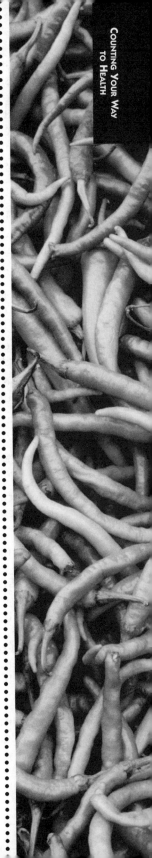

COUNTING YOUR WAY TO HEALTH

Quite a bit has changed in the American diet in the past several decades. We used to dine in steak houses, feasting on fatty prime rib, baked potatoes buried under mountains of sour cream, and pies slathered with whipped cream. Nobody worried too much if they were overweight or ate the wrong foods, and only exercise fanatics worked out. But today we line up at salad bars and flock to gyms. We fret that we'll develop heart disease or cancer if we eat fatty foods. And more than ever, we want to be slim. There is a stigma in our culture attached to those who are obese. Slim folk, on the other hand, are generally considered healthy, successful, and attractive. And we've taken this message to heart: at any given time, some 40 percent of women and almost a quarter of men are on diets.

Yet, despite our national obsessions with healthful eating, dieting, fitness and thinness, we're not slimmer and healthier than before. In fact, we're even *heavier*. The statistics are alarming:

- The average American adult has put on eight pounds in the past ten years
- The incidence of obesity in adults has increased from one in four to one in three[1] in the past decade.
- Adolescent obesity has increased by a whopping 40 percent since 1980.[2]
- Despite the "fitness craze," we burn over 200 calories a day *less* than people did thirty years ago.

The discouraging and frightening result: obesity in the United States has taken on epidemic proportions, and there's no end in sight.

Obesity has traditionally been defined as being at least 20 percent above the recommended weight limit for your height, frame size, and sex. In June 1998, two divisions of the National Institutes of Health issued new guidelines, using the Body Mass Index (BMI) to help us determine whether or not we're obese. The BMI, which works the same for men and women, measures the relationship between height and weight. It's not a perfect tool; heavily muscled football players or weight lifters, for example, may register as being obese according to the BMI, even though they have little fat on their bodies. For most of us, however, the BMI is a good indicator of our "fat status."

According to the latest guidelines, those with BMIs over 25 are overweight, and are classified as obese once their BMI hits 30. There's a table showing a range of BMIs in Chapter Five. Here are some quick numbers to give you an idea of what constitutes being overweight:

- If you stand 5 feet 1 inch and weigh 132 pounds...
- If you stand 5 feet 4 inches and weigh 145 pounds...
- If you stand 5 feet 7 inches and weigh 159 pounds...
- If you stand 5 feet 10 inches and weigh 174 pounds...
- If you stand 6 feet 1 inch and weigh 189 pounds...

...your BMI is 25 and you are overweight. About ninety-seven million American adults fall into this category.[3] Unfortunately, it doesn't take many more pounds to move from the overweight to the obese category:

- If you stand 5 feet 1 inch and weigh 158 pounds...
- If you stand 5 feet 4 inches and weigh 174 pounds...
- If you stand 5 feet 7 inches and weigh 191 pounds...
- If you stand 5 feet 10 inches and weigh 209 pounds...[4]
- If you stand 6 feet 1 inch and weigh 227 pounds...

...your BMI has hit 30 and you're obese. And adults aren't the only ones with girth problems. Sadly, one quarter of our children are already obese, and many of them will never know what it's like to be in the peak of health. Obesity is a "package deal," full of unwanted "bonuses" such as an increased risk of heart disease and stroke, high blood pressure, elevated cholesterol, osteoarthritis, adult-onset diabetes, and cancer (especially of the breast, prostate, colon, and uterus). The statistics quite clearly show that being obese increases your odds of dying early. That's right—carrying too much body fat can actually kill you! If you are more than 30 percent overweight, your odds of dying early shoot up by 42 percent (compared to persons of normal weight).[4] All told, an estimated three hundred thousand deaths each year are directly related to obesity. The new overweight and obesity guidelines issued by the National Institutes of Health note that obesity is the second leading cause of preventable death in the United States today. (Smoking is number one.)

Too Much and Too Little

Why are we continually growing heavier? The answer is simple: we eat too much fat and not enough fiber. Let's begin with our fat intake. The average American takes in 85 grams of fat per day, the equivalent of about one half cup of butter—and many of us consume even more than that. The fat that we feed ourselves makes our bodies fat in several ways:

1. *Fat is the most concentrated form of calories, so it's easy to gobble down more than your body needs without knowing it.* One piece of pecan pie tops off your dinner with a hefty 575 calories, a taco salad from Wendy's packs a whopping 640 calories, and

Boston Market's Chunky Chicken Salad Sandwich with mayo and dijon serves up a gut-busting 980 calories! That's because they're all extremely high in fat: 32 grams of fat in the pecan pie, 30 grams in the taco salad, and an incredible 65 grams in the chicken salad sandwich! Most of us could probably eat an entire portion of these foods without feeling too uncomfortable because the concentrated calories from fat don't take up much space in the stomach. The unfortunate result: we can pack away large amounts of fatty foods with ease.

2. *The fat on your plate is easily converted to body fat.* Calories come in the form of fat, protein, carbohydrate, and alcohol. Every single excess calorie we take in is used to make fatty tissue, but it's easier for the body to turn the fat from food into body fat. The body "spends" about 30 calories converting 100 calories of carbohydrate or protein to body fat, but it takes only about 5 calories to convert 100 calories of dietary fat to body fat.

3. *Fatty foods usually don't have much fiber, so you don't feel full.* You could probably eat a regular-sized order of French fries (300 calories, 14 grams of fat) and still have room for more. But to get the same amount of calories by eating a low-fat, high-fiber food like barley (100 calories, 0 grams of fat and 5 grams of fiber per cup), you'd have to eat almost three cups. Most likely, you'd be full long before you get through half a cupful.

As for fiber, we have the opposite problem: we don't eat nearly enough. The average fiber intake in the United States is only about 10–15 grams per day. You get much more on ***The 20/30 Fat & Fiber Diet Plan***, which encourages you to eat unlimited amounts of fruits, vegetables, whole grains, and beans.

- High-fiber foods are bulky, so they fill you up and leave you feeling satisfied for a long time.

- High-fiber foods take a long time to digest. This means that their sugars are released slowly into your bloodstream, preventing sharp rises and falls in blood sugar and ensuring that you have plenty of energy throughout the day.

- Fiber adds bulk to your stool, speeding the transit time of undigested wastes through your lower intestines. This rapid passage helps prevent constipation, irritable bowel syndrome and other digestive problems, and colon cancer.

- Fiber lowers cholesterol by binding up bile acids, the building blocks of cholesterol, and carrying them out of the body.

Many people embarking on weight-loss programs know that they should cut back on their fat consumption, and they do so. Unfortunately, they tend to replace the fat on their plates with refined carbohydrates and sugar, or special "low-fat" foods. Simply eating low-fat foods is not enough, for they are usually composed of carbohydrates that have had the fiber stripped away (for example, the refined flour in pastries). In other words, they're stuffed with the calories that cling to the waistline, but none of the fiber that cuts down on overall consumption by giving a comfortable feeling of fullness. As a result, these dieters often take in *even more calories than before*. It's no wonder they can't lose weight—and that sometimes they wind up even heavier. The key to safe and permanent weight loss is to reduce fat consumption *and* eat more fiber.

It's easy to increase your fiber intake with a few little changes: eat the whole fruit instead of drinking the juice; use whole grains in place of white rice, pasta, or bread; reach for whole grain cereal instead of refined cereal; put beans on your plate rather than meat or chicken; limit your intake of processed foods and animal products (the latter of which never have any fiber.)

There Is a Way to Lose Weight Permanently

The evidence is clear: the only way to lose weight permanently, without risking your health, is to cut back on your fat intake while eating more fiber. Years of experience with patients and people from all walks of life have shown this to be true. The *20/30 Plan* is simple, satisfying, and easy-to-follow. It has been successfully used by thousands of people, male and female, young and old, all over North America. There are just five simple rules to start:

1) Eat all the fruits, vegetables, whole grains, and beans that you want.

2) Eat no more than 20 grams of fat per day (see ☺ on page 6).

3) Eat at least 30 grams of dietary fiber each day.

4) Limit foods made with refined flour, and other low-fiber foods.

5) Reward yourself. If you follow the program faithfully for nineteen out twenty-one meals, enjoy two "free" meals. Have reasonable-sized portions of anything you want (but don't binge and stuff yourself).

Following these guidelines you don't have to buy special diet foods, skip meals, drink your lunch from a can, or measure your portions. You can eat when you're hungry and keep eating until you feel satisfied. All the foods you enjoy, every single food you can think of, is included in the plan. Use the food lists in Chapter Ten to help you select your foods. You'll find that each item is marked with a convenient symbol:

☺ means you can eat all you want of these low-fat, high-fiber foods, *even after you've reached your 20 grams of fat limit for the day.* The foods in this category—fruits, vegetables, whole grains, and beans—should comprise the bulk of your diet. They're loaded with fiber, vitamins, minerals, phytochemicals (described in Chapter Four), and water, but are low in fat. (A few fruits, such as avocados and coconuts, are listed as foods to avoid because they are relatively high in fat.)

👍 indicates items such as spices and seasonings that have fewer than 10 calories per serving. Although not nutritional standouts, seasonings, spices, and condiments help make food taste good, and some contain helpful phytochemicals. Use them as often as you like.

✂ means you should cut way back on these foods. Although low in fat they also lack fiber, so they don't fill you up. Pasta, bread, fat-free cookies and chips, sugar, juices, soft drinks, alcoholic beverages—in fact, all fat-free but low-fiber foods made from refined grains and refined sugars—should be used only occasionally, for variety. Select the ones that are important to you, and cut back to no more than two to three servings (100 calories each) per day. Seafood and fat-free dairy products contain some important nutrients, but no fiber to fill you up. Limit your dairy servings to two to three per day, and your seafood to two to three servings per week. If you want to follow *The 20/30 Plan* as a strict vegetarian, you can substitute soy milk or other vegetarian sources to make sure you get adequate amounts of vitamin B12, calcium, and vitamin D.

💣 is reserved for the foods that should be avoided, for they have more than 2 grams of fat per serving. But you needn't give them up completely. Remember, if you follow the program for nineteen meals a week, you can have whatever you like for the other two, including foods marked with the 💣.

Keeping Track with the Key Chain Counter

The fat and fiber wheels on the "gram counter" key chain that came with this book will help you keep track of your daily intake of fat and fiber. Begin each day by setting the Fat Counter and Fiber Counter to zero. Use the food counts in Chapter Ten to tally up the fat grams you eat at breakfast, then turn to the corresponding number on the dial. Every time you eat something, add the fat grams to your running total. When you reach 20 grams, you've consumed your daily fat allotment. The Fiber Counter works the same way. But with fiber there is no limit. Instead, you want to reach, and preferably exceed, 30 grams per day.

It's as easy as that. Simply limit your fat and increase your fiber intake. When you do, you will lose weight safely, improve your overall health, and lower your chances of developing the major life-threatening illnesses that strike us down.

Beware the Fat-free Food Hype

There are numerous low-fat or fat-free pastries, snacks, or other foods available these days, but don't be swayed by their "good health" hype. Most of these foods are filled with empty calories—refined flour and sugar with little or no nutritional value. They have very little fiber, and even though they may help you cut down to 20 grams of fat per day, they still have plenty of calories—and all excess calories consumed are converted to fat. So we recommend that you count each 100-calorie serving of a low-fat, low-fiber food as 2 grams of fat on your daily fat counter, as a way of limiting the amount of these foods you eat. (You can defeat *The 20/30 Plan* by eating these fat-free foods. Remember that even if its fat has been removed, junk food is still junk food.)

Menu Planning

When planning your daily or weekly menus, remember that variety is key. Yes, you can meet the less-than-20 and more-than-30-gram rules for fat and fiber by eating the same few foods over and over again. But while consuming nothing but apples and barley all day long may technically fulfill the requirements of the program it's not a good idea, for no single food or small group of foods contains all the nutrients and phytochemicals you need for optimal health. (See Chapter Four for a discussion of the health-enhancing phytochemicals in foods.) Here are some simple ideas for planning your meals.

- *For breakfast*, try whole grains or whole-grain cereal, nonfat milk or nonfat yogurt, and fruit.
- *For lunch*, choose two or three of the following:
  - fruit salad
  - green salad and raw vegetables
  - bean/vegetable/whole grain casserole, soup, or salad (prepared with nonfat ingredients)
  - baked potato with salsa
  - nonfat yogurt
  - whole grains or whole wheat pasta
  - fat-free canned or instant soup
  - tuna fish (packed in water) with fat-free mayonnaise
  - fresh fruit
- *For dinner*, try mixing and matching vegetables, grains, and beans in a soup or casserole and serving them with a green

salad and fruit for dessert. Or enjoy whole-meal salads of seafood, beans, grains, vegetables, or fruits.

■ *Any time at all*, feel free to snack on fresh vegetables, fruits, cereal, or leftovers from your other meals.

You will finds numerous delicious, easy-to-make recipes in Chapter Nine to help you plan your meals and snacks.

The Nineteen Meals Rule

You may think that you just can't live without fatty and sugary junk foods. But you're in for a great surprise. The more you eat fresh, whole, healthful foods, the more you'll enjoy them. Fresh, unprocessed foods taste great. They make you feel comfortably satisfied instead of stuffed or bloated, and they boost your energy levels higher than you may have thought possible. Excess pounds begin to drop away and you begin to glow with radiant good health. One day you may find yourself wondering: "Who needs fatty foods anymore?"

Still, you're only human. Occasionally you may crave certain favorite foods or special meals. Or maybe you're going to a friend's house for dinner and don't want to ask him or her to prepare something special. That's when the "Nineteen-Meals Rule" can come in handy. Each week, if you follow the program faithfully for nineteen out of twenty-one meals, you can enjoy two "free" meals. Have anything you want for these two meals. Don't go overboard and stuff yourself, of course. But feel free to enjoy a restaurant meal or a special snack without counting the fat and fiber grams. Just knowing that you can have whatever you want twice a week makes it even easier to stick with the plan.

Not a Diet, It's a New Way of Living

The 20/30 Fat & Fiber Diet Plan is a straightforward, easy-to-follow program that has helped thousands of people lose weight, keep it off, and greatly improve their health. But it's not just a diet that you go on for a few weeks or months, then discard. Instead, *The 20/30 Fat & Fiber Diet Plan* is a lifelong program.

In the chapters that follow, we'll discuss the scientific basis behind the program, look at the health-enhancing phytochemicals you'll be getting with your foods, teach you how to set up your kitchen, and otherwise prepare you to shed pounds and gain great health. Let's begin our exploration of the program with a look at the scientific rationale behind *The 20/30 Fat & Fiber Diet Plan.* ■

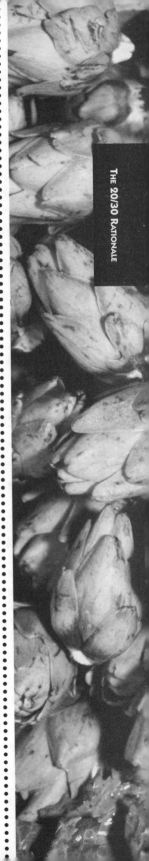

THE
20/30
RATIONALE

- *Dr. Atkins' New Diet Revolution* insists we should eat a high-protein diet.
- *Bodyfueling* says that you must fuel your body with the right mental approach.
- *Dr. Abravanel's Body Type Diet* divides us into thyroid, adrenal, pituitary, and gonadal types, with special programs for each.
- *The New Cabbage Soup Diet* and similar approaches claim that the key to weight loss is focusing on a single food.
- *Eat Right 4 Your Type* argues that your blood type determines which foods you should be eating.
- *Fit For Life* maintains that foods should be eaten in specific combinations at certain times, or else they'll rot in your gut.
- *The Rotation Diet* favors eating different amounts of calories in three stages.
- *The Scentsational Weight Loss Diet* claims that sniffing foods or special food scents can curb your appetite.

Is it any wonder that people are so confused about diets, dieting, and nutrition?

Yo-Yo Dieting

You can lose weight on any of these diets—at first—because you'll probably eat less than you're accustomed to, and the mere fact that you're on a diet will encourage you to watch what you eat. But, when you tire of following the latest fad diet, you'll probably gain back all the weight you lost, plus more. Meanwhile, these diets can harm your health by restricting important food groups and by turning you into a "yo-yo" dieter, with your weight bouncing up and down as you try one diet after another. Food restriction doesn't work in the long run because it leaves you hungry; eventually you'll give in and quite likely binge on unhealthful foods.[1] This yo-yo dieting is even more harmful than being overweight, for it increases the risk of developing heart disease, high blood pressure, and diabetes.[2] In fact, yo-yo dieters who repeatedly lose and gain weight have double the risk of suffering heart attacks and dying prematurely.[3] New research indicates that repeatedly losing then regaining weight may even trigger cancer of the breast, uterus, and prostate![4] Rapid weight loss all by itself can also be dangerous, even if you don't pack the pounds back on, because every time you quickly shed pounds you increase the odds of developing gallstones.[5]

High Protein Diets Are Dangerous

Many people have turned to high-protein diets such as Dr. Atkins' Diet Revolution, Protein Power, and the Stillman Diet. Eating large amounts of protein means, of course, that you consume lots of meat, fish, poultry, eggs, and dairy products, but relatively few fruits, vegetables, and whole grains. In other words, you get lots of protein, plus the fat that comes along with it, but only small amounts of fiber and even fewer phytochemicals.

You will lose weight on a high-protein diet, since it works on the basis of lowering your calorie intake, but the weight will quickly return when you go off the diet. While on a high-protein diet, starved of fiber and flooded with fat, you will be at increased risk of heart disease, stroke, certain cancers, diabetes, constipation, diverticulitis, and hemorrhoids. And high intakes of protein can also leach calcium from your bones, contributing to osteoporosis.

The liquid protein diets popular in the 1970s are extreme versions of the Atkins and Stillman diets. They caused a great deal of illness and are associated with more than 50 deaths.

Beware the Danger Zone

The popular diet known as "The Zone" restricts carbohydrates to 40 percent of one's daily intake. (Which means, of course, that the bulk of the diet has to come from fat and protein.) You may or may not lose weight on "The Zone," but you may also lose your health because virtually every study on diet and health conducted in the past quarter century has shown that eating carbohydrates in the form of vegetables, fruits, whole grains, and beans is the key to good health and weight loss. You certainly want to avoid the refined carbohydrates in white bread, pasta, and bakery products, but you should be eating more — not less — of health-enhancing unrefined carbohydrates.

The best way to lose weight safely and permanently is to eat less fat and more fiber.

Good Fats and Bad Fats

Trying to figure out fats can be difficult. There are saturated fats, monounsaturated fats, polyunsaturated fats, trans fats, and hydrogenated fats. We hear that saturated fats cause heart disease but monounsaturated and polyunsaturated fats reduce cholesterol. Or is that the omega-6s?

Just as proteins are made by linking together various amino acids, fats are created when fatty acids "come together."[6] Fatty acids are essentially chains of carbon atoms, lined up like pearls on a necklace, one after another. As the diagram below shows, each carbon has four "arms." The rules of the body's chemistry dictate that all four of these arms *must* hold on to something. One arm links it to the carbon atom ahead, one to the carbon behind. That leaves two arms free. Either they each grab onto a hydrogen atom and hold it out to the side, or they latch onto the carbons directly ahead or behind.

Fatty acids are said to be either saturated or unsaturated. The simplest way to cut through the scientific jargon and confusion is to remember that "saturated" means "filled." Fatty acids can be saturated with hydrogen atoms, just as the paper towel you use to clean up the kitchen counter can become saturated with water.

Here's the key structural difference between saturated and unsaturated fatty acids. If each carbon "pearl" in the necklace (except the last carbon atom, linked to two oxygen atoms) is holding onto two hydrogen atoms the fatty acid is saturated, it can't possibly hold any more. If not, the fatty acid is unsaturated.

Saturated Fatty Acid

H—C—C—C—C—C—C—C—C—C—C—C—C—C—C—C—C—C—C—O—H

Monounsaturated Fatty Acid

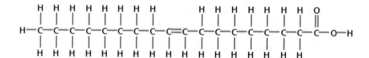

Polyunsaturated Fatty Acid

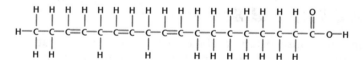

Saturated fatty acids have their "arms" filled with hydrogen atoms, unsaturated fatty acids do not.

The unsaturated fats are further broken down into two categories: monounsaturated and polyunsaturated. These long names simply tell you whether one or more sets of carbon atoms can hold on to additional hydrogens. If only one set of carbons is holding on to each other, instead of a full set of hydrogens, the fat is monounsaturated ("mono" means "one"). If two or more sets of carbons are holding on to each other, rather than to a full compliment of hydrogens, it's polyunsaturated ("poly" equals "many").

Dietary Fat	Cholesterol (mg/tbsp)	Breakdown of Fatty-Acid Content
Safflower Oil	0	10% — 77% — Trace— 13%
Sunflower Oil	0	11% — 69% — 20%
Corn Oil	0	13% — 61% — 25%
Olive Oil	0	14% — 8% — 1% — 77%
Soybean Oil	0	15% — 54% — 7% — 24%
Margarine	0	17% — 32% — 2% — 49%
Peanut Oil	0	18% — 33% — 49%
Vegetable Shortening	0	28% — 26% — 2% — 44%
Palm Oil	0	52% — 10% — 1% — 37%
Coconut Oil	0	92% — 2%— 6%
Beef Fat	12	52% — 3%— 1% — 44%
Butter Fat	33	66% — 2%— 2% — 30%

■ Saturated Fatty Acid　　■ Polyunsaturated – Alpha-Linolenic Acid – Omega 3

■ Polyunsaturated – Linoleic Acid – Omega 6　　□ Monounsaturated Fatty Acid

There's an important step we still have to understand: getting from fatty acids to fat. This is accomplished by lumping many fatty acids together. The fat on a steak, for example, is composed of various fatty acids, some saturated, some monounsaturated, and some polyunsaturated (linoleic and linolenic acid). In general, meat, fish, milk, butter, and palm and coconut oils tend to have more saturated fatty acids, while vegetables, fruits, and whole grains generally contain more unsaturated fatty acids. To keep things simple, we designate a fat according to the characteristics of the majority of fatty acids in it. Since slightly more than half of the fatty acids in meat are saturated, we call the fat from meat saturated fat.

That's the essential skinny on fat. It's made up of fatty acids, which are "necklaces" of carbon atoms strung together, each carbon holding hydrogen atoms out to the side. If it's filled up with hydrogen, it's saturated. If not, it's either monounsaturated or polyunsaturated.

Hydrogenated oils or trans fats means that extra hydrogen atoms have been artificially forced onto an unsaturated fatty acid "necklace" in order to make it saturated. Unsaturated fats tend to spoil relatively quickly, so manufacturers who use them in their foods often hydrogenate them to prevent spoilage. Unfortunately, what's good for food processors is not good for you. Hydrogenated fats have been shown to raise the "bad" LDL cholesterol and lower the "good" HDL cholesterol; this two-pronged attack on your body's chemistry can cause heart disease. Partially hydrogenated oils are also linked to the current epidemic of breast and prostate cancer. Hydrogenated fats turn up in all kinds of snack foods, bakery products, and other processed foods, and so these foods are best avoided.

There's one more concept to understand: the omega fatty acids. We use omega, which is the last letter in the Greek alphabet, to designate the carbon at one end of a fatty acid "necklace."[7] If we say that a polyusaturated fatty acid is an omega-3 fatty acid, we mean that the third carbon from the end is unsaturated. If we designate it as an omega-6 fatty acid, then the sixth carbon from the end is unsaturated.

Most vegetable oils contain large amounts of omega-6's, while fish, whole grains and soybean oil have omega-3s. The omega-3 fatty acids became well known and wildly popular back in the late 1970s when researchers discovered that Eskimos who consumed large amounts of omega-3s had very little heart disease, despite eating an incredibly high-fat diet based on fish, whale, and seal blubber. Eager medical scientists soon learned that the omega-3s helped guard against heart disease by preventing the formation of blood clots that could lodge in the tiny arteries in the heart, triggering heart attacks. (Although many thought that eating fish every day would eliminate heart disease once and for all, it turns out that eating fish two or three times a week provides the maximum benefit.)

The Bottom Line on Fats

When you're trying to lose weight or lower your cholesterol, cut back on all fatty foods and avoid added fats, for they are the most concentrated sources of calories. You will get all the "good" fat you need by eating a wide variety of whole grains, vegetables, and beans. Eat the whole food, not its oil; corn, not corn oil, olives rather than olive oil, and soybean products instead of soybean oil. When you eat the whole food you get all the vitamins, minerals, fiber, and phytochemicals that nature pairs with the "good" fats.

Don't worry about not getting enough fat. That's not possible, unless you eat nothing but refined carbohydrates. Fashion models who exist on diets of bagels, pretzels, soft drinks, and coffee may be fat deficient, but if you eat any reasonable variety of foods, you will get all of the essential fatty acids your body needs. Even onions, celery, and shrimp contain some fat; the only truly fat-free "foods" are salt, refined sugar and refined grains.

How Much Fat Are We Eating?

The average person needs to consume between 1,800 and 2,500 calories per day. Those calories can come from fat, protein, carbohydrate, or alcohol.

- A gram of fat has 9 calories.
- A gram of alcohol adds about 7 calories to your intake.
- A gram of either protein or carbohydrate gives you 4 calories.

Gram for gram (and ounce for ounce), fat is the "fattiest," the most calorie laden of our energy sources.

The average American chows down about 85 grams of fat per day, accounting for 765 calories. Assuming you're taking in a total of 2,000 calories daily, those 85 fat grams equal 38 percent of your total caloric intake. If you tend to dine in fast food restaurants, you can breeze through 85 grams of fat in no time, leaving you relatively little "dietary room" for the nutritious foods your body needs.

Although the typical American diet gets 38 percent of its calories from fat, many consume much more fat than that. Think of a hungry teenager whose daily diet looks something like this:

Breakfast at home
Swanson Breakfast Burrito with bacon—11 grams

Midmorning snack
Hershey's milk chocolate bar, 1.55 ounces—13 grams

Lunch at school
Beef hot dog—16 grams
Pillsbury crescent rolls, 2—12 grams

Afternoon snack
Hostess frosted Donettes, 3—12 grams

Dinner at McDonald's
Quarter pounder with cheese—28 grams
Small French fries—10 grams
Chocolate shake—5 grams

Late night snack
Hostess Ding Dongs—18 grams
Whole milk, 1 cup—8 grams

That comes to an astonishing 133 grams of fat! But you needn't be a voracious teenager to "inhale" fat. We often don't realize how much fat is in our foods. Here's what a harried office worker on a "diet" eats:

Breakfast at home
Kellogg's Corn Flakes, 1 cup—0 grams
Grapefruit, $1/_2$—0 grams
Low-fat milk, 1 cup—2.5 grams

Midmorning snack
Chee-tos, 1 ounce—10 grams

Lunch (heated in lunch room at work)
Stouffer's Vegetable Lasagna—20 grams
Carrot cake, 1 regular slice—15 grams

Afternoon snack
Sunchips, 1 ounce—6 grams

Dinner at home
Salad with iceberg lettuce—negligible
Hidden Valley Ranch dressing, 1 tablespoon—14 grams
Lean ground beef, 3 ounces—16 grams
Campbell's baked New England style beans, $1/_2$ cup—3 grams

Late night snack
Planters dry roasted peanuts, 1 ounce—13 grams

The total is an amazing $99^1/_2$ grams of fat! The fat in those foods accounts for 900 calories, or almost half the total on a 2,000 calorie per day diet.

"But how can that be," the office worker protested. "I'm eating plain cereal, vegetable lasagna and carrot cake, I'm having just a little bit of Sunchips and peanuts for a snack, and I'm hungry all the time! How bad can that be?" Who would think that a vegetarian meal would have 35 grams, a single tablespoon of dressing 14 grams, and a "little bit of peanuts"—one ounce—would have 13 grams of fat?

Fat is the "magic ingredient" food manufacturers add to their products to get us to buy them. And it works, because we like the taste of fat. But we don't realize how fatty so many of the foods we buy in markets and eat at restaurants really are. We don't realize that the average person swallows 38 grams of fat per day, well over the 20 or less that we actually need.

Now that we're conversant with "fat terms" and facts, let's look at fiber.

All About Fiber

Americans have long been fascinated by fiber. Back in the 1820s and 1830s, a minister named Sylvester Graham preached about the virtues of fiber. In the 1870s, Dr. John Kellogg went on a fiber crusade at a health sanitarium in Battle Creek, Michigan. Convinced that many of our health problems could be traced to poisons in the bowels, he fed all his patients bran. And in 1897 a fiber cereal called Grape-Nuts—possibly the first successful commercial health food—was developed by Charles W. Post.

Although throughout the twentieth century numerous scientists and laypeople have echoed the early claims made for fiber, it wasn't until the 1970s that we began accumulating hard scientific data to prove that large amounts of fiber are indeed necessary for good health. Key discoveries began in Africa, when a British physician noticed a marked difference between the stool of rural Africans, who ate a very high-fiber diet, and that of the British, who did not. (The African stool was almost twice as heavy as the British, and tended to be softer and more fluid.) Knowing that the Africans did not suffer from hemorrhoids, diverticulitis, colon cancer, appendicitis, constipation, and other "Western" diseases of the gastrointestinal tract, the observant doctor began to investigate the link between fiber and health.

Thanks to the early enthusiasm of Graham, Kellogg, and Post, and the modern research conducted over the past twenty-five or so years, we now know that large amounts of dietary fiber are absolutely essential for good health. Dietary fiber is composed of various substances found in the walls of plant cells, which the body cannot digest. Fiber has absolutely no nutritional value in and of itself—it simply goes in and comes out. Despite that fact, fiber is a powerfully medicinal food.

■ Fiber absorbs water in the intestines, making elimination easy by enlarging and softening the stool. Lack of fiber causes the stool to become small, hard, and difficult to eliminate with out the intense straining that can cause ailments such as hemorrhoids, diverticulitis, and varicose veins.

■ Eating large amounts of fiber has been linked to a reduced risk of developing colon cancer.

■ Fiber also helps prevent heart disease, gall bladder disease, high blood pressure, elevated cholesterol levels, and obesity.

■ Fiber aids diabetics by slowing the absorption of glucose from the small intestine.

■ Because fiber gives you a feeling of satiety, it helps you lose weight.

Fiber is classified as either *soluble* or *insoluble*. Both types are beneficial, but for different reasons. In a nutshell, soluble fiber reduces cholesterol and guards against heart and gall bladder disease, while insoluble fiber protects against colon cancer, constipation, hemorrhoids, diverticulitus, and varicose veins. Here's a simple way to remember the key distinction between the two: *soluble* fiber *sops up* cholesterol to help prevent heart disease, while *in*soluble fiber goes *in* and out of the body, thus guarding against diseases of the digestive and waste tract, and filling you up without contributing calories.

Where do you find the two types of fiber? Both are present in most whole plant foods. This means that you don't have to worry about eating certain foods to get a specific type of

White Flour Is Like Sugar

As far as your body is concerned, eating white flour is almost the same as eating sugar. Food has three main sources of energy: carbohydrates, fats, and proteins. Carbohydrates contain single sugars or combinations of sugars. Glucose is an example of a single sugar. Sucrose or common table sugar is a double sugar. Starch contains thousands of sugar molecules bound together, while fiber contains millions of sugars bound together so tightly that your body cannot break them down.

Only single sugars can pass from your intestines into your bloodstream. Double, triple, and other combinations of sugars and starches must first be split into single sugars before they can be absorbed. These reactions occur so rapidly in your intestines that most starches cause rises in blood sugar that are not

much lower than those of single sugars. On the other hand, the sugars in fiber are so tightly bound together that they cannot be separated from their parent molecule and therefore cannot be absorbed in the small intestine. They bind to and delay absorption of sugars that are in the intestines at the same time, which helps to prevent the steep rises in blood sugar levels that cause aging and nerve damage.

Ideally, you do not want your blood sugar level to rise too high because it causes sugar to attach to the outer surface membranes of cells. Sugar, by itself, is harmless, but after being attached to membranes, sugar is converted to sorbitol, which damages cells. That's why diabetics who carry high blood sugar levels can suffer extensive nerve damage, which causes blindness, loss of hearing and fiber. Instead, eat plenty of fiber-filled foods and you'll get enough of both.

Remember, fiber comes from plants, not animals. Fruits, vegetables, whole grains, and seeds have fiber. Meat, fish, poultry, and dairy products do not. Neither do refined (white) breads, rolls or pasta, bagels, pretzels, cookies, crackers, corn chips, "kid's" cereals, couscous, cornmeal, grits, cakes, pies, or other foods made from grains from which the fiber has been removed.

The Bottom Line on Fiber

If you eat lots of fruits, vegetables, and whole grains, you'll get all the fiber you need and all the benefits of fiber. But if you don't eat these foods, consuming only ground-up fiber in the form of bran cereals or supplements won't help much. That's because the real benefits of fiber come from eating fiber-rich foods, not fiber in isolation.

feeling, burning feet, a feeling that bugs are crawling over you, amputations, and even kidney damage.

Nowhere in nature do you find sugar or starch without fiber. Humans take whole grains, remove the outer husk, and grind the inner endosperm to make white flour—just as they take sugar beets, sugarcane, maple sap, apples, and grapes and extract the sugars, leaving the fiber, vitamins, and phytochemicals behind. Do your body a favor and eat mostly foods that have not been refined to remove the fiber and valuable nutrients.

This chart illustrates the effects of fiber particle size on blood sugar. Unprocessed whole wheat grains cause blood sugar to rise gently, then sink back down slowly, providing a steady stream of energy over

a long time. Cracked wheat, with each grain broken into a few pieces, prompts a more sudden rise. Coarse flour, where the grains have been ground but no fiber has been removed, causes a dramatic, sharp rise. Worst of all is the refined white flour, with fiber removed, which sends blood sugar soaring and then brings it crashing back down. Eating white flour has almost the same effect as eating table sugar.

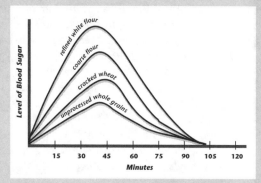

The fiber in fruits, vegetables, and whole grains binds to water, carbohydrates, and other nutrients in your food, slowing digestion and giving you a feeling of comfortable fullness. Ground-up fiber won't absorb nearly as much water or slow digestion to the same extent. There's a simple test you can do to see the difference between whole and ground-up fiber. When you cook a cup of whole wheat pasta, you get two cups of cooked pasta. But if you cook one cup of dry wheat berries in water, you get four cups of cooked wheat berries. The natural, unprocessed, whole grain form of wheat binds to twice as much water, giving you more of a feeling of fullness when you eat it. And unrefined grains take much longer to

Are Complex Carbohydrates Best?

You may have heard that you should avoid simple sugars and that complex carbohydrates are good for you. That's not true. Complex carbohydrates (long chains of sugars) are better than sugar only if they take your body a longer time to break down and digest, and if they are paired with other nutrients such as vitamins and minerals. White flour and other starches that have been removed from their fiber are broken down in your body just as quickly as table sugar. They have also been stripped of the protein, vitamins, and other nutrients found in whole grains.

All carbohydrates (both sugars and starches) are always paired with fiber in nature. The important point is not whether the carbohydrate is simple or complex, but whether you are getting the complete package—loaded with vitamins, minerals, and phytochemicals as well as fiber and energy—or a stripped down, refined version that gives you only calories. Get your complex carbohydrates in whole grains, fruits, vegetables, and beans that have their fiber intact.

We certainly recommend that you avoid refined sugars as much as possible, but the sugars in fruit are also simple sugars, and if you eliminate them, you miss all the other benefits of fruit. On the other hand, when you separate fruit sugars from their fiber, they are no better than table sugar; "all fruit" jams and juices, sweetened with concentrated apple juice or grape juice, are no better than those sweetened with sugar from sugarcane or sugar beets. That's why you should eat apples instead of apple juice or apple jelly, and grapes or raisins instead of grape juice or wine. Fiber slows down the absorbtion of sugar and provides bulk. You can delay the digestion of sugar in fruit even longer if you combine it with other foods. Diabetics should always eat fruit with whole grains or other food to slow the rise in blood sugar.

digest, slowly releasing their sugars into the bloodstream to provide steady, longer-lasting energy. Finally, a significant portion of the whole grain will pass through your colon undigested, keeping your stool soft and preventing constipation.

Eat "Real" Fiber

Delighted to hear that there's an easy way to reduce the risk of heart disease, certain cancers, constipation, and other ailments, many people have eagerly added fiber to their diets. Unfortunately, they've often added it in the form of bran cereals or fiber supplements.

Sprinkling bran into your food certainly increases your fiber intake, but there's a crucial difference between the fiber in food and "fiber in a jar." And the fiber in fiber supplements has been separated from the carbohydrates, protein, fat, vitamins, minerals, and phytochemicals in the foods from which it came, and has been ground up into small pieces. It has some value, but doesn't compare to fiber in food, the fiber still wrapped up in nature's nutritious "package." Get your fiber from the original and best sources: fruits, vegetables, whole grains, and beans.

How Much Fiber Are We Eating?

Most of us are eating only 10–15 grams of fiber per day,[8] not nearly enough for optimal health. Let's see how much fiber our hypothetical teenager consumes:

Breakfast at home
Swanson Breakfast Burrito with bacon—1 gram

Midmorning snack
Hershey's milk chocolate bar, 1.55 ounces—1 gram

Lunch at school
Beef hot dog—0 grams
Pillsbury crescent rolls, 2—0 grams

Afternoon snack
Hostess frosted Donettes, 3—1 gram

Dinner at McDonald's
Quarter pounder with cheese—2 grams
Small French fries—2 grams
Chocolate shake—1 gram

Late night snack
Hostess Ding Dongs—0 grams
Whole milk, 1 cup—0 grams

How Much Fat, How Much Protein, How Much Carbohydrate?

On **The 20/30 Plan**, you get approximately:

- 10–20 percent of your calories from fat
- 15–20 percent of your calories from protein
- 60–75 percent of your calories from whole food carbohydrates

You'll get plenty of fat and protein—more than enough to feed your body's needs, but not too much. Carbohydrates will be your major source of energy, as they should be. But most of the carbohydrates you eat are bound up with fiber, which means they will be digested slowly and will not cause sharp rises in blood sugar. You can stay on this plan for the rest of your life, enjoying the benefits of eating the most healthful possible diet.

That comes to a mere 8 grams of fiber daily. Here's what the harried office worker gets:

Breakfast at home
Kellogg's Corn Flakes, 1 cup—1 gram
Grapefruit, $1/_2$—6 grams
Low-fat milk, 1 cup—0 grams

Midmorning snack
Chee-tos, 1 ounce—0 grams

Lunch (heated in lunch room at work)
Stouffer's Vegetable Lasagna—3 grams
Carrot cake, 1 regular slice—3 grams

Afternoon snack
Sunchips, 1 ounce—2 grams

Dinner at home
Salad with iceberg lettuce—1 gram
Hidden Valley Ranch dressing, 1 tablespoon—0 grams
Lean ground beef, 3 ounces—0 grams
Campbell's baked New England style beans, $1/_2$ cup—3 grams

Late night snack
Planters dry roasted peanuts, 1 oz—2 grams

A total of 21 grams of fiber daily, which is better than the fast-food-loving teenager but not nearly enough for great health. These two people are not unusual. Like most of us, they are eating way too much fat and not nearly enough fiber.

20/30, the Formula for Safe and Permanent Weight Loss

Twenty grams of fat represents about 10 percent of your daily caloric intake, assuming you eat 2,000 calories per day. But in fact, you'll get more than 20 grams of fat daily. In addition to the 20 grams you track on your counter, you'll get another 10 grams or so from foods that are listed as having 0 grams of fat. (They all have some fat, which adds up.) If you eat a variety of whole grains, fruits, vegetables, beans, and nonfat dairy products, you will get more than enough fat to satisfy your body's need for essential fatty acids.

As for fiber, 30 grams per day is a very modest goal: when you check the fiber counts of our delicious recipes, you'll see how easy it is to exceed that total. If you take in less than 30 grams of fiber daily, your diet is bound to be deficient in the vitamins, minerals, and other nutrients that accompany fiber in nature (and you won't be taking full advantage of fiber's natural appetite-suppressing effect). We encourage you to eat more than 30 grams of fiber per day—way more if you are getting your fiber from whole grains, vegetables, and fruits, rather than from fiber or bran supplements.

When you eat the same amount of food you've always eaten, but substitute high-fiber foods for the old fatty, low-fiber parts of your diet, you lose weight automatically. Not only that, but your cholesterol will fall and you'll feel more energetic. So start counting.

20/30 Works!

In October 1997, the *American Journal of Clinical Nutrition* published a series of articles penned by top nutrition researchers from around the world.[9] Although each had his or her own favorite approach to diet, the consensus was that the most healthful diet is one filled with vegetables, fruit, whole grains, and beans. It also has you eating fish or shellfish twice a week, is low on meat and chicken, and has few refined grains (such as pastries and white bread).

Laboratory studies are always interesting, but they are no substitute for real-life experience. Fortunately, our program has made the leap from laboratory to the daily lives of many happy dieters. Here's what some successful *20/30* dieters have said:

"This is a great deal! I've lost 15 pounds in one week! I've got more energy and feel great!"

—MH, Brawley, CA

"I've lost over 10 pounds on the program and am so happy with the results. I am 65 years old and losing weight at my age is really difficult."

—CC, Springfield, VA

"Following the program has been wonderful for myself and my boyfriend. I have lost a total of 13 pounds. I'm finally down to 101 and loving it! My boyfriend has lost 22 pounds, down to his high school weight of 160! He's thrilled that he didn't have to give up eating to lose weight."

—JB, Abington, PA

A Bowl a Day Keeps the Fat Away

Researchers at Australia's University of Sydney have shown that beginning your day with a bowl of high-fiber cereal helps you stay slim and healthy. Their study found that eating high-fiber, low-fat cereal in the morning fills you up. With a comfortable feeling of satiety, you're less likely to reach for snacks or other foods, and you eat less fat during the day.[10]

Check the ingredient list on your breakfast cereal to make sure that it's made from whole grains and has at least 3 grams of fiber (per 50-gram serving). Avoid cereals with added fats or a lot of added sugar.

See page 69 for tips on picking a good cereal.

"I have lowered my blood pressure. I have lost weight, from 163 150 pounds and still losing! I eat right and food tastes better! I feel great and am very proud!"

—JB, Bowie, MD

"I lost 22 pounds (12 $1/4$ inches)."

—JB, Middletown, OH

"I have lost a tremendous amount of weight (34 pounds) in two months. I went from a 43-inch waist to a 34-inch waist and I feel GREAT! I've tried many diet programs with little success."

—CC, Phoenix, AZ

"Seventy pounds down—30 to go!"

—SS, Manassas, VA

The safest, easiest, and most permanent way to lose weight is to eat less fat and more fiber. The scientific theory is valid and practical experience proves that it works. You'll lose weight on *The 20/30 Fat & Fiber Plan*. And, as a "side effect," you'll also gain great health. ■

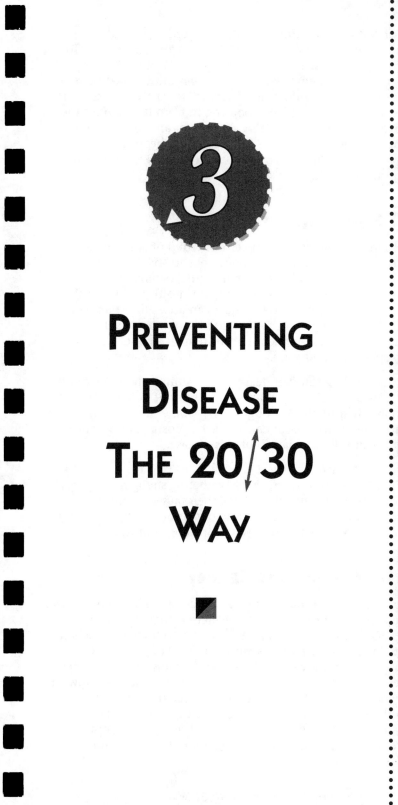

3

PREVENTING
DISEASE
THE 20/30
WAY

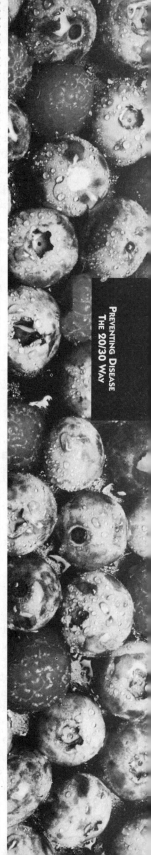

Cancer, heart disease, stroke: these very words can send chills down our spines as we think about their devastating effects. To combat these and other ailments, many Americans submit to surgery, radiation, chemotherapy, and other drastic treatments, while consuming a bewildering variety of drugs. And these "cures" often don't work. But evidence pouring in from laboratories the world over has shown that eating more fiber and less fat are two of the best medicines available for preventing heart disease, cancer, stroke, diabetes, impotence, and other common diseases, as well as aiding in their treatment. Let's see how.

20/30 Fights Cancer

Rather than a single disease, cancer is a group of ailments with one thing in common: it causes body cells to shuck off their constraints and live too long, snatching up resources (such as nutrients and oxygen), and squeezing out healthy cells and tissues as the cancerous tumor grows. Cancer can arise almost anywhere in the body, from the brain to the blood to the bowels. It may be aggressive or slow growing, content to remain in one place or eager to spread far and wide.

The second leading cause of death in the United States, cancer is an ever growing problem, despite the billions of dollars spent on research and treatment. Although many women fear breast cancer and many men worry about cancer of the prostate, lung cancer is actually the deadliest variation of this disease.

Cancer can be difficult to detect early, with its cells lying in wait in the body for months or years, slowly gathering strength until they have grown powerful enough to make their presence known. By then they are pressing on neighboring organs or tissues, destroying crucial white blood cells or otherwise impeding your health.

Less Fat Equals Less Cancer

We've long suspected that eating too much fat could contribute to the development of cancer.[1] Early suspicions that some cancers may be related to poor dietary habits were given credence when it was noted that cancer patterns among groups of people tended to change when they moved from country to country and adopted new diets. For example, the incidence of prostate cancer is low in Japan, where the traditional diet contains relatively little fat, but high in the United States, where we eat a high-fat diet. However, when Japanese men move from Japan to Hawaii and adopt the fatty Western diet, their odds of developing the disease shoot up.

Other studies have backed up these observations. For example, Chinese-Americans living in San Francisco have four times the risk of developing colorectal cancer compared to Chinese of similar age living in the People's Republic of China.[2] The authors of this study, which appeared in the *Journal of the National Cancer Institute*, argued that the American diet, which is high in fat and protein but low in fiber, was a key cancer culprit.

Many studies published in prestigious scientific journals have identified excess fat and a lack of fiber as chief factors in the causation of cancer.[3] Indeed, the National Academy of Sciences has estimated that up to 60 percent of the cancer in women, and 40 percent in men, are related to these and other dietary factors. Let's take a quick look at some of the studies linking excess dietary fat and lack of fiber to cancer.

Low Cholesterol Does Not Cause Cancer

Some people fear that eating a low-fat, high-fiber diet will reduce their cholesterol to the point that they will get cancer.

It's true that some cancer patients have low cholesterol levels. However, the drop in cholesterol is the result, not the cause, of cancer. Cancer begins silently; you don't realize that it's quietly growing in your body. Long before you recognize its symptoms, or your doctor stumbles across it in a routine examination, it may be affecting you in very subtle ways. Many patients with hidden cancers lose their appetites and their cholesterol levels fall as a result of their changed eating habits.

- **Breast cancer:** A review of twelve studies published in the *Journal of the National Cancer Institute* showed that breast cancer in postmenopausal women could be cut by 25 percent if dietary fat were reduced.[4]

- **Colorectal cancer:** Nine hundred six Chinese suffering from colorectal cancer were compared to over 2000 who did not. Analysis of their diets showed that the more saturated fat they ate, the greater their risk of developing the cancer.[5] Fat is being linked more and more closely to this terrible cancer. A 1998 study presented in the *American Journal of Epidemiology* described how researchers followed over 900 people aged fifty to seventy-five. They found that obesity, weight gain, and unstable adult weight were all associated with colorectal cancer.[6] And studies on animals have shown that saturated and partially hydrogenated fats in meat, chicken, dairy products, and "doctored" vegetable oils increase the risk of colon cancer.[7]

- **Ovarian cancer:** When the dietary practices of 455 Italian women suffering from ovarian cancer were compared to those of 1,385 in control groups, the high-fat diet was found to be a cancer-causing culprit. (Those women eating lots of green vegetables, carrots, whole grains, and fish had the lowest risk of developing the cancer.[8]) A large-scale study of over 16,000 Seventh-Day Adventist women linked consumption of fatty fried foods and eggs to ovarian cancer. Those who ate eggs (which are relatively high in fat and have absolutely no fiber) at least three times a week had three times the risk of developing the cancer than those who consumed eggs less than once a week. Fried fish, fried chicken, fried potatoes, and fried eggs were also linked to the development of fatal ovarian cancer, with fried eggs being the worst culprit.[9]

Just how does excess dietary fat contribute to cancer? Nobody really knows. Each normal cell in your body is programmed to go through a certain amount of doubling, and then die (e.g. skin cells live for 28 days, the cells lining your intestines live for 48 hours, and red blood cells live for around 120 days). Cancer means that old cells do not die, but continue growing until they invade and destroy other natural tissues. If breast cancer cells, for example, invade the bone marrow and prevent it from making red blood cells, you could die of anemia. A number of substances can damage the genetic material that tells a cell to die, including chemicals, ultraviolet rays, viruses, X-rays, cigarette smoke, and excess dietary fat.

Fiber Fights Cancer

As for fiber, a great deal of evidence taken from large population studies suggests that fiber guards against breast cancer and colorectal cancer, and possibly other forms of the disease as well. If you look at the numerous fiber-cancer studies conducted at hospitals and research centers all around the world, you'll see the link between a high fiber diet and a lessened risk of developing many kinds of cancer.[10]

Fiber may protect against cancer of the breast by influencing the metabolism of estrogen, the female sex hormone.[11] Breast cancer is most likely estrogen-dependent, which means that it needs a plentiful supply of estrogen in order to flourish. A high-fiber diet helps the body excrete excess estrogen through the feces, which may be why such a diet is linked to a reduced risk of breast cancer.[12] Together, the high-fiber, low-fat diet packs a powerful punch against breast cancer. A four-year study conducted in Israel of almost 1,000 women matched for age and other factors found that those who ate a high-fat, low-fiber diet were twice as likely to develop breast cancer once they passed menopause as women who ate less fats and more whole foods.[13] Clearly, eating plenty of fiber and relatively little fat is preventive medicine for this terrible scourge.

How does fiber shield you from cancers of the colon and rectum? There are several possible means. Fiber may serve as a diluting agent to "water down" the concentration of dangerous substances that can initiate or activate cancer cells. In fact, simply by bulking up the stool and helping push it through the intestinal tract more quickly, fiber reduces the amount of time during which potential cancer-causing substances are in contact with the body. And of course, fiber fights cancer by displacing fat in the diet.[14]

Other Elements of the 20/30 Program That Help Fight Cancer

Low fat and high fiber are just two of *The 20/30 Plan's* weapons against cancer. Remember, the fruits, vegetables, and grains you'll be eating are filled with vitamins, minerals, and phytochemicals that strengthen the body's resistance to the disease. Let's look at some of the studies showing how *The 20/30 Plan* foods can act as shields against cancer:

■ **Less risk of cancer death:** The link between consumption of vegetables and the risk of getting cancer was examined in 1,271 people age sixty-six years or older. Those who ate the most carotene-containing vegetables were 70 percent less likely to die of cancer than those who ate the least.[15]

■ **Bladder cancer:** When 163 people suffering from bladder cancer were compared to 181 people hospitalized for other reasons, it was found that eating more green vegetables and carrots reduced the risk of developing this cancer.[16]

■ **Breast cancer:** The dietary histories of 1,108 women suffering from breast cancer were compared to those of 1,281 hospitalized for other reasons. The results made it clear that eating fewer green vegetables increased the risk of developing breast cancer.[17] A healthful diet and lifestyle is very important in combating breast cancer. Your risk rises with cigarette smoking, alcohol drinking, and being overweight. On the other hand, it decreases with exercise and eating foods containing carotenes (vitamin A), including fruits and vegetables.[18]

■ **Cervical cancer:** Ranging in age from twenty to seventy-four, 189 women suffering from cervical cancer were compared to 227 controls. The more frequently the women ate dark green vegetables, yellow vegetables, and fruit juices, the less likely they were to develop this cancer.[19]

- **Endometrial cancer:** Comparing the diets of 168 women with endometrial cancer to controls showed that eating carrots, spinach, broccoli, cantaloupe, and lettuce protected against this cancer.[20]
- **Lung cancer:** A study of 763 white men suffering from lung cancer (compared to 900 controls) found that frequent consumption of vegetables, especially yellow-orange vegetables such as carrots, was linked to a low risk of developing the disease.[21]
- **Vulvar cancer:** Comparing the diets of 201 cancer patients with controls showed that when the consumption of deep yellow-orange vegetables and alpha carotene drops, the risk of vulvar cancer rises.[22]

Finally, *The 20/30 Plan* fights cancer by helping you to slim down. The relationship between obesity and the incidence of cancer, known for over four decades, has been upheld in study after study.[23] Simply slimming down on the program is a "medicine" against cancer.

20/30 Shields the Heart

Frightening as cancer is, it is only the second deadliest disease in our country today. Top "honors" go to heart disease, which will end over five hundred thousand lives in this year alone.

Although, technically speaking, "heart disease" can refer to any ailment afflicting the heart, we generally use it to identify the problems that arise when all or part of the heart muscle dies because the arteries that should supply it with blood become clogged or blocked.

The heart pumps the blood that brings oxygen and nutrients to every part of the body—including itself. When freshly oxygenated blood leaves the heart, the bulk of it flows through the massive artery called the aorta into smaller arteries and finally the capillaries, where it passes oxygen and other nutrients to the body's cells and takes up waste products to carry away for disposal. A small portion of the blood exiting the heart is routed right back into the heart muscle itself—not into the four chambers of the heart, which serve as collecting stations and "pumping platforms," but right back into the heart muscle, the strong band of fibers that contract rhythmically to keep the blood circulating.

Just like the muscles in your arms and legs, the heart muscle must be continually supplied with freshly oxygenated and nutrient-rich blood. An intricate series of arteries tunnel through the heart muscle, serving as the highways along which the fresh blood travels to every nook and cranny of the organ. Called the coronary arteries, these narrow arteries can easily become blocked by years of accumulated "debris" we call plaque. Made up of dead immune-system cells, fat, cholesterol, and other elements, plaque can form a dam across an artery, slowing the flow of blood. The dam itself may not cause a serious problem, if enough blood still manages to get through. But suppose a blood clot drifts through arteries and gets stuck at the dam: now the passage is completely blocked. Starved of oxygen, the part of the heart muscle fed by this artery will die. Laypeople call this a heart attack; physicians refer to it as a myocardial infarction or a coronary.

If only a tiny portion of heart muscle dies during the attack, you may not notice anything other than some chest pain. But if a more substantial portion of the heart is stricken you'll certainly feel the pain, and probably experience difficulty breathing, some sweating, and fatigue. If a large enough chunk of heart muscle dies, you will probably go along with it.

Many risk factors can bring about clogged arteries, including these:

- Elevated "bad" LDL cholesterol
- High blood pressure
- Smoking
- Obesity
- Diabetes
- Lack of exercise

At first glance, the list of risk factors is intimidating. There are so many things to worry about. But look at it again from the *The 20/30 Plan's* point of view. Starting right now, you can lower your "bad" LDL cholesterol, take steps to lower your blood pressure if it's elevated, lose weight, combat diabetes, and begin exercising. In other words, you can shrink your list of risk factors down quickly and easily. All you need to do is *follow the program.*

A Quick Look at Cholesterol

We'll look at the studies proving that eating less fat and more fiber reduces the risk of heart disease in just a moment. But first, let's define two more terms: *cholesterol* and *triglycerides.*

Cholesterol is a perfectly natural, health-enhancing substance manufactured by the body. It's used to make hormones such as estrogen and testosterone, is found in the cell membranes, and has other duties within our cells. The problem arises when we have too much cholesterol, or imbalances among two of its "types": the "bad" LDL cholesterol, and the "good" HDL cholesterol. (LDL stands for low-density lipoprotein and HDL for high-density lipoprotein.)

Simply stated, the "bad" LDL cholesterol ferries fat and cholesterol to the artery walls where it can adhere, adding to the dams that block the flow of blood. But if LDL is a delivery truck, the "good" HDL cholesterol acts like a garbage truck, collecting cholesterol molecules and carting them off for safe disposal.

Most health experts advise that your LDL should be under 100 and your HDL above 35. The key is to have enough good HDL to counteract the harmful LDL. If you have lots of LDL clogging up your arteries, you must have a correspondingly large amount of HDL cleaning them out. Use this chart to find out if you have enough HDL to clean up after your LDL.

Keeping Your HDL and LDL in Balance

If your LDL is:	You need an HDL of at least:
90	35
100	40
110	45
120	50
130	60
140	65

If your LDL is over 140 you need to follow a low-fat high-fiber diet regardless of your HDL level.

Your blood fat level, technically known as your triglyceride level, indicates the amount of fat in your bloodstream at any given time. This fluctuates through the day, especially as fat from your food enters your bloodstream. Ideally, your triglycerides should be under 150; more than that can make the blood sludgy and more likely to clot. An interesting experiment conducted many years ago showed how fat affects the blood. Medical students were given a fatty meal. Then, some time later, a special device was used to look into the tiny blood vessels in their eyes. Normally, the red blood cells move easily through these blood vessels. But as fat from the food got into the bloodstream and gunked things up, the blood cells began to slush together. This is called the Rouleau Effect. Up to nine hours later, in some cases, the medical students' blood cells were still stuck together in misshapen clumps. It's not just in the eyes that fat can cause trouble by turning blood into sludge. Excess blood fat contributes to heart disease, stroke, gangrene, and other diseases associated with the clogging of the arteries.

Chicken Is a Fowl Substitute

Many people concerned about their cholesterol levels switch from red meat to chicken, believing that it will help them lower their cholesterol.

It's true that chicken has less cholesterol-raising saturated fat than red meat does. However, much of the extra saturated fat in meat is in the form of stearic acid, which has little effect on cholesterol.[25] That's why switching from beef to chicken won't lower your cholesterol much, and opting for beef instead of chicken won't cause it to go much higher. Restrict your intake of both red meat and chicken while eating plenty of fresh vegetables and fruits, whole grains, and beans.

Fortunately, the odds are great that your total cholesterol and LDL will fall, your HDL will rise slightly, and the balance between your LDL and HDL will adjust to a proper level as you follow *The 20/30 Plan*. You needn't do anything but watch with pleasure as your risk of heart disease recedes.

20/30 Protects the Brain

A loss of blood flow to the heart muscle triggers a heart attack. Now suppose the same thing happens up in the brain: the result would

The Brainy Way to Eat Fish

Scientific studies have shown that eating fish is a good idea. We know, for example, that it helps prevent both colon and breast cancer and reduces the risk of heart attacks. But you needn't go overboard in your quest for good health. Rather than consuming fish or downing fish oil every day, limit yourself to two to three servings per week. Those few fish meals are all you need to enjoy the "good" fat and other benefits of eating fish. Eat a variety of fish, including, if you like, shellfish. (Shellfish has been accused of raising cholesterol, but some of its sterols may actually lower it.)

be a "brain attack," also known as a stroke. And the unfortunate consequence is the death of some portion of brain tissue. Depending upon which part of the brain is affected and to what degree, the symptoms can range from a tiny loss of memory or fine motor skills all the way up to death.

There are other causes of strokes, including ruptured blood vessels and elevated blood pressure. But hardened or blocked arteries and blood clots plugging small arteries or lodging in "plaque dams" are major problems, caused by the same factors that bring about heart disease. The good news, though, is that you can help protect yourself from strokes with a sensible diet.

20/30 Helps Keep Blood Pressure Under Control

It's a frightening idea: a disease that can seriously damage your cardiovascular system, trigger a stroke, damage the kidneys, or cause various other, potentially serious problems, yet produces no symptoms, no warning bells, or flashing red lights to warn you of its existence. That's why elevated blood pressure (hypertension) is called the "silent killer." It can go unnoticed for years, quietly doing irreversible damage to your vital organs long before you know it's there. And by the time you find out, it may be too late.

It's estimated that more than fifty million Americans have hypertension, but only two-thirds of them have been diagnosed. Here are the definitions of good and dangerous blood pressure readings, according to the 1993 report by the National High Blood Pressure Education Program:

Optimal: *lower than 120/80*   **Normal to high:** *up to 139/89*
Normal: *up to 130/85*   **Hypertension:** *140/90 or more*

About 90 percent of those with elevated blood pressure have essential hypertension, also known as primary hypertension. It seems to come on its own, perhaps because of problems with the heart or blood vessels. The rest have secondary hypertension, so called because it's due to something else, such as obesity, kidney disease, hormonal disorders, certain drugs, or excessive alcohol consumption. It may even be "white coat" hypertension, the temporary rise in blood pressure caused by the stress of being in the doctor's office.

Your blood pressure is determined by two key factors: how hard your heart beats and how easily the blood flows through your arteries. Your blood pressure will rise if your heart is shooting blood out of its chambers by pumping forcefully and/or your arteries are clogged or too stiff to easily expand and contract with the flow of blood. Your blood pressure will fall if your heart is in a relaxed mode, gently squeezing the blood out and/or your arteries are wide open, and your artery walls can easily expand and contract with the flow of blood.

The *20/30* approach helps to lower blood pressure by clearing away the plaque that clogs arteries and makes them too stiff to open wide

A Low-fat Rather Than Low-salt Diet Lowers Blood Pressure

For years, physicians have been advising their patients with elevated blood pressure to eat less salt. That's good advice for those who are salt sensitive, but it won't do the trick for most.[26] An even better approach is to go easy on the salt and switch to the 20/30 way of life.

Salt "holds" water in the body, so increasing your salt intake can expand your blood volume and raise your blood pressure. Thus, it is reasoned, a low-salt diet should lower blood pressure. However, the facts do not support the theory. Low-salt diets are relatively ineffective when it comes to lowering blood pressure. Severely restricting salt intake can actually push blood pressure up even higher, increase cholesterol and even trigger a heart attack. All told, people on very low-salt diets have a higher death rate than those who eat average amounts of salt.[27]

For most people, the key to lowering blood pressure is adopting a low-fat diet containing lots of fruits and vegetables [28], exercising, losing excess weight, restricting alcohol consumption, and reducing stress.

then contract efficiently. And it combats obesity, which has been associated with elevated blood pressure.

The added fiber you'll be eating on the *20/30* plan is also effective at reducing blood pressure. In one fiber/blood pressure study, forty-six patients with blood pressures averaging 157/97 were given either tablets containing 7 grams of fiber or a placebo that had no fiber.[29] Three months later, the average blood pressure had dropped to 147/92 in the fiber group, but remained constant among those who took the placebo. These positive results were limited by the small amount of fiber the patients took in (only 7 grams a day), and the fact that it came in pill form, rather than from real food. Just think how much better the results will be when you're eating even more fiber and it comes from real food.

Another experiment grouped ninety-four volunteers, ranging in age from eighteen to sixty, according to how much fiber they ate.[30] Here are some of the findings:

- Those who ate high-fiber diets had lower blood pressures than those who consumed low-fiber diets.
- When eleven who had been eating high-fiber diets switched to low-fiber diets for four weeks, their blood pressures rose.
- When thirty-one who had been eating low-fiber diets consumed more fiber, their blood pressures dropped.

Findings like these are not surprising. We've known for several years that among populations eating lots of fiber, blood pressure does not rise with age, as it does here in the United States, where relatively little fiber is consumed.

20/30 May Help Prevent a Major Form of Impotence

Viagra, the "wonder drug" men are snatching up like candy, is in the news as this book is being written. With some 50 percent of men age sixty-five suffering from impotence to one degree or another, it's no wonder that a pill that promises to restore sexual function is flying off pharmacy shelves.

Like heart disease and strokes, impotence can be caused by clogged arteries. In this case, however, the blockage lies in the arteries that normally swell with blood at the appropriate times, holding the fluid there in order to make the penis erect. In fact, clogged arteries are responsible for more than 60 percent of impotence.

For those suffering from this problem, the solution may be this simple: use the *20/30* approach to begin clearing out clogged arteries and improve your circulation.

20/30 Keeps the Immune System Strong

Like small fish in the ocean, we're constantly surrounded by danger, but instead of fearing sharks and eels, we have to watch out for bacteria, viruses, fungi, toxic chemicals, and other substances that, once inside our bodies, can make us ill — or even kill us. Fortunately, we've evolved a multilayered, highly complex defense system called the immune system.

Like any modern army, the immune system has specially trained "soldiers" equipped to handle specific attacks. Macrophages literally surround and engulf the enemy; T cells called natural killer cells grapple with invaders and cancer cells in hand-to-hand combat; B cells produce antibodies specifically designed to seek out and destroy targeted germs; neutrophils serve as the foot soldiers for this internal army. Lightly armed, the neutrophils are often among the first to enter the fray en masse, sacrificing themselves in large numbers to keep the body healthy. There are also helper T cells to assist in "combat control," and suppressor T cells to help calm things down once the battle has been won.

Although they possess tremendous power, the immune system soldiers are absolutely dependent on their supply system. Without the proper nutrients to keep it strong, our internal army would quickly weaken and be overrun. What do our immune soldiers require? The same vitamins, minerals, phytochemicals, and other substances that keep the rest of the body healthy—the same nourishing items found *The 20/30 Plan*. A deficiency of even a single vitamin or mineral can hamper the immune system, reducing the production of T cells, impairing the ability of macrophages to ingest foreign bodies, interfering with the manufacture of antibodies by the B cells, or otherwise weakening our internal army.

Like most of the rest of the body, the immune system works better when not plagued by excess fat. In one study proving this fact, seventeen healthy young males were asked to reduce the amount of fat in their diets. Three months later, there was more natural killer cell activity in their blood.[31]

By reducing your fat intake *The 20/30 Fat & Fiber Diet Plan* can help you strengthen your immune system.

But be careful not to swing to the other extreme, to very low-calorie eating, in an attempt to lose weight or strengthen your immune system. That can be just as dangerous. A study in the *European Journal of Clinical Nutrition* reported that severely restricting food intake reduces the blood levels of gamma globulins and natural killer cells, two very important components of the immune system.[32]

20/30 Helps Defeat Diabetes

Diabetes mellitus type II is another ailment intimately related to diet. Although its causes are varied, quite often it is the result of poor diet and sedentary lifestyle—too much fat and too many refined carbohydrates on the plate, leading to too much fat on the body.

As food is digested and glucose (sugar) released into the bloodstream, your blood sugar rises. The pancreas responds by pumping out insulin, which helps drive the blood sugar into the body's cells for use as energy or to be stored for later use. Unfortunately, with diabetes mellitus type II, your body becomes resistant to insulin, "ignoring" its attempts to push the glucose into the cells. The pancreas continues sending out insulin, but to no avail. The sugar remains in the blood, its level rising. The sugar by itself is harmless, but it can stick on cell membranes, causing nerve damage leading to heart attacks, strokes, blindness, deafness, kidney damage, impotence, and amputations. In addition, the excess insulin pumped out by the pancreas can constrict arteries, increasing the risk of heart attacks and strokes. It also makes you hungrier than usual, causing you to eat more and gain more weight, exacerbating the problem.

Dietary fat encourages high blood sugar levels by slowing the cell's absorption of blood sugar, thus allowing it to build to high levels.[33] And if you have diabetes, the high-protein Western diet is doubly dangerous. A major European study has shown that eating too much protein damages the kidneys in diabetics.[34] Another recent study demonstrated that diets rich in refined carbohydrates harm diabetics, while consuming the monounsaturated and polyunsaturated fats in vegetables, and the omega-3 fatty acids in fish, helps to reduce insulin requirements.[35]

Unchecked, diabetes can do the the following:

- Encourage the buildup of plaque in the arteries, resulting in heart disease, stroke, impotence, infections, poor wound healing, and gangrene.
- Impair the immune system, leading to increased infections and other problems.
- Harm the small blood vessels in the eyes, causing vision problems and blindness.
- Trigger kidney failure by damaging the blood vessels in the kidneys.
- Damage nerves, causing pain, tingling, reduced sensation in the hands and feet, weakness in the legs, and many other problems.

Fat is a major contributing factor to this metabolic disorder: 80–90 percent of those with type II diabetes mellitus are obese. Many diabetics who slim down to normal weight, exercise regularly and keep their blood sugar under control become nondiabetic, no longer needing insulin shots or other medications. Diet and exercise are crucial components in the fight against diabetes. Excess fat prevents insulin from attaching to receptors, forcing the body to pump out more insulin to "shove" the fat into the appropriate cells. That extra insulin can cause serious damage to the body. Reducing your fat intake, and consequently your total body fat, lessens the problem.

The key to treating diabetes is to prevent blood sugar levels from rising too high after meals. It is far safer to let your blood sugar remain slightly elevated for a long time after eating than to allow it to rise rapidly to high levels, then crash down to unnaturally low levels. Develop the following eating habits to keep your blood sugar generally stable:

Type I Versus Type II

Diabetes mellitus type I, like the more common type II, is caused by the failure of insulin to drive blood sugar into the cells. But while those with type II make sufficient amounts of insulin, perhaps even more than normal, those with type I make little or none at all.

Only about 10 percent of those with diabetes mellitus have type I, which tends to develop before the patient is forty years old. We're not quite sure why the insulin-making cells in the pancreas are destroyed with type I; it may be due to genetic errors or viruses.

- Severely restrict your consumption of dietary sugar and refined carbohydrates. Refined carbohydrates—such as white bread, pasta, bagels, cookies, crackers, rolls, and white rice—cause almost the same rise in blood sugar as granulated sugar.
- Eat lots of whole grains, which break down slowly, releasing a slow, steady stream of glucose. The fiber in whole grains binds to the starch, delaying the entry of sugar into the bloodstream and keeping blood sugar from spiking.
- Only eat fruit when you're eating other foods that will slow sugar absorption, such as whole grains.

A recent study has shown that while eating lots of refined carbohydrates harms diabetics, the monounsaturated and polyunsaturated fats in vegetables, as well as the omega-3 fatty acids in fish, help combat the problem by reducing the need for insulin.[36] And a study conducted with laboratory animals has demonstrated that adult-onset diabetes can be prevented by restricting caloric intake and preventing excessive weight gain.[37]

Many Type II diabetics can eliminate their symptoms and get off all medications by employing just three strategies: consuming a high-fiber, low-fat diet, losing excess weight, and exercising regularly.

Diabetes, cancer, heart disease, stroke, high blood pressure, impotence, and other ailments: *The 20/30 Plan* helps guard against them all. And as you'll learn in the next chapter, the foods you'll be eating contain special substances, called phytochemicals, that also help boost health in many ways. ■

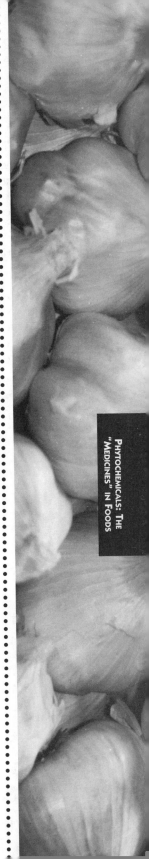

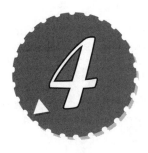

PHYTOCHEMICALS: THE "MEDICINES" IN FOODS

The use of food to cure ills is an ancient art garnering modern attention. For centuries, for example, the Polish people treated various ailments with onions. Today, studies have shown that eating onions can help lower cholesterol, prevent unnecessary and dangerous blood clots, ease breathing difficulties, and fight both cancer and heart disease.

Long before the Europeans came to the New World, Native Americans were drinking a beverage made from willow bark to ease aches and pains. Today we know that willow bark contains salicylic acid, the main ingredient in aspirin.

Hundreds of years ago, women in Mexico ate yams to prevent pregnancy. Today, a widely used contraceptive medication is derived from yams.

Residents of the Shizuoka Prefecture in Japan have long consumed copious quantities of green tea—and they also have much lower rates of stomach cancer than those who live elsewhere in Japan. Today, researchers have discovered that green tea contains *catechins*, which strengthen the body's resistance to cancer.

Quick Definitions: Free Radicals and Antioxidants

Free radicals are formed during most chemical reactions in your body. They can damage the genetic material in your cells to cause aging and increase your chances of getting cancers. Anything that increases chemical reactions in your body increases the production of free radicals including the following:

Diabetes	Immune reactions
Obesity	Injuries
Air pollution	Tobacco smoke
Excessive vitamin C	Radioactive emissions
Some trace minerals	Asbestos
Ultraviolet light rays	Some herbicides

To protect your cells from free radical damage, your body produces **antioxidants** such as superoxide dismutase. The fruits, vegetables, and whole grains you eat are loaded with antioxidants, such as vitamins A, C, and E; minerals such as selenium; and phytochemicals such as carotenoids, flavinoids, and genistein.

Hippocrates, the "father of modern medicine," praised the use of food as medicine all the way back in 400 B.C. when he said "Let food be your medicine and medicine be your food." But with the advent of modern medicine, of X-rays, antibiotics, and surgery, food remedies fell out of favor. Technically minded twentieth-century Western physicians deemed such approaches too simple and old-fashioned to be effective against complex diseases. The evidence linking diet to health and disease was discounted, or simply ignored. And there was, in all fairness, reason to believe that drugs and surgery would soon cure all diseases. Why bother examining the medicinal potential of foods when you could kill germs with penicillin or surgically bypass clogged coronary arteries?

But in the past twenty or so years, as we've come to realize that while modern medicine can perform wonders it can not cure all our ailments, medical scientists have again turned an inquisitive eye to foods. Thanks to modern research techniques, we've discovered that numerous foods contain powerful substances that fight deadly diseases, control free radical damage, lessen the body's inflammation response, strengthen the immune system, ease pain, and otherwise improve and maintain health in countless ways. What substances perform these miracles? *Phytochemicals.*

What Are Phytochemicals?

Neither vitamins nor minerals, phytochemicals are naturally occurring substances in plants that trigger beneficial chemical reactions within the body ("phyto" means "plant"). There are thousands of phytochemicals in the foods we eat, many of them not yet identified or studied. We do know, however, that they can help us become healthier—and stay that way.

The many phytochemicals with which we are familiar are found in fruits, vegetables, and whole grains. This means that you get them "free" while on *The 20/30 Fat & Fiber Diet Plan*. You don't have to eat any exotic foods or take supplements; phytochemicals are already there in the foods you'll be eating. Here are twenty-seven of the better-known of these "food medicines":

- **Adenosine** is a blood thinner that guards against stroke and heart disease by preventing the formation of unnecessary blood clots. These clots may get stuck in the tiny arteries of the heart or brain: Just like logs and debris in a river, they can "dam" the flow of life-giving blood. If this happens in the heart, the result may be a heart attack; if in the brain, a stroke. Adenosine is found in garlic, onions, and black mushrooms.
- **Ajoene** is another blood thinner. It's found in garlic.

- **Allicin**, which acts as an antibiotic and antifungal, also helps prevent the formation of cancer-causing nitrosamines in your stomach. Allicin is found in garlic.

- **Bioflavonoids**, a group of two hundred–plus substances found in plants, give citrus fruits their orange and yellow colors. Strong antioxidants that help the body ward off heart disease and cancer, they also strengthen the tiny blood vessels called capillaries, and reduce allergy-driven inflammation. The outer layers of fruits and vegetables are good sources of bioflavonoids, as are green leafy vegetables. The catechins in green tea and the quercetin in red grapes are among the better known bioflavonoids.

- **Capsaicin**, which gives chili peppers their heat, helps us keep cool by reducing inflammation and pain. It also aids in easing cluster headaches, clearing blocked breathing passages, protecting cells from cancer-causing chemicals, reducing the "bad" LDL cholesterol, and lowering blood fat (triglyceride) levels.

- **Catechins**, part of the bioflavonoid family, are in the news thanks to the increasing popularity of the green tea in which they are found. These bioflavonoids can help fight cancer, lower cholesterol and high blood pressure, combat bacteria, reduce high blood glucose, and slow the aging process. But you won't find many catechins in black tea, for they're destroyed in the processing.

- **Coumarins**, like adenosine and ajoene, help prevent heart disease and stroke by "thinning" the blood, and aid the body in the battle against cancer. You'll find coumarins in many whole grains, fruits, and vegetables.

- **Ellagic acid** is a quiet soldier in the battle against cancer, helping to neutralize carcinogens before they complete their assault on healthy cells. Ellagic acid is a "sweet" phytochemical found in grapes, strawberries, cherries, and other fruits.

- **Genistein** is at least partially responsible for the anti-cancer properties attributed to tofu and other foods made from soy. This phytochemical helps to fight diseases (especially cancers of the breast and uterus) by hindering the flow of blood to tumors.

- **Glutathione** is an antioxidant found in tomatoes, watermelons, strawberries, and other foods. It fights free radicals, protects against cancer and heart disease, and delays the appearance of some of the signs and symptoms of aging.

- **Indoles** are part of the "crucifer" family of vegetables' armament against cancer. The crucifers (including broccoli, Brussels sprouts, cabbage, and cauliflower) have long been noted for their ability to help guard against colon cancer, breast cancer, and other forms of the disease.

- **Isoflavones** use their resemblance to estrogen, the female hormone, to fight cancer. Some breast and other tumors are "strengthened" by estrogen. Isoflavones fit into the estrogen receptors on these tumor cells, preventing the real estrogen from interacting with the cell. Deprived of estrogen, the tumors cannot grow. Isoflavones are found in legumes (peas, lentils, and beans), sweet potatoes, and whole grains.

- **Lignans** fight cancer by "deactivating" the estrogen that seeks to feed tumors. They're also antioxidants that guard against free radical damage. Lignans are found in most plants.

- **Limonene**, named for the lemon, is found in the skins of citrus fruits. This little-noticed phytochemical may help retard the development of cancer.

- **Linolenic acid**, an essential fatty acid and powerful antioxidant, aids in the battle against heart disease, cancer, inflammation, and other ailments, including, many believe, the symptoms of premature aging. It's found in fish and most seeds (including whole grains and beans).

- **Lycopene**, a relative of beta-carotene found in watermelon, tomatoes, ruby red grapefruit, red peppers, and other red fruits or vegetables, may help guard against cancers of the prostate, colon, lung, bladder, and cervix. Researchers have also found that people with the highest stores of lycopene in their bodies were only about half as likely to suffer heart attacks as those with the lowest levels. That's because it's a potent antioxidant, keeping LDL in the bloodstream from being oxidized to form plaque.

- **Phenols** are a large group of compounds that promote health in many ways, including helping to fight viruses, control excessive bleeding, and neutralize carcinogens. The phenols' strong antioxidant effect protects the body against heart disease, cancer, and the deleterious effects of aging. Garlic, soybeans, some seeds, potatoes, citrus fruit, and green tea all contain phenols.

- **Phytoestrogens** shield us against certain cancers by "pretending" to be estrogen. They bind to special receptors on estrogen-dependent tumors, preventing the "real thing" from nourishing the unwanted growths. Eating large amounts of beans and soy products, which contain phytoestrogens, has been linked to lower rates of breast cancer, as well as fewer deaths from cancer of the pancreas and prostate.

- **Protease inhibitors** help prevent the digestion of excessive amounts of protein. Too much protein can encourage the growth of certain types of cancer, so preventing unnecessary protein from entering the body can help inhibit the growth of these cancers. Protease inhibitors also assist in keeping cellular DNA from mutating and turning a cell line cancerous. These cancer-fighting phytochemicals are found in soybeans (and tofu), beans, chick peas, oats, and seeds.

■ **Quercetin**, an antioxidant found in red grapes, broccoli, onions, and other fruits and vegetables, helps to deactivate certain strong carcinogens and tumor promoters. When combined with vitamin C, it can also help fight off viruses.

■ **Resveratrol**, like adenosine and other blood-thinning phytochemicals, helps to ward off heart attacks and strokes. It also may help to keep healthy cells from becoming cancerous, while inhibiting the spread of cancerous growths that have already started. Resveratrol is found in red and white grape skins, wine, and grape juice.

■ **Sulfides** work to keep the cardiovascular system healthy by helping to keep blood pressure under control and thinning the blood. You'll find them in garlic, cabbage, broccoli, Brussels sprouts, and other vegetables.

■ **Tannins** are acids found in tea. They can help inhibit inflammation, as well guard against unnecessary and dangerous blood clots.

■ **Triterpenoids**, found in licorice root and citrus fruits, can slow or prevent the growth of certain kinds of cancer by deactivating steroidal hormones.

■ **Zeaxanthin** is a carotenoid, which makes it a cousin to beta-carotene. Found in dark green, leafy vegetables such as spinach, it may play an important part in preventing some of the ailments associated with aging, including the macular degeneration that can rob you of your sight. ■

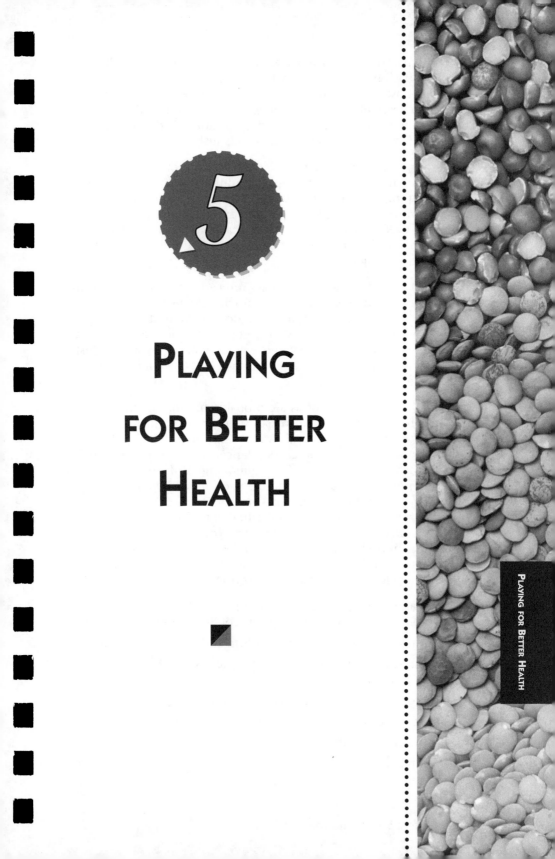

5

PLAYING
FOR BETTER
HEALTH

Think back to when you were a kid: remember how much fun it was to dash back and forth with your friends, playing tag? How about those endless hours spent jumping rope, turning cartwheels, playing baseball, riding your bike, belly-boarding at the beach, or scrambling over the rocks? Dancing for hours at the high school prom? It wasn't exercise, was it? It was just fun.

We were made to move; it's programmed into our genes. Unfortunately, our natural love of running, jumping, skipping, and leaping is often ruined by formal physical education classes, where running laps, climbing ropes, and doing push-ups become chores, even punishment for bad behavior. It's no wonder that so many people become convinced that exercise is uncomfortable, tiring, and a big bore.

But it doesn't have to be like that. You can recapture the youthful joy you used to experience when moving. Remember, you're not in Phys. Ed. class anymore and you don't have to do something just because the teacher says so. You can run and play just because you enjoy doing it, just as you did when you were younger. Just as you were made to—for the fun of it—and get slimmer and healthier in the process.

Today, of course, most of us are probably not terribly interested in playing tag or kick the can. But there are a number of terrific "adult" ways to play. You can walk briskly, jog, swim, cycle, play tennis, racquetball, or soccer, ski, dance, or engage in any number of fun activities that will keep you moving. And while you're at it, you can pretend you're leading the pack at the Olympic races, leaving your buddies behind as you cross-country ski toward buried treasure, or dancing a breathtaking solo on stage at the Met. Or, if you're not into fantasy and you'd like to take a more serious approach that allows you to determine just how hard you're playing and at what level, you can use various machines, including electronic bicycles and rowing machines.

Forget about exercise—it's time to play. Regular playing can benefit you in at least six different ways. You'll develop the following:

1. A faster, more efficient metabolism and decreased body fat

2. Improved efficiency of the heart, lungs, and circulatory system; increased fitness

3. Protection from cardiovascular disease

4. Improved emotional and psychological states

5. Increased flexibility and strength

6. Improved health for life

Let's take a closer look at each of these six points.

1) A faster, more efficient metabolism and decreased body fat

It's not news to most weight-watchers that the best way to burn off extra calories, and the only way to convert soft, fat, flabby bodies into trim, muscular ones, is to "play." Think of weight loss as an equation: if calorie output is greater than calorie input, you lose pounds. If the reverse is true, you gain weight. Obviously, the longer or harder you play, the more calories you'll burn. Running fast for ten minutes will certainly burn more calories than jogging slowly for ten minutes. But there's also evidence showing that the harder you play, the more calories you'll continue to burn *for hours afterwards*.

Here's why this works the way it does. We all need a certain number of calories to support basic bodily functions (respiration, digestion, cardiovascular action, for example). This number, known as the *resting metabolic rate*, increases after intense play, and can remain high for as many as eighteen hours after a play session. Think about what happens when you take your car out for a spin, then park it in the garage. Even though you turn the car off, it may remain warm and continue to emit heat for hours. Your body also emits extra heat after vigorous play, which is why your temperature may run slightly higher and you'll continue to burn calories at a faster rate after a workout.

When "Fat" Is not Fat

A guy who stands six feet tall and weighs 230 pounds is fat, right? And woman who is five feet five inches and weighs 100 pounds is skinny, right?

Maybe, maybe not.

Many football players and other bulky athletes tip the scales at alarmingly high weights without actually being "fat." They're simply very muscular, and muscles weigh a lot. On the other hand, some people who appear to be slim have very little muscle and a surprisingly high amount of fat, making them quite "fatty." Some fashion models are much "fattier" than athletes.

As a general rule of thumb, men should carry 10–15 percent of their body weight as fat. This means, for example, that 18 to 27 pounds on a 180-pound man's body should be made up of fat, while the rest is made up of lean body tissue (bone, organs, and muscles).

For women, 18–22 percent body fat is considered healthy.

And that's just the beginning. Your metabolic rate is also affected by the amount of muscle tissue you've got. Since muscle tissue is more metabolically active than fat, it burns more calories just to "stay alive," aside from the calories it uses to do the "work" of contracting. People who have greater amounts of muscle tissue automatically burn more calories, even when they're not exercising. This means that engaging in regular, intense play that tones and builds your muscles can help you lose weight and keep it off even when you're doing *nothing*!

This is particularly important when dieting because weight loss *without* play causes you to lose both fat *and* muscle. Just as a gain of muscle drives your resting metabolic rate *up*, a loss of muscle pushes it *down*. The unfortunate result, as many dieters can tell you, is that you wind up burning calories more slowly after a diet than you did before. This, in turn, means you can gain weight even though you're eating *less* food than before. You can actually wind up fatter *after* dieting than you were before you started! The solution is simple: play. Playing prevents the loss of muscle tissue and keeps your body humming along, burning calories at a good clip.

2) *Improved efficiency of the heart, lungs, and circulatory system; increased fitness*

For our purposes, fitness simply refers to the strength of your heart muscle. If your heart is strong, you're fit; if it isn't, you're not. The only way to become more fit is to strengthen your heart. You do this the same way you strengthen any other muscle—by exercising it against increasing resistance. To make your biceps stronger, you have to lift increasingly heavy weights. To make your thigh muscles stronger, you have to bicycle up increasingly steeper hills. To make your heart muscle stronger, you have to make it beat increasingly faster and harder through intensive aerobic play activities.

Aerobic means "with oxygen," and aerobic exercises are designed to get you breathing—hard! When performed for at least thirty minutes at a stretch, aerobic play activities such as running, walking quickly, biking, or aerobic dancing will improve the ability of your heart, lungs, and circulatory system to carry oxygen through-out the body. When you engage in some form of aerobic play three to five times a week for at least twenty to thirty minutes each session, you'll strengthen your cardiovascular system and make it much more efficient. Your heart will begin to pump more blood with each beat, your resting blood pressure and resting heart rate will decrease. The number of red blood cells (the oxygen-bearing cells) in your bloodstream will increase, as will the amount of blood that's delivered to the tissues. All this happens because your heart, lungs, and circulatory system are

Measuring Percent Body Fat

No matter what your height or weight, you're better off if you have just enough body fat, not too much or too little. As we said earlier, for men 10–15 percent body fat is ideal, for women, 18–22 percent. There are several means of measuring your percent body fat. You may have seen people being measured with the "pinch test." A small device called a skinfold caliper is used to pinch the skin at various points on your body. With each pinch, the tester jots down a measurement. These numbers are used to figure your body fat percentage. It's a simple, inexpensive means of getting a quick reading, but it's not perfect. If the tester is good, pinching properly and at the right spots, your result will be fairly accurate. If not, it may be off by as much as four to five points, which means that a reading of 15 percent body fat could actually mean anywhere from 10 to 20 percent.

Bioelectrical impedance is a high-tech approach to measuring percent body fat in which a mild electrical current is sent through your body. The current travels more quickly through lean body tissue than through fat, so the machine analyzes the speed with which the current travels, then plugs the results into a mathematical formula. You can have this test performed at some doctors' offices, or your gym may offer it. You can also purchase home models that look like bathroom scales for between $125 and $250 (depending on the type). These may not be completely accurate, but they will give you a consistent reading to help you track your progress.

The most accurate method of determining your body fat percentage is underwater weighing. Since fat floats and muscle sinks in water, "dense" people who have relatively large amounts of muscle and other lean body tissue but little fat will be heavy underwater. Conversely, "fatty" folk with lots of body fat and comparatively little lean body tissue will be relatively light. In other words, a lower amount of body fat means you'll weigh more underwater, while a higher amount of body fat means you'll weigh less. This test has a fairly small margin of error, but is expensive, time consuming, and requires that you completely submerge yourself in a tank of water.

becoming better at what they do, so they'll be working less than before to attain the same results.

In this respect, fitness is more a product of how hard you play than of how long. You won't get a lot of benefit by just stretching, or shuffling through a long list of play activities that don't get you breathing hard. You can increase your fitness level more by working at it intensely for shorter periods—for example, running fast a couple of times a week rather than running slowly several times a week. (Note: Beginners should start slowly and cautiously. See "Before You Begin" on page 54.)

3) Protection from cardiovascular disease

Cardiovascular disease, the clogging of the coronary arteries that leads to heart attacks, is currently the number one cause of death in the United States. Every year, 1.5 million Americans suffer heart attacks; the disease claims another life every thirty-four seconds. In 1992, the American Heart Association added "sedentary lifestyle" to their list of risk factors for cardiovascular disease, putting it right up there with smoking, high blood pressure, and harmful cholesterol levels. They did this because medical science learned just how important regular play is for maintaining heart health.

Besides strengthening and improving the efficiency of the cardiovascular system, regular play can lower the levels of blood fats (triglycerides) and "bad" LDL cholesterol. Lower levels of blood fats and LDL cholesterol means there will be less fatty gunk (plaque) building up in your arteries. At the same time, play raises your levels of "good" HDL cholesterol slightly. Some studies with animals also suggest that play can help widen the blood vessels, making it even harder for these vital bloodways to become blocked. Energetic play is great for lowering high blood pressure, eliminating excess weight, preventing or controlling diabetes, and releasing stress. Play combats all of these risk factors for heart disease at once.

4) Improved emotional and psychological states.

Playing is a terrific way to deal with stress, decrease the appetite, and enjoy the euphoria that comes from smacking the tennis ball right in the center of the racquet, perfectly executing a dance step, or jogging through the park on a beautiful day. The release of endorphins and certain brain neurotransmitters that occurs during vigorous play can bring about a sense of joy and overall well-being. And play appears to help people stick with their eating plans. A research paper published in the *American Journal of Clinical Nutrition*[1] showed that overweight people who began a play program at the same time they started dieting were much more likely to stay with their regimen than those who dieted without exercising.

5) Increased flexibility and strength.

In addition to improving cardiovascular health, a good play program increases overall muscle tone and joint flexibility. Many health problems can be traced to a lack of muscular strength—

Beware the False Promises of Protein

Many fitness buffs and instructors praise the muscle-building prowess of protein, insisting that you must drink high-protein shakes or take protein pills if you want to bulk up, develop "cuts," or have rippling muscles.

We certainly need protein to build muscles, but most of us are getting way too much of it, not too little, and that can be bad for your bones. If you live long enough, you will probably end up suffering from some degree of osteoporosis, the weakening and thinning of the bones that makes them unusually susceptible to breakage. Excess protein, however, exacerbates the problem by increasing the excretion of calcium. This, in turn, hastens the loss of bone.[2] Studies have shown that high-protein diets loaded with meat weaken the bones of post-menopausal women. Knowing that excess protein encourages osteoporosis, researchers looked into whether eating less protein would reverse the problem. The answer is yes. A study reported on in the New England Journal of Medicine *found that osteoporosis could be prevented by reducing protein intake to moderate levels.[3]*

You're better off passing on the excess protein and loading up on low-fat, high-fiber foods. In the 20/30 program, you'll get plenty of protein for muscle building as well as lots of complex carbohydrates for energy.

back pain, for example, is often due to weak back or abdominal muscles. "Bad knees" may be caused by weak joint supporting structures. Neck problems may arise from chronically poor posture due to lack of muscle endurance. Keeping muscles well-toned and well-stretched can help prevent these problems, as well as strains, sprains, stiff joints, and pain caused by overusing other muscles to compensate for the weak ones.

6) Improved health for life.

Play can help prolong your life. People who play regularly are less likely to develop the disabling and deadly diseases we associate with aging, including heart disease, stroke, high blood pressure, diabetes, osteoporosis, and even cancer. A recent paper appearing in the *New England Journal of Medicine* reported on a study that followed over twenty-five thousand women aged twenty to fifty-four for an average of thirteen years. The researchers found that the women who engaged in regular physical activity at least four hours per week had a 37 percent lower risk of developing breast cancer.[4]

Exercisers tend to look and feel younger, sleep better, keep their weight within normal limits, fend off memory loss, suffer less arthritis, fewer back problems and muscle strains, and remain in better spirits than nonexercisers. And, within certain limits, it seems that the more you play, the better. One study looking at nonsmoking retired men over a twelve-year period found that those who walked two miles a day were half as likely to die as those who walked only one mile per day. [5]

Before You Begin

If you're not already working out, how do you get started? In a word, slowly. Most people who begin an ambitious play program, (especially those who haven't exercised in a long time), quit in the first few weeks, either because they're injured or it's just too hard. Give yourself a break and start slowly. It may have taken you years to get into your current shape. Getting fit can't be accomplished overnight.

If you're over the age of thirty and not already exercising regularly, or if you want to intensify your workout routine, begin by seeing your physician. Tell your doctor what you'd like to do and ask him or her to examine you to make sure there is no reason why you shouldn't.

Aerobic Exercises of All Types

The bulk of your play session (twenty to thirty minutes) should be devoted to aerobic activity, continuous play that increases your heart rate and leaves you breathing heavily. To get aerobic benefits, you must increase your heart rate by at least 20 beats per minute over your resting rate. (Take your pulse when your body is at rest to get this number.) Many enjoyable sports—including tennis, baseball, golf, basketball, volleyball, football, and weight-lifting—are beneficial but not truly aerobic, for they don't keep you moving vigorously enough for a long enough period. On the other hand, fast walking, cycling, running, jogging, rollerblading, ice skating, rowing, and aerobic dance do provide aerobic benefits when they're done energetically and without stopping for twenty to thirty minutes.

The challenge is to find forms of play that you really like, because you're much more likely to continue to do something fun. And doing it, of course, is the real goal.

Strength Training

Exercises that develop muscular strength and endurance fulfill an important role in any fitness program. Good muscle tone is essential for the maintenance of correct posture, prevention of osteoporosis, ease of movement, and the look of a lean, healthy body. Strength training exercises also help you preserve your muscle condition as you grow older. With age, many muscle fibers die off and are not replaced. In order to stay strong, you must strengthen and enlarge the remaining muscle fibers to avoid the weakness and frailty seen in so many of the elderly. (Most older folks can't get out of a chair without using their hands to push off because their thigh muscles are so weak.) And of course, toned muscles help you stay slim by burning calories even when you're not working out.

You're All Wet — and Should Be!

If you want to take a "supplement" to help you become stronger and more fit, try H_2O.

The human body is over 75 percent water; even the "dry" bones are 20 percent H_2O. If your water reserves drop too low, your blood, bowels and other parts of the body can suffer. We lose water constantly, even though we're not always aware of it, as it goes out with our breath, sweat, and wastes.

A good rule of thumb is to drink eight 8 ounce glasses of water a day and be sure to drink while you exercise to avoid dehydration. Don't wait until you're thirsty. By then you've already lost two pints of fluid.

To build muscle strength and size, you must play against resistance — that is, use your muscles to exert a force against a countering force. Free weights, exercise machines, or even your own body weight can provide resistance. But whether you choose free weights or machines, it's essential that you find a good instructor to help you learn how to use exercise equipment correctly. This person should also help you design a safe training program, tailored to your needs, that gradually increases the amount of work your body does over time. Your coach or trainer should then stay with you at least through your first few sessions to make sure you are holding the equipment properly and executing each movement with correct form.

Start out with one to three sets of ten repetitions, using a weight you can lift ten times in a row without losing form. When that weight becomes easy for you, move up to the next heavier level. You build stronger muscles by working with increasingly heavier weights, not by doing more repetitions. Eight or ten exercises using different machines is plenty. Your entire weight training session should last no more than ten to fifteen minutes, unless you spend a lot of time resting between sets.

Lifting weights increases blood pressure significantly, so check with your physician before beginning a weight training program or significantly increasing your existing routine.

How Flexible Are You?

Your goal needn't be to be able to hook your ankle around the back of your neck or put your nose to your knees while sitting with your legs straight out in front of you, but good flexibility does make it easier for you to perform daily chores and exercises, while reducing the risk of strain and injury. The more flexible you are, the more you can move a joint through its full range of motion, and the better able you will be to take advantage of the movement potential built into your body.

You can use devices such as a goniometer, which works something like a protractor, to precisely measure the degree to which you can bend and flex. But unless you're an athlete with dreams of Olympic gold, or an aspiring ballerina, some simple do-it-yourself estimates will suffice. Try these:

- **Toe touch**—Stand with your feet together, barefoot. Bend over and reach for the floor right in front of your feet. Keep your knees gently straight, but not locked.

  ▶ *Very good:* You can touch the floor with your palms, feeling little or no discomfort. This means you have good flexibility in your lower back and the back of your thighs.

  ▶ *Not bad:* You can touch your toes with your fingertips with only a little discomfort.

  ▶ *Needs work:* It's difficult to touch your toes even with your fingertips, or you can't reach them at all.

- **Behind the back clasp**—Put your left hand behind your back then reach up toward your right shoulder. Lift your right hand straight up in the air then bend your arm and lower your right hand to the back side of your right shoulder. Try to grab hold of the fingers of one hand with the other hand. Repeat, switching sides.

  ▶ *Very good:* You can easily grab hold of the opposite hand on each side. This means you have good shoulder flexibility.

  ▶ *Not bad:* You can touch or almost touch your fingertips together.

  ▶ *Needs work:* You cannot bring your fingertips close to each other.

- **Knee clasp**—Lying on your back, lift your right knee up to your chest. Pull it as far in to your chest as possible, holding on to your shin with your hands. Keep your left leg straight, resting on the ground. Repeat, switching sides.

  ▶ *Very good:* You can hug one knee to your chest with little or no discomfort, while the other leg stays straight and flat to the floor. This means the top front part of your hips and your buttocks are flexible.

  ▶ *Not bad:* You can almost pull your knee to your chest with the opposite leg pulling up or to the side just a little bit.

  ▶ *Needs work:* You cannot bring your knee close to your chest and your opposite leg pulls up or to the side significantly.

- **Heel to derriere**—Lying on your stomach, bring your right heel up to your derriere. Grab hold of your foot with your hand and try to touch your heel to your derriere. Repeat with your left leg.

  ▶ *Very good:* You easily touch your heels to your derriere. This means you have good flexibility in the front of your thighs.

  ▶ *Not bad:* You can almost touch your heels to your derriere.

  ▶ *Needs work:* You cannot bring your heels any closer than a few inches from your derriere.

These are not the only flexibility tests you can perform. You can devise more on your own by simply working your way through a series of common stretches, gauging to see if you can perform them fully, properly, and with ease, or if you struggle a bit, can't quite make it, or aren't even close.

There are no winners or losers in these tests. If you're very flexible, great. Keep working at it so you don't lose it. If you're not particularly flexible, work toward improving your stretch a little at a time, during each of your play sessions. It won't be long before you see some good results.

Play Program

A good play program includes aerobic exercise three days a week, strength training twice weekly, and two days off. That makes five sessions per week.

An aerobic play session includes:
      Ten minutes of warm-up
      Twenty to thirty minutes of aerobic activity
      Five to ten minutes of cool-down and stretching

The strength training session includes:
> Ten minutes of warm-up
> Ten minutes of strength training
> Five to ten minutes of cool-down and stretching

Work up to these times gradually, stopping if you feel tired or sore. If it's been a long time since you've exercised, it may take you six weeks or even six months to reach your goals. Don't worry if you start slowly—just keep playing away.

Avoiding Injury

The best way to avoid injury is knowing when to quit, and that's simple: if you feel pain, distress, or a "funny feeling," stop! Don't be a martyr. "Going for the burn" was popular in the 1980s, but not very wise. And beginners certainly don't want to start out that way. Out of shape muscles can easily become strained or torn, especially if you are older. If you feel pain or simply feel that something isn't right, stop for thirty seconds, then try again. If you notice the same sensation right away, move on to another play activity. But if the discomfort builds up gradually, just play until you feel it, then rest. Alternate these short periods of play and rest until you begin to strengthen your muscles and can play continuously.

If You Do Injure Yourself...

Should you suffer a muscle injury, think ***RICE*** — *Rest, Ice, Compression,* and *Elevation.*

> *Rest*—Immediately stop exercising.

> *Ice*—Place a bag of ice or chill pack wrapped in a towel on the affected area.

> *Compression*—Wrap a bandage around the ice bag, but don't make it so tight it is constricting.

> *Elevation*—Raise the injured area above heart level. If your back is injured, lie down.

After icing the injured area for ten to fifteen minutes, remove the ice bag and reapply once every hour for the first several hours. Unfortunately, there are no effective drugs or treatments for muscle injuries other than rest. Don't subject the injured part to any play activity until the pain is gone. When you do start exercising that area again, start slowly and easily, gradually building up to your former level of intensity and duration. If you feel any pain whatsoever, stop and don't use the area in a play activity again until all pain has disappeared.

Stepping up the Pace

Once you get into better condition, you'll need to play vigorously in order to increase your fitness level. Vigorous play—movement that causes you to breathe heavily, become tired, and feel no more than slightly sore the next day—is necessary to move you up to the next level but, once again, be careful not to push yourself too hard. Your muscles respond to the extra demand placed on them by becoming thicker and stronger. But if you demand too much, you can do damage that might leave you sidelined for weeks, if not permanently. (And even minor injuries that take you away from your activities for just a few days or weeks can be discouraging.)

Even if you're in great shape and not overdoing it, you should not use the same muscle groups in vigorous play activities every day. Intense play breaks down muscle fibers, causing them to become frayed like an old piece of rope. The muscle fibers actually bleed and the "Z bands" that hold muscle filaments together are temporarily disrupted. This is normal and natural, but your muscles will need at least forty-eight hours to heal. If you continue to stress them while they're healing, they can tear. Competitive athletes know this, so they avoid working the same set of muscles at high intensity day after day. Instead, they may work out vigorously one day, then do easy workouts on subsequent days until their muscles feel "fresh" again, all traces or soreness having vanished. You should do the same.

Combine Your Sports for Maximum Fitness

The ideal play program would include at least two different sports or activities; one that targets the lower body (such as running) and one that works the upper body (such as rowing). Play intensely in each sport once a week, do easier workouts the rest of the time, taking off one or two days a week. Here's an example:

> **Monday:** Aerobic dancing (lower body), moderate pace
> **Tuesday:** Rowing (upper body), vigorous pace
> **Wednesday:** Aerobic dancing (lower body), moderate pace
> **Thursday:** Rowing (upper body), moderate pace
> **Friday:** Aerobic dancing (lower body), vigorous pace
> **Saturday:** Day off.
> **Sunday:** Day off.

With this program, you only stress the major muscle groups to the extreme once a week—those in the upper body on Tuesday and the lower body on Friday. You are never working the same muscle groups two days in a row. And you're taking a complete rest for two days to give your body a chance to recover.

Alone, with a Friend, at the Gym, or with a Trainer?

Should you work out on your own or with a friend, in a gym or a club? Or is it best to hire a trainer? Here's a look at the pros and cons of each option.

__Alone__—You'll be able to work out whenever and in any way you desire, without worrying about anyone else's schedule or preferences. You'll also be able to watch television while stretching or read a book while riding a stationary bicycle if you feel like it. On the other hand, you may get lonely, need companionship, or wish for some encouragement to get yourself going. And procrastination is a big problem for all but the most highly motivated. You'll also have to devise your own workout program and purchase any equipment you need, but some people work out alone very successfully.

__With a friend__—You'll have company and someone to cheer you on, but you'll also have to accommodate your friend's schedule and wishes. But remember, a friend can also encourage you to be lazy or give up sooner than you should, if he or she is unmotivated. And the two of you will have to design your own exercise programs and buy all needed equipment.

__At a gym__—You'll have access to lots of equipment, as well as advice on how to use it and how to structure your program. The gym may also offer aerobics, stretching, or other classes, as well as babysitting services, lockers, and showers. However, you can only work out when the gym is open, and you may have trouble getting to the machines you need during prime time. Also, gym memberships cost money—sometimes a lot—and you'll have to make a special trip to get there.

__With a trainer__—You'll have someone to help you design your workout routine, to make sure you're doing everything safely and properly, and to motivate you to keep going, especially when you'd like to quit. But you'll have to exercise at a specific, prearranged time, your workout will only be as good as your trainer, and it costs plenty of money.

Which approach is best? Whatever style works best for you is the best one, and the best exercises are the ones that you will do consistently. The choice is yours.

Exercising Away Excess Weight

Exercising to lose weight and exercising to increase fitness are practically the same thing. The same three elements are required: aerobic play activity, regularity, and intensity.

Aerobic play activity—This means continuous play (moving without stopping) for twenty to thirty minutes. Aerobic play activity is the best way to raise your metabolic rate. It's also the best way to burn fat, since fat is the primary fuel source for this kind of playing.

Note: Although swimming is an excellent aerobic activity, it may not be the best approach to weight loss. Water conducts heat away from your body, which means that you won't experience the rise in body temperature that signals an increase in metabolism. As a result, you'll miss out on the calorie-burning aftereffects that other aerobic exercises can provide. When exercising on land, however, air insulates the body, allowing its temperature to increase. So for maximal weight loss, consider doing your aerobic exercises on land rather than in the water.

Regularity—For weight loss as well as overall fitness, you should play at least three times a week, including twenty to thirty minutes of aerobic play activity in each session. Five days a week is even better, if you alternate the kinds of sports or activities you do.

Intensity—You have to play hard enough to raise your pulse before you'll see aerobic benefits. To strengthen your heart, you must increase your heart rate at least twenty beats per minute above your resting heart rate. You needn't check your pulse while you're playing, however. You'll be able to tell when your heart rate is high enough by your breathing; it will be deeper and faster than usual. You'll still feel comfortable and able to talk, but you'll have trouble singing. If you begin gasping for breath and are breathing as hard as you can, you've reached your maximal heart rate. That's too much; ease off a little. To improve your fitness and "burn" away fat, work up to the point where you can exercise continuously while breathing deeply and more rapidly than normal, but not to the point where you're short of breath.

Body Mass Index

The results of regular play combined with healthful eating will soon be evident in your Body Mass Index (BMI). Remember, a BMI greater than 24 means it's likely that you're overweight, while 30 or greater signifies that it's likely you're obese. Here's a chart showing BMIs at typical heights and weights.[7]

	HEALTHY		OVERWEIGHT			
BMI	**23**	**24**	**25**	**26**	**27**	**28**
Height	**Weight**					
5'	118	123	128	133	138	143
5'1"	122	127	132	137	143	148
5'3"	130	135	141	146	152	158
5'5"	138	144	159	156	162	168
5'7"	146	153	159	166	172	178
5'9"	155	162	169	176	182	189
5'11"	165	172	179	186	193	200
6'1"	174	182	189	197	204	212
6'3"	184	192	200	208	216	224

If you prefer, you can use this formula to figure your BMI: Multiply your weight (in pounds) by 703, then divide the result by your height in inches, squared. That may sound complicated, but it's not. Plug your weight and height into this formula:

Step 1: My weight_____ times 703 = _____

Step 2: My height in inches _____ times my height in inches _____ = _____

Step 3: My answer from Step 1 _____ divided by the answer from Step 2_____ = _____

You want your BMI to be 25 or less for optimal health, but remember that the BMI alone is not the ultimate guide, and that people with "safe" BMIs may still be at risk. Even if your BMI is in the low to mid–20s, if you carry your excess weight around your waist (as men tend to do), it's more dangerous than packing it onto your hips (as women typically do). Also, if you've gained ten or more pounds as an adult, your risk of heart disease and other problems will automatically be higher than if you had maintained your weight.

If you're not slim, fit, flexible, and strong, don't worry—it's never too late to start. There are no perfect results that you must attain. The most important thing is to start playing—today! And keep playing regularly throughout your long and healthy life. ■

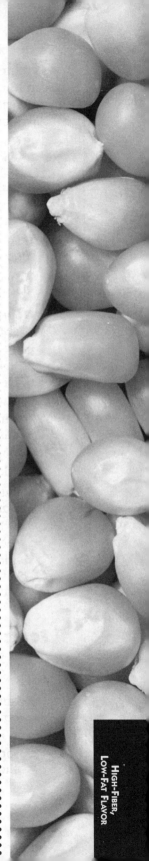

6

HIGH-FIBER, LOW-FAT FLAVOR

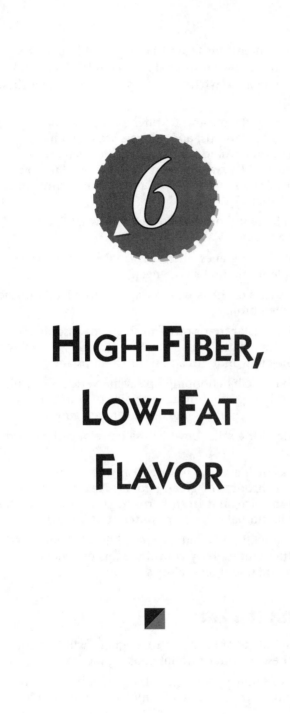

Nothing kills good intentions faster than plain, dull food. You can learn to bring out the great natural flavors in food and add different, exciting flavors to whatever you prepare. Consider these flavor-boosting tips:

- Combine as many flavors and textures as possible. Beans cooked with garlic, onions, and peppers are much more palatable than they would be plain. Cut up several fruits into a fruit salad. Mix two or three kinds of cereal in your breakfast bowl. The more variety, the more interesting and the more nutritious the meal.
- Freeze peeled bananas for use as delicious low-fat "popsicles" or as a tasty addition to "smoothies."
- Freeze blueberries or grapes, then use in salads or as snacks. They're wonderful natural sweeteners.
- Sprinkle fish steaks or fillets with a Cajun spice blend or other seasonings, then broil.
- If you have extra cilantro or other fresh green seasoning herbs, blend them with a small amount of water and freeze as ice cubes. They're wonderful additions to soups and sauces.
- Make fruit compote by chopping up several varieties of fruit, garnishing with a sprig of mint, a sprinkle of cinnamon, or a dash of lime juice. Or add some diced candied ginger.
- Rub the inside of the salad bowl with a clove of garlic before adding the salad.
- Put fish steaks or filets in a baking dish with some sliced onion and mushrooms or green peppers. Season with black pepper, lemon juice, and fresh herbs to your taste, seal the dish with foil and bake 20–30 minutes at 400°–450°.
- Add tomato-based liquids (sauce, puree, juice) to soups, bean dishes, or other sauces. They contribute lots of delicious flavor with zero fat and few calories.

Ferreting Out the Fat

Keeping your daily intake of fat down to 20 grams will be a lot easier if you use these low-fat or no-fat cooking methods:

- Saute, stir-fry, or simmer your vegetables, fish, or beans using bouillon, broth, or wine instead of butter, margarine, or oil.
- If you need to fry, use a quick spritz of vegetable cooking spray on the pan and keep the food moving so that it doesn't stick. You can also brown food this way.

- Steaming is a great, no-fat way to cook vegetables, grains, or even fish. Just make sure the water doesn't boil away completely, or you may burn up your pan! Even easier, use an electric countertop steamer.

- Dips or toppings that call for sour cream can be made with nonfat yogurt instead. It tastes great on a baked potato!

- Skip the dollop of butter on your vegetables, using a squirt of fresh lemon juice instead. It really enhances the natural flavor.

- You can make delicious sauces, soups, or gravies by using oatmeal or pureed cooked vegetables as thickeners, rather than the traditional flour and butter mixture. (A handheld blender makes pureeing easy.)

Favoring the Fiber

You'll do yourself and your body a big favor by exchanging the refined grains in your kitchen for whole grains. That will greatly improve your chances of stepping up your fiber intake. To get even more fiber, try the following:

- Eat vegetables and fruits in their whole, natural state whenever possible. Consume all edible peels and seeds, since they contain valuable fiber, vitamins, minerals, and phytochemicals.

- The fiber that you can recognize as part of a plant is more beneficial than fiber that has been removed from the plant or ground up. That's why whole wheat berries (seeds) are better than whole wheat flour, whole corn is better than whole cornmeal, and so on. To get the maximum appetite-suppressing and constipation-preventing benefits of fiber, use the whole foods instead of the ground-up versions whenever you can.

- Cooking, freezing, canning, or drying does not destroy fiber. This means you can enjoy your vegetables and fruits in any form that is appealing, convenient, and/or economical.

- Instead of drinking juice, eat the whole fruit or vegetable. Juicers that extract the liquid for you to drink and throw away the pulp are criminal. If you want a fruit or vegetable drink, use your blender and make a thick smoothie that contains all the fiber and nutrients.

- Use whole grain cereals at lunch or dinner, as well as for breakfast. Oatmeal is a great thickener for soups and vegetable stews. Crispy cereals make good snacks, by themselves or with nonfat fruit yogurt. Grape-Nuts and other crunchy cereals can be used as substitutes for nuts.

- Many of the vegetables we usually cook are also good raw. Try cutting a raw sweet potato into thin slices to use as "chips" for no-fat dips. Freshly washed raw green beans make a good crunchy snack. Slice a small zucchini right into your green salad. Many people prefer the taste of raw turnips, cabbage, cauliflower, and broccoli to their cooked versions.

■ On the other hand, vegetables that are usually eaten raw can be cooked, too. Lettuce, radishes, Chinese cabbage, and most other salad vegetables can be "stir-fried" or steamed in a little bouillon.

Introducing the Whole Grains

Whole grains are the seeds of grasses, which grow on all continents including Antarctica and have always been a major food source for the human race as well as for many other animals. Whole grains were the first food humans learned to cultivate, marking our transition from hunter-gatherers to agricultural societies. The various grasses that grew in different parts of the world—rice, corn, wheat, rye, quinoa, amaranth, teff, millet— became the "staff of life" for ancient societies. Our ancestors relied heavily on grains because they are easy to grow and store and they are excellent food, providing lots of carbohydrates for energy plus protein, fat, vitamins, and minerals.

We know that people began to process whole grains very early in our history. Why would they take a perfect food and break it apart, often discarding the fiber and the valuable nutrients found in the germ? Dry whole grains are as hard as rocks, and they must cook a long time to make them soft enough to chew. Until the twentieth century, cooking fuel was as scarce and precious as food. So our ancestors had little choice: they had to grind their grains into small particles and remove their hard outer coverings; then the grains could be eaten raw in liquid (gruel) or cooked quickly into porridge or flat breads. They learned to discard the germ, because once the seed is broken open, the germ begins to turn rancid almost immediately, while the starchy parts keep a long time without refrigeration.

Today we have easy access to cooking fuel and refrigeration, so the practices of our ancestors are now just customs, not necessities. But there's more to the story. Our ancestors' biggest concern was finding enough food to stay alive and have enough energy to do all the work that was required for simple survival; they needed concentrated sources of calories. Today, our lifestyles are very different. We have abundant food and sedentary habits. Most of us consume far more calories than we burn. The custom of removing fiber and nutrients from our staple foods, passed to us by our ancestors, is killing us.

Anatomy of a Grain

When you eat whole grains you are eating viable seeds — you can sprout them if you wish. As shown in the diagram, each grain or seed has four parts:

Husk: The hull, or husk, is a papery outer covering that is always removed. Many grains fall out of their husks when they are harvested. A few grains (such as barley and buckwheat) have very hard hulls; these must be ground away. Grains that have only the husk or hull removed are considered whole grains (and will still sprout) if the bran layers and the germ are intact.

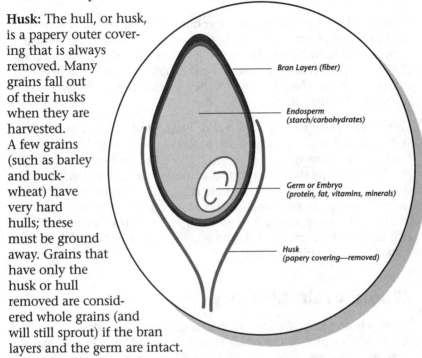

Bran Layers (fiber)

Endosperm (starch/carbohydrates)

Germ or Embryo (protein, fat, vitamins, minerals)

Husk (papery covering—removed)

Bran layers: Each seed is protected by an outer coating that is several layers thick. The bran layers are rich in fiber, vitamins, and minerals.

Germ or embryo: This is the part of the seed that becomes a new plant if it is allowed to sprout. The tiny germ contains protein, fat, vitamins, and minerals. If the seed is broken open, the germ begins to turn rancid almost immediately, so it is removed when grains are ground into flour.

Endosperm: The largest part of the seed feeds the growing embryo if the embryo is allowed to sprout. It is virtually 100 percent starchy carbohydrates. The calorie-rich endosperm is all we eat when grains are refined to remove the coarse bran layers (the fiber) and the quick-spoiling germ.

Refined Grain Products to Avoid

Virtually all grains that are ground into flour and kept, uncooked, for any length of time have had the germ and most or all of the fiber removed. Breads, crackers, and most baked products are made with refined flour, even if they say "whole wheat," "seven-grain," "rye," or any other term that implies that a whole grain was used. Manufacturers are allowed to use these terms even if they have used only a tiny percentage of the original fiber and/or germ of the grains listed in the ingredients.

Almost all corn products have also had the germ and fiber removed: grits, hominy, corn meal, and corn flour (masa harina) are refined grains. The term "stone ground" does not mean it's the whole grain. Most rice products—cereals, rice cakes, crackers, and the like—are made from white rice unless they specifically list brown rice as the main ingredient.

When you shop for a new cereal or grain product such as whole wheat pasta, read the labels. Try to find at least 3 grams of fiber and 0 or 1 grams of fat per serving. More fiber is better! Less fiber probably means that the product is made from refined grains. If the fat content is higher but there is no added fat in the list of ingredients (as in oatmeal), go ahead and use the product but make it one of several different kinds you use. If you eat a wide variety of whole grains and whole grain products, you will get the nutritional benefits of them all.

Whole Grain Glossary

Most whole grains are oval-shaped and light tan to dark brown in color. If it's white or has fewer than 3 grams of fiber per 50-gram serving, the outer seed coat (the fiber) has been removed. The oval-shaped grains are interchangeable in recipes; use whatever you can find and try different ones to see which you like best. They all take about 60–75 minutes to cook. Some whole grains are small round seeds. These take less time to cook and have a distinctive texture, like tiny pasta. Products made from broken or ground grains may or may not contain all of the fiber and nutrient-packed germ. Check the fiber content; it should be close to the amount of fiber in the original whole grain.

> **Oval-shaped whole grains:**
> Barley
> Kamut (a variety of wheat)
> Oats or oat groats
> Brown rice
> Wild rice
> Rye
> Spelt (a variety of wheat)
> Triticale (a hybrid of wheat and rye)
> Wheat or wheat berries

How to Pick a Breakfast Cereal

The very best breakfast consists of whole grains. You can have any cooked whole grains, adding raisins, cinnamon, vanilla, or a little brown sugar to your taste. Packaged hot whole grain cereals such as oatmeal are also fine.

If you prefer cold cereal, there are plenty of good whole grain choices. Many of the old standbys, such as shredded wheat and puffed wheat, are precooked, shaped, and toasted whole grains. Don't rely on the nutritional information on the package label to guide you in your choice of breakfast cereals. They make it hard to compare one to another by using different serving sizes and weights. Instead, look at the list of ingredients. The first item should be a whole grain or combination of whole grains. Avoid milled corn, white rice, and other refined grains. Reject any cereals that contain a lot of added sugars or any partially hydrogenated oils.

*Oat cereals may have 3 grams of fat per serving. Don't let that worry you, for whole grains contain "good" fat. The trick is to make sure the cereal doesn't contain any **added** fats. Cereals with raisins may have as many grams of sugar as a frosted cereal, but sugar bound to the fiber in fruit is not a concern in the **20/30 Plan**.*

Cereals made with whole grains will have at least 3 grams of fiber per 50-gram serving. All-bran or high-bran cereals will have more fiber, but may cause digestive discomfort. For this reason, you may want to mix different kinds of cereals together in your bowl.

Small, round whole grains:
   Amaranth
   Buckwheat
   Whole kasha (toasted buckwheat)
   Millet
   Quinoa
   Teff

Broken or ground grains:
   Bulgar (wheat that has been steamed, dried, and crushed)
   Cracked wheat (uncooked, broken wheat berries)
   Whole grain polenta or corn meal (ground corn)
   Kasha, medium or fine (ground toasted buckwheat)

Where to Buy Whole Grains

Most larger supermarkets carry wild rice, barley, and brown rice. They may all be in the section with white rice and pasta, or you may find barley in the international section (with Jewish specialties) and wild rice in the gourmet food section. Your supermarket may have a health section with various other whole grains (the selection varies widely from store to store and region to region). You'll probably need to go beyond your supermarket to find some of the less common whole grains. Try the health food stores, specialty gourmet shops, and food co-ops in your area. Or you can order grains by mail through the Get Healthy Shop at (800)420-4726 or by writing to P.O. BOX 613, Great Falls, VA 22066.

How to Store Whole Grains

Uncooked whole grains keep a long time in canisters or other airtight containers. Leftover cooked grains should be refrigerated and will keep about a week in a covered container. If you don't have plans to use them up in a few days, put your leftovers in small freezer containers or zip-style bags and freeze them. They're ready to serve after a minute or two in the microwave.

How to Cook Whole Grains

Ignore the instructions on bags of whole grains — use the charts on pages 71–72 instead. You do not need to presoak whole grains. Do follow the directions on boxes of whole grain pasta, whole grain couscous, bulgur, or polenta; they vary from brand to brand.

Any of the whole grains can be cooked in a pot on the stovetop just as you would cook white rice, but they take a long time and you have to stand around watching the pot. After you've done this once or twice, you'll want to get a countertop steamer or whole grain cooker. Stovetop directions are on page 71. If you're comfortable using a pressure cooker, it will work just fine for whole grains. Follow the stovetop cooking chart and adjust the cooking time as you would for any other food (usually about half the regular time).

If you are serious about following a low-fat, high-fiber diet, invest in an electric countertop steamer such as the Black and Decker "Flavor-Scenter Steamer Plus" (with an 8-cup capacity rice bowl and 75-minute timer). The chart on page 71 gives you full instructions.

Cooking Whole Grains in a Steamer

Fill the steamer base with water to the top line. (Do not use the drip tray). Place the steamer basket on the base. Place the grains and bouillon (use amounts from chart below) in the rice bowl and set the rice bowl in the steamer basket. Cover, plug it in, and set the timer. When the timer rings, let the grains sit until cool enough to handle. Drain the grains in a colander if there is excess liquid. Leftovers can be reheated in a microwave or used chilled in salads.

The first time you cook a new grain, check it 5–10 minutes before the end of the cooking time to make sure the grains are not getting mushy. If they aren't tender enough to suit you at the end of the recommended time, cook them a little longer.

For 2½ cups (1 pound) grain:	Amount of bouillon	Cooking time
Wheat berries, Kamut, or Spelt	4 cups	75 minutes
Rye	4 cups	75 minutes
Triticale	4 cups	75 minutes
Oat groats	4 cups	75 minutes
Barley	4 cups	75 minutes
Brown rice	4 cups	65–75 minutes
Wild rice (1/2 lb.)	4 cups	75 minutes
Millet	4 cups	40 minutes
Quinoa	4 cups	30 minutes
Amaranth	4 cups	30 minutes

Cooking Whole Grains on the Stovetop

Use a medium-sized pot with a tight-fitting lid. Bring the bouillon (see chart below for amounts) to a boil in the pot, stir in the grains, and return to boiling. Reduce the heat to low, cover the pot, and simmer until the grains are tender and most of the water is absorbed.

For 2½ cups (1 pound) grain:	Amount of bouillon	Cooking time
Wheat berries, Kamut, or Spelt	6 cups	60 minutes
Rye	6 cups	60 minutes
Triticale	6 cups	60 minutes
Oat groats	6 cups	60 minutes
Barley	6 cups	60 minutes
Brown rice	5 cups	40 minutes

Continued ➡

Wild rice (1/2 lb.)	6 cups	60 minutes
Millet	5 cups	30 minutes
Quinoa	5 cups	10-15 minutes
Amaranth	5 cups	20 minutes

A Simple Way To Cook Grains

The Fiber-Magic™ Whole Grain Cooker, developed by Gabe Mirkin, M.D., provides you with a quick and easy way to cook nutritious grains—without having to stand over a boiling pot for forty-five minutes! All you do is put a scoop of grains into the cooker, add water to the fill line, microwave uncovered for three to three and a half minutes, seal the cooker with its stopper, and shake to blend. Let it sit for two to three hours (or overnight) and your grains will cook themselves. When you're ready to eat, just pour off any excess water, heat the cooked grains in a microwave (if necessary), and enjoy! Full instructions come with the cooker.

Bean Basics

Beans are an excellent low-calorie source of protein and they are loaded with fiber. The recipes in Chapter Nine call for canned beans, but you can always cook your own from scratch if you prefer. One can of beans equals about two cups of cooked dried beans. You can always substitute different varieties in any recipe that calls for beans.

Some people are bothered by excessive gas when they eat cooked dried beans (canned beans usually do not cause severe gas problems because the cannery uses a process similar to the following). To solve this problem try this special pre-soaking method: put the beans in a large pot and cover them with water. Bring them to a boil and take them off the heat. This breaks the skin surrounding each bean to allow stachyose, verbascose, and raffinose, the gas-causing sugars, to escape into the water. Add two tablespoons of baking soda to make the water alkaline, and let the beans soak overnight. Drain the soaking water off the beans and rinse them thoroughly. Cover them with fresh water, bring back to a boil, and simmer them until they are tender.

Time Savers

Some people complain that "It takes too long to prepare the food. I'm in a hurry, so I just grab whatever is there." Fortunately, with a little planning and foresight, you can make sure that "whatever is there" is good for your body and part of the *20/30* program. The following tips will help you save time, as well as your health and sanity:

- Keep containers of precooked whole grains in your refrigerator and freezer.

- Take a weekend afternoon to make up two or three big pots of a vegetable stew or soup. Refrigerate some for the next few lunches and dinners, and freeze the rest in individual-serving containers to build up your own collection of "fast food."

- Two or three times a week, wash and cut up cauliflower, green beans, celery, peppers, and other of your favorite sturdy vegetables. Store them in a covered container in your refrigerator where they will be handy for snacking, packing lunches, or tossing into a green salad.

- Keep bags of frozen vegetable mixes on hand for last-minute meals. Frozen pepper-onion mix can be used in any recipe that calls for chopped onions and peppers. Most supermarkets carry lots of other inspiring mixtures. (Avoid the ones with sauces or pasta.)

- Make sure you always have plenty of carrots, celery, apples, bananas, oranges, and other snacks right at hand. You can even prewash foods such as apples and celery, so there's no time wasted when you're hungry—and no excuses about not having the energy to prepare your snack.

- Use freezer-to-oven style cookware or microwave dishes to avoid having to wash two containers.

- Make your own instant cocoa mix by combining $1/3$ cup nonfat dry milk, 1 teaspoon unsweetened cocoa powder, and 1 packet Equal. Just pour the dry mix into a cup, add $3/4$ cup boiling water and stir. Make up several of these dry packets to take to work or school.

- Create weekly menus, figure out what you'll need to buy, then do your shopping all in one trip. This will save you from those time-wasting "quick trips" to the grocery store at the last minute before preparing a meal. Although planning may seem time consuming, you'll actually spend fewer hours on food preparation in the long run, while eating more nutritiously.

That's all there is to it. Use the easy, delicious recipes in Chapter Nine, or invent your own. Be sure to look up the fat and fiber content of everything you eat, then dial it into your key chain counter, making sure you take in no more than 20 grams of fat per day and eat at least 30 grams of fiber. (Attach the fat and fiber gram counter to your key chain, or carry it in your pocket or pocketbook so it will always be at hand.) ■

SETTING UP
FOR A SLIM
NEW YOU

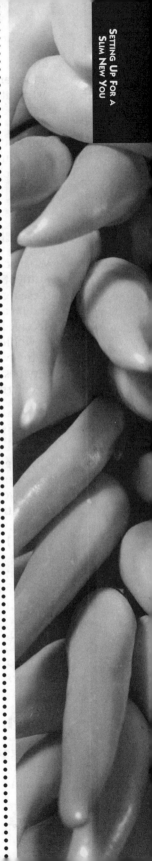

In order to live the *20/30* way, you need the right tools. The most important, of course, are nutritious foods that are free of unwanted extras like the fat, sugar, and other refined carbohydrates that pile on extra pounds and devitalize your body. But even if you fill your kitchen with high-fiber, low-fat foods, if you've still got a box of chocolate-covered cupcakes lurking in the cupboard, or a cheese-cake buried in the freezer, sooner or later you'll probably give in and gobble them up. It's much better to get rid of the offending foods and "go clean."

Cleaning Out Your Pantry and Refrigerator

What should you get rid of? Any ready-to-eat foods that aren't nutrient packed and health enhancing. You'll recognize some of these right away; cookies, cakes, pies, pastries, sugar-coated cereals and bread made from refined flour lead the pack. And don't be deceived by "health foods" such as granola, whole wheat muffins, or whole grain cakes that can have more fat and sugar than many of the worst kid's cereals. If you want to ensure you're eating the very best foods, you'll need to become an expert at reading labels to determine just what's in them.

Reading the Labels

Although much of what you'll be eating is whole, "live" food, you should become adept at reading the labels of any packaged foods you consume. The Food and Drug Administration (FDA) insists that all ingredients be listed on the back or side of the label in descending order, beginning with the one that makes up the largest percentage of the product. Also listed are serving size, servings per package, total calories, calories from fat, total fat, saturated fat, cholesterol, sodium, total carbohydrate, dietary fiber, sugars, protein, vitamin A, vitamin C, calcium, and iron.

The key items on the food labels are the amounts of total fat and fiber, which are listed in grams. Each serving should have no more than two grams of fat and *at least* two grams of fiber.

Watch for Tricky Labels

Reading the labels is a good idea, but remember that their primary goal is to entice you to buy the product. Manufacturers use several tricks in order to sell their products, including these common ones:

- **Distorting the portion size**—Hoping to fool you into thinking that their foods are low in fat or high in fiber, some manufacturers divide their products into absurdly small servings.

  While the average candy bar has about 220 calories and 14 grams of fat, the label of a certain "lite" candy bar boasts that it has only 100 calories and 8 grams of fat. The "lite" candy bar was a similar size to other candy bars, but if you look closely, you'll see that the label says "Servings per package: 2." When was the last time you considered a candy bar to be two separate servings?

! **Fight-back strategy:** Make sure the serving size is realistic for you before choosing the product.

- **"Lite" or "light" foods**—These terms are used so universally throughout the food retailing industry you might believe that they actually mean something. They don't. There is no federal standard for the use of either of these words, so the manufacturer may be referring to the color of the product, the amount of calories, the weight of the product, or nothing at all.

! **Fight-back strategy:** Check the label for fat, fiber, and calorie content before purchasing.

- **"Zero" grams of fat**—A listing of "0" grams of fat on the label means that the food has less than 1 gram of fat, not necessarily that the food is totally fat free. If the portion sizes are tiny, and if you can eat all or most of the food in the package at one sitting, you're probably taking in a fair amount of fat. The saturated fat number is also likely to be deceptive.

! **Fight-back strategy:** The real information you need is found in the list of ingredients: if the food contains partially hydrogenated oils, animal fats, and tropical oils (such as palm or coconut oil), don't put it in your shopping cart.

- **Fortified foods**—Although fortified foods may sound like a great deal ("all the vitamins and minerals you need for an entire day in one bowl of cereal"), they are generally refined foods with some of the vitamins added back to keep them from being totally worthless. Remember that sugary orange drink fortified with vitamin C advertised as the drink that astronauts took into space? Without the C, it was essentially sugar water.

! **Fight-back strategy:** When you eat foods that are plucked straight off a tree or out of the ground, you won't need expensive fortification. You'll already be getting a superior source of nutrition.

- **Natural or organic foods**—"Natural" is another one of those unregulated, meaningless words you'll find plastered on the labels of foods. "Organic" foods are not more nutritious and may not even be more free of chemical pesticides than "regular" fruits and vegetables.

❗ **Fight-back strategy:** Buy fresh fruits and vegetables from any store that's convenient for you. All produce is "natural" and nutritious.

Out with the Old

Now that you know what to watch for in food labels and packaging, prepare for a new way of eating by cleaning out your kitchen. First of all, get rid of those sugary, fatty, and low-fiber foods.

Sugary foods — You can spot a food that's high in sugar by checking to see if any of the first three ingredients on that label are sugar, dextrose, dextrin, sucrose, fructose, honey, brown sugar, turbinado sugar, raw sugar, corn syrup, high fructose corn syrup, corn sweeteners, maple syrup, concentrated fruit juice, or molasses.

If one or more of these sugars shows up in the first three ingredients, the product is probably primarily empty calories — it can pile on the pounds, while doing very little for your health. If you check the labels, you'll see that most cakes, pies, cookies, muffins, sugary cereals, certain soups (i.e., tomato), baked beans, soft drinks, and fruit drinks or juices that contain concentrates all fall into this category. Low-fat cakes and cookies are especially high in sugar.

Fatty foods — The easiest way to spot a high-fat food is to look at the "Total Fat" listing on the label. Generally speaking, if a food has more than 2 grams of fat, you should look for a different food. (The exceptions are beans, seafood, and whole grains that will be your major sources of protein. Some have more than 2 grams of fat.) Remember, you only have 20 grams of fat for the whole day, and you can reach your limit very quickly. Get rid of all oil, butter, margarine, shortening, lard, salad dressings, cream cheese, sour cream and mayonnaise (except fat-free), cheese and yogurt (except fat-free), milk (except nonfat), eggs (except whites), baked goods, potato chips, avocados, nuts, peanuts, seeds, coconut, packaged convenience foods containing more than 2 grams of fat per serving, and meats. (Yes, that includes chicken and turkey.)

Low-fiber foods — You will probably have tossed out most of these foods already under the guise of "sugary foods" or "fatty foods," but don't forget to clear out all products containing refined (white) flour, including breads, crackers, cereals, rolls, breadsticks, and pasta, for example — anything that isn't 100 percent whole grain. It's also a good idea to limit your intake of juices, since they have very little fiber. Eat the whole fruit or vegetable instead.

Read the labels on *everything* that's currently in your cupboard or refrigerator. You'll be surprised at what's in some of your favorite foods! Then gather up all of the offending foods and give them to your friends or neighbors, or to a food bank. Throw them in the trash if you like, but find a way to get them out of your house. And once you've done so, promise yourself you won't bring them back in again. When unhealthful foods are out of sight, you'll enjoy the more healthful choices.

In with the New

Now you've just gotten rid of half (maybe three-quarters!) of your food supply. So what do you replace it with? Look for all the foods with the ☺ symbol in the food lists in Chapter Ten. You'll stock your pantry with lots of fruits, vegetables, whole grains, and beans and in Chapter Nine you'll learn new tricks to make them taste great.

How To Avoid Partially Hydrogenated Oils

The only way to find out if a food contains partially hydrogenated oils (trans fats) is to read the list of ingredients. Zero grams of fat in the nutrition information does not mean the food has no trans fat, because the manufacturer can claim zero grams for anything less than .5 grams per serving, and a serving size can be as small as one teaspoon or one cookie. That adds up to a lot of trans fat by the time you finish the whole package.

Check the list of ingredients on any new food you plan to buy (not just the obviously fatty foods such as margarine, chips, pastries, or cookies). Trans fats show up in bread, cereals, "fat-free" candies, sauces, frozen entrees and desserts, and just about every other kind of processed food. Bread and cereal makers often add trans fats to make their new higher-fiber products more palatable; for example, Multi-Grain Cheerios are made with partially hydrogenated oil, while regular Cheerios are not. Be sure to read the list of ingredients even if the product name includes "healthy" words such as "light," "fat-free," or "whole grain."

Be particularly careful with claims made for butter substitutes. One supposedly "healthy" margarine label boasts "No Trans Fats," yet partially hydrogenated oil is the second ingredient. They say there's a "dietetic insignificant amount" that has been rounded to 0 grams. We say it's a bald-faced lie. If a product has the words "hydrogenated" or "partially hydrogenated" in the list of ingredients, put it back on the shelf and look at another brand.

Tips for Healthy Eating When You're Not In Your Kitchen

Okay, you've got everything perfectly set up in your kitchen. The pantry is stuffed with low-fat, high-fiber whole grains and other foods. The refrigerator is bursting with a delicious assortment of fresh fruits and vegetables. A tasty array of dishes have been carefully cooked and frozen, awaiting inclusion in one of your wholesome, satisfying meals. But what happens when you have to leave your controlled environment and venture out into the world of cheese-laden Mexican enchiladas, French dishes oozing with cream sauce, or double-decker hamburgers paired with chili-cheese fries? How do you manage to stay with *The 20/30 Plan*?

Luckily, you may not have to worry about dining out because of the Nineteen Meals Rule. If you've eaten nineteen healthful meals in a week's time, you have two "free" meals coming to you; you can go out to eat and enjoy yourself (within reason, of course). But if you go out a lot, or you have slipped up too often during the week, you'll need to know how to eat out while following the program. Here are some helpful tips:

- Avoid fast-food restaurants. Not only is most of their food loaded with fat and very low in fiber, you may tend to gobble it down quickly so you can get out in a hurry, or even worse, you might eat it while driving. Because you're not really concentrating on what you're eating, you can end up chowing down a lot of unhealthy junk food, while still feeling unsatisfied.

- Bring a companion along when you go out to eat. Engaging in conversation encourages you to eat more slowly, so you'll feel filled up faster.

- Don't eat the bread, rolls, or chips while waiting for your main dish. Have them taken off the table!

- Avoid anything prepared with cheese, butter, cream, or oil.

- Stay away from anything fried.

- Start out with soup. Tomato-based vegetable and seafood soups (like Manhattan clam chowder) are good choices. Avoid any cream soups.

- Have fish, but ask for it baked, broiled, or poached without butter or added fats.

- Order your salad plain, then add only vinegar, lemon, tomato juice, or fruit juice as a dressing. (You might want to bring your favorite fat-free dressing with you.) Stay away from croutons, sunflower seeds, Chinese noodles, bacon bits, or any of the other fatty extras that restaurants like to add to salads.

- Ask for your vegetables to be cooked and served without butter or added fats.
- Restaurant bean dishes usually contain meats, fats (as in refried), cheese, sugar, or a lot of other ingredients you're trying to avoid. Unless you know that the bean dishes on the menu don't contain these items (minestrone soup is usually a good bet), don't order them.
- Order potatoes baked rather than fried, mashed, or scalloped. Top with salsa or veggies (but not sour cream or butter).
- Don't drink alcoholic beverages, since the loosened inhibitions they bring about can derail even the most conscientious dieter. And remember, all extra calories, including those from alcohol, are converted to fat.
- Don't get discouraged if you "fall off the wagon." The most important thing is to get back on immediately.

A Final Word

A wise old sage once pointed out that getting organized is 90 percent of the battle. This is surely the case with good eating. Once you've gotten rid of the old, unhealthful foods and replaced them with fresh, whole foods, you're certain to begin eating better, feeling better, and looking better. And by coupling this new way of eating with a moderate exercise program, you can change your looks and your life in ways you'd never imagined! It just takes a little organization and the decision to go for it. ∎

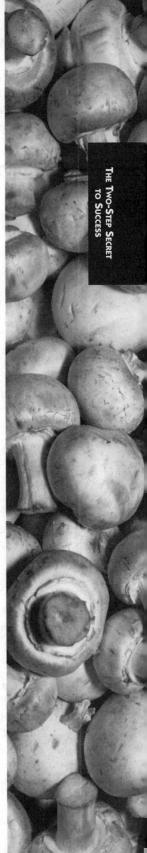

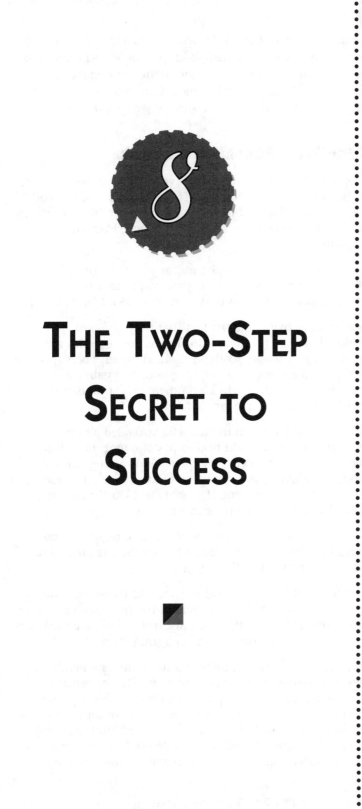

8

THE TWO-STEP
SECRET TO
SUCCESS

You've mastered the *20/30* philosophy, looked at the relationship between diet and health, learned about phytochemicals and foods that can help you heal, prepared your kitchen and exercise regimen. Now it's time to take the most important step, one that some people find the hardest—actually doing it.

The Two-Step Secret to Success

Some people feel that they shouldn't even bother to begin a diet because they're doomed to failure. "There's no way I'll succeed," such a person may claim. "I haven't got the discipline, I've never stuck to anything before, I'm not good enough. Everything is stacked against me."

Perhaps the outlook doesn't look rosy for you right now. Maybe there's some good reason to believe that you'll have trouble sticking with the program. Even if that is the case, *don't let it stop you!*

Many people have overcome the fact that they "obviously" couldn't do what they wanted to do. Things looked grim for a poor boy raised in a tough Scotland slum. He spent years working as a coffin polisher, cement mixer, lifeguard, and baby-sitter. Tommy Connery was clearly headed nowhere, yet managed to become rich and famous as Sean Connery.

The future was bleak for two friends who struggled along with whatever little jobs they could find to pay the rent. Both were voted "Least Likely to Succeed" by their fellow acting students at the Pasadena Playhouse. Both were rejected time and time again in their bids for roles. Yet Gene Hackman and Dustin Hoffman became Academy Award–winning movie stars.

Radio talk show host Rush Limbaugh overcame regular firings, harsh personal criticism, and ridicule to become the king of radio. Like him or not, he's still riding high.

Actor Pat Morita of the Karate Kid movies and television's *Happy Days* spent nine of his childhood years in the hospital recovering from spinal tuberculosis, getting out just in time to be tossed into a Japanese-American internment camp during World War II.

Name an obstacle, a disaster, a tragedy, a hardship, or an embarrassment. Pick any terrible thing you can imagine: it's happened to some of the most successful people in the country. Poverty, personal tragedy, horrible family circumstances, lackluster education, not-so-hot looks, lack of connections, even lack of talent: nothing stopped these people who were determined to succeed. They were certainly no smarter or better than you are. But they were unstoppable because they knew the two-step secret to success: To succeed you must want to succeed and you must get started.

Step #1: Wanting to Succeed

It can be difficult to change your dietary and exercise habits if you have only vague notions of what these changes will bring you in the distant future. That's why it's important to decide what you want and visualize it, then keep that great desire in your mind at all times.

With your mind's eye, see yourself slim and trim, looking great in your new clothes. See yourself smiling modestly as your friends and family compliment you on your wonderful new look. See yourself in your doctor's office getting a clean bill of health, your doctor marveling at how strong your heart is and what good results your blood tests show. Keep reminding yourself of what you really want:

I can't wait to lose the extra weight that makes me unhappy and unhealthy.

I can't wait to drop my total cholesterol, "bad" LDL cholesterol, and blood fats down to safe levels.

I can't wait to reduce my risk of cancer, diabetes, constipation, hemorrhoids, immune system dysfunction, and other problems.

I can't wait to eat lots of different, great tasting foods, instead of the same couple of things over and over again.

I can't wait to find out how wonderful "real" foods and spices taste, now that their tastes are not hidden by globs of fat and added sugar.

I can't wait to feel energetic all day long.

I can't wait to cut down on the medicines I'm taking for high blood pressure, diabetes, high cholesterol—or to get off them altogether.

I can't wait to be so fit that I can climb the stairs, romp with my kids or grandchildren, run for a bus, or shovel snow without feeling exhausted.

I can't wait to save so much money on food that I'll be able to take a vacation or buy a new wardrobe.

Most people look upon diets as terrible things that force them to surrender their favorite foods and suffer in many ways. That may be so with other programs, but not with *The 20/30 Fat & Fiber Diet Plan.* You don't give up anything. Instead, you *gain* good health and vitality. Look at it this way:

■ You're not surrendering sweets and good tasting foods. Instead, you're gaining the ability to enjoy the sweet tastes of fruit and the wonderful flavors of natural foods and spices. (You've probably never noticed these tastes before because they were buried under piles of refined sugar and fat.)

■ You're not losing the right to eat meat. Instead, you're gaining freedom from the stiflingly repetitive and dull habits that had you eating meat and just a few other foods over and over again. Now you can enjoy tremendous variety and taste sensations as you partake of the numerous fruits, vegetables, whole grains, and beans available — plus occasional meat, poultry, and fish dishes, if you like.

■ You're not giving up the convenience of fast foods. You're going to learn how to make your own!

■ You're not giving up satisfying portions of food and forcing yourself to eat tiny amounts. When you eat mostly whole grains, vegetables, and fruit, you can have as much as you want, as often as you want, until you are comfortably full and satisfied. You need never feel hungry.

■ You don't have to give up any foods forever. You're going to learn to use the fatty or low-fiber foods you really love as occasional treats, replacing the ones you don't care about so much with delicious new, healthy choices.

Going on *The 20/30 Fat & Fiber Diet Plan* is a "win-win" situation. You win once when you lose weight, then win again when you gain health. And it all starts with your desire to be slim and healthy.

Step #2: Getting Started

There's a story told about a man who knew exactly how to get started. Known as "Doc" Wiley, he was a messenger boy back in the 1940s. His job wasn't very important, he wasn't paid much, but he performed his duties with pride and joy. Every time he handed a letter or message to a customer, he also gave that customer one of the many little slips of paper he kept in his pocket with positive messages like *"Keep Your Chin Up!"* or *"The Sun Is Always Shining!"*

When World War II broke out, Doc went to the draft board to sign up to fight for his country, but they wouldn't take him. "You're too old," they said.

Eager to help and absolutely undeterred, Doc volunteered at a hospital. Nothing was going to stop him from helping his country in its time of need.

Soon, Doc Wiley found himself pushing a gurney. But one thing troubled him greatly. Every time he had to wheel a soldier or a sailor who had died down to the morgue, he felt terrible. He wanted to do something to help, but what? He wasn't a doctor or nurse, he didn't have any medical knowledge or skills. What could he do? Then it hit him.

The next morning, the entire hospital was abuzz about the strange thing that had happened in the ward where Doc Wiley worked. Someone had written on the walls! In giant letters, the message read *"No One Dies On This Ward."* Doc admitted that he had done it.

Well, the hospital heads were furious. They wanted to kick Doc out right then and there but the doctors and nurses on the ward said "Wait a minute. This may not be so bad. The men in that ward are sitting up in bed, talking about that slogan, laughing and taking bets as to who will live the longest. It may not be such a bad thing after all."

And so the slogan was left up, where everyone could see it. Six simple words: *"No One Dies On This Ward."* And you know what? The patients all vowed to each other that they would not die, because they did not want to be the one who broke the "magic" spell created by Doc's slogan. Days passed, yet no one died on that ward. They died in the other wards as usual, but not in Doc's ward, not where he had written those magic words on the wall.

Eventually, of course, someone died—some soldier or sailor whose wounds were simply overwhelming. But the sick and wounded men on his ward did better than those anywhere else in the hospital.

What's the point of this story? What do Doc's slogans have to do with your losing weight? The point is that Doc knew what he wanted—happiness for his customers and health for the hospitalized soldiers—and he took steps to turn his desires into reality. His slogans were only small steps, but they were a start. He didn't worry about doing everything at once, or whether his approaches would work, whether or not people might laugh at him or get mad. He just got started. He did what he was capable of doing. He took the first step.

> Your kitchen isn't fully stocked yet?
> You're not sure you can reduce your fat intake enough?
> You don't know the difference between kasha and kamut?
> You can only do two push-ups?
> You wonder if you can stick with the program?
> Just get started.

If you rise early on the morning of your first *20/30* day to go shopping, cut back "cold turkey" on excess fat, fast foods, and fiberless meals and jump right into the full program, that's wonderful; you're on your way to success. But if you do nothing more on the first day than write a slogan on your mental blackboard, an exhortation that says "No one stays fat in this body," that's great. You, too, will be on your way to success.

Now you've got to get started. If you can't follow the program three meals a day, seven days a week, start with one day. Which day do you have the most control over your food? That is, which day do you eat at home or otherwise prepare your own meals? Start with that day. If tackling an entire day seems too much to handle at once, start with one meal. Eat the *20/30* way every day at breakfast, lunch, or dinner, beginning with the meal over which you have the most control.

If you can't do that, start with one food. Put down the French fries you were going to eat and have a piece of whole wheat bread instead. Grab an orange instead of a candy bar when you're snacking. There, you've gotten started.

Computer visionaries Steven Jobs and Steve Wozniak began Apple Computers in a garage. Inventor Charles Goodyear performed in his kitchen the experiments that led to the manufacture of vulcanized rubber. International soccer sensation Pelé began kicking a ball in a tiny, poor Brazilian village. They all began small, against overwhelming odds. But they got started, and that made them unstoppable.

Watch Out for "Doom & Gloom" and "Wrong Reasons"

Two "diseases" make it difficult for some people to lose weight: "doom & gloom" and "wrong reasons."

"Doom & gloom" is a condition that causes people to sabotage their efforts to slim down by focusing on what they can't do, rather than on what they can do. Take this quick quiz to see if you have "doom & gloom."

Do you do the following:

❑ Spend a lot of time thinking about your weight problems?

❑ Enjoy telling people how hard it is for you to lose weight?

❑ Often find yourself in the company of others who have problems with their weight or diets?

❑ Spend more time talking about your problems than doing something about them?

❑ Know that your back hurts because you're overweight, or that your elevated cholesterol increases your risk of heart disease, but aren't doing anything about it?

- ❏ Take medicines for elevated blood pressure or cholesterol rather than handle the same problems by eating more healthfully?
- ❏ Tell people how high your cholesterol is, even as you're eating foods that push it higher?
- ❏ Sit in front of the TV for hours on end, wondering why you're not energetic anymore?

If you've checked two or more items, you may be attached to being overweight. For one reason on another, you may be drawing some form of comfort from your extra pounds. Although serious cases of "doom & gloom" may require counseling, most "doom & gloomers" can "cure" themselves. Just remind yourself of what you want, be determined to get it, and get started—now!

People with **"wrong reasons,"** like those suffering from "doom & gloom," also tend to undermine their efforts to adopt a health-enhancing approach to eating. Those with "wrong reasons" tend to eat for the wrong reasons. There's really only one good reason to eat: your body has signaled its need for nourishment by turning on the hunger signal. If we only ate in response to our automatic internal cues, obesity would not be the terrible problem it is. Unfortunately, we eat for numerous other, often unhealthy, reasons.

Do you suffer from "wrong reasons?" Find out by taking this quiz.

Do you eat for some of the following reasons?

- ❏ You're unhappy.
- ❏ You're celebrating.
- ❏ You're angry.
- ❏ You're stressed.
- ❏ Things are going well.
- ❏ Things are not going well.
- ❏ Your team is winning.
- ❏ Your team is losing.
- ❏ You have to make a big decision.
- ❏ You've just made a big decision.
- ❏ You're watching TV (you always eat while watching the tube).
- ❏ Seeing a food advertised on TV or on a billboard makes you want to have it, right now.
- ❏ Someone offers you food.
- ❏ You see your favorite food.
- ❏ You're at the movies and it's part of "the movie experience."

❑ You're planning on dieting, and want to get in the last "good" foods before the diet starts.

❑ Because it feels good.

❑ Because it's easier to stop at a fast-food place than to cook at home.

❑ There's no reason at all to eat; you simply feel like doing so.

If you've checked off two or more items, you are eating for the wrong reasons.

Fortunately, it is possible to overcome this problem. Here's what one successful *20/30* dieter, a woman from Virginia, wrote.

"I have been struggling with weight problems since childhood, and many of my issues were and are emotional and psychological (i.e., overeating as a defense against pain, loss, or neglect in my alcoholic family of origin). I am continuing to work on those issues, but I found myself in my fortieth year weighing 260 pounds (at 5' 3") and struggling to get up and down the stairs in my house or walk in a mall. Last July 13th, I began following The 20 Gram Diet, as well as exercising. In September, I joined a fitness club, and am now working out 4–5 times per week. After nearly six months maintaining 20 grams of fat or less, and concentrating on increasing my consumption of fruits, vegetables, grains, and beans, I am happy to report that I have lost nearly 70 pounds. I feel great and look better than I have in years. Although I still have a way to go to get to my ideal weight, I am confident that I will do so, and that I can maintain this new life style and eating habits forever."

If she can do it, *you* can! Here are some tips to help you stop eating for the wrong reasons:

■ Separate your perception of food and your perception of emotional satisfaction. Eating chocolate cake may feel good for a moment or two, but it does nothing to really bolster positive feelings.

■ Constantly remind yourself that food is not love. Eating for comfort when you are lonely only adds guilt to your feelings of need. And being overweight makes you feel less lovable.

■ Remember that when you eat because you're angry, you're hurting yourself, not the person who has angered you.

■ If you're eating because you're anxious or depressed, look for help in dealing with the underlying problems rather than masking the feelings with food.

- If you eat because the food advertisements look so good, ask yourself who is in control of your life, you or unknown hucksters who have absolutely no interest in your health?

- If you eat everything on your plate because your mother told you about the poor starving children in Armenia, make a contribution to your favorite charity instead of stuffing yourself.

- If you cook the way your mother taught you, remember that she (or her mother, who taught her) was probably feeding family members who were doing hard physical labor. You need to learn some new recipes and cooking techniques that fit your modern lifestyle.

- If you eat and drink junk foods because they're there at the office, at a party, or available when you go out with friends, bring your own snacks or eat ahead so you're not ravenous. Then sip a noncaloric drink and concentrate on talking to people.

- If you eat fast food because you just don't have time for anything else, consider your priorities. You won't be able to do your work or enjoy your hobbies and other satisfying activities if you lose your health. Besides, it really doesn't take any longer to prepare your own food once you get organized.

- If you eat just because food is nearby, or placed in front of you, remind yourself that we eat to live, we do not live to eat.

Keep track for a few days of what, when, where, and why you eat,. "What," "when," and "where" are self-explanatory. As for "why," think about what is prompting you to eat. Are you hungry, really hungry? Or is it simply time to eat? Are you eating because your buddies are? Because you love the taste of your favorite foods, even if you're stuffed? Examining the reasons why you eat can help you overcome "wrong reasons."

You **Can** Succeed!

It doesn't matter how much weight you have to lose, how many times you've "failed" at diets, or how many diets have failed you. Plenty of people have overcome terrible adversity to find themselves sitting on top of the world. There's no reason why you can't be one of them.

Pat Morita, who went from the hospital to an internment camp, said, "If one dwells only on the hardships in life . . . that's all you will get in life. No matter what happens to a person, you have to rise above it and at least hope or dream there is a better existence."

British playwright George Bernard Shaw noted that, "The people who get on in this world are the people who get up and look for the circumstances they want and, if they can't find them, make them." Or, in the words of H. E. Jansen, "The man who wins may have been counted out several times, but he didn't hear the referee."

You're reading this book, which means you're ready to become a winner. You can do it; all you have to do is get started! ∎

LOW-FAT, HIGH FIBER RECIPES

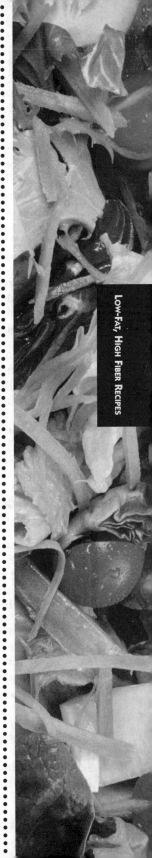

First of all, relax! It's hard to go wrong when you cook with fruits, vegetables, whole grains, and beans. You don't need to worry about precise measurements, cooking times, or ingredient preparation. The recipes give you general guidelines, but if you do things a little differently, chances are your dishes will still be delicious!

Chop, slice, dice, mince: Lots of recipes for fruits and vegetables instruct you to cut the ingredients up. How you do it is up to you. A knife and cutting board work fine, but if you want to use a food processor or other favorite cutting device, go right ahead. Chop or dice means $1/4"$–$1/2"$ chunks; anything smaller than bite-sized is fine. Slice usually means cutting the ingredient crosswise into about $1/4"$ pieces. Mince means the pieces should be really small—$1/8"$ or so. For minced garlic, you may want to use a garlic press.

Measurements: Recipes have to list measurements to give you some idea of what the author has in mind but you can use your eyes and taste buds for most measuring. Taste as you go and adjust the seasonings to suit yourself.

When a recipe calls for ingredients such as an onion, a potato, an orange, or a green pepper, use average-sized vegetables or fruits. If you like an ingredient, feel free to add more; if you're not crazy about it, add less or leave it out (see substitutions below).

Cooking times: Cooking times in recipes are approximate. Your taste testing is far more important then the clock. Learn about long-, medium-, and short-cooking vegetables from the list on pages 96–97 so you can add ingredients in the general order that makes sense, but the ultimate test is "doneness." Check a carrot or a potato and see if it's tender. The general goal is to cook a dish long enough to blend the flavors but not so long that it turns to mush.

Covered or uncovered? Keep pots uncovered unless the recipe specifies covered. Soups and stews thicken when the lid is off; put the lid on when you want to retain liquid.

Substitutions: All of the recipes can be used as springboards for new inventions. Be creative! You may want to make changes to use up ingredients you have on hand; you may not be able to find an ingredient in the store; or you may just prefer some other ingredient or seasoning. Make a note of your substitutions if you like the results. Do be brave about trying things you "don't like"; new combinations and seasonings can change your mind.

To Peel or Not to Peel?

Vegetable and fruit skins are loaded with fiber and nutrients. You don't want to throw them away unless you must. Peeling is time-consuming and wasteful. Recipes in lots of other cookbooks tell you to peel potatoes, apple, eggplants, and everything else, whether you need to or not. Use this "rule of thumb": if you can put your thumbnail through the skin, use it! (That eliminates thick or tough skins like those on winter squash, bananas, and oranges).

Potatoes and carrots just need to be scrubbed. Apple and pear skins add color and crunch. Cucumbers look pretty in salad if you score the skin with a fork before slicing instead of peeling. If you think peeling is important for the texture or appearance of your dish, go ahead, but at least consider leaving the skins on before you automatically throw away valuable fiber and vitamins.

Whole Grains and Salt

Most doctors now agree that salt restriction does not significantly lower blood pressure and it certainly won't cause you to lose weight. Unless you are salt sensitive, there is no need to seek out low-salt foods.

A little salt is necessary to make whole grains and vegetables taste good. Without it, they are flat and boring. Use salt in moderation and enjoy your tasty whole grains!

Bouillon and Other Flavored Liquids

When a recipe calls for bouillon, here's what to use:

Bouillon cubes, granules, pastes, and concentrates —Chicken or vegetable bouillon granules have a natural flavor that goes well with all grains and vegetables. Beef, ham, or fish flavored bouillons have stronger flavors that can be used in hearty recipes such as chilies or soups. Try several brands of bouillon until you find some you like. Most bouillons include some salt. If you use a low-salt version, add salt to the recipe to your own taste. If the recipe calls for "bouillon granules," add them dry without additional water.

Homemade stock—Classic chefs swear by homemade stock, and believe that using canned bouillon or bouillon cubes is a mortal sin. The traditional stockpot is based on lots of gelatin-rich, flavorful bones and meat scraps, which of course you will not have in a low-fat kitchen. You will need to decide whether it's worth your time, and whether you have the refrigerator space, to keep a stockpot going. There's no set recipe; you start with boiling water, add the vegetables and scraps, and simmer as long as you like — at least an hour — and strain.

Other Choices—You can use fat-free canned broth or consommè in any recipe that calls for bouillon. You can also use tomato or vegetable juice, bottled clam juice, wine, beer, or citrus juice and the liquids left over from soaking dried mushrooms, or from cooking shrimp; just add more water and bouillon granules to get the amount you need for your recipe.

About Fat-Free Mayonnaise and Salad Dressings

Many of the salad recipes use fat-free mayonnaise or bottled salad dressings. Some of the bottled fat-free salad dressings are quite tasty while others are just plain awful.

Many of them are very sweet and make a good dressing for cole slaw, but if you're looking for a substitute for oil and vinegar, you will want to search out an unsweetened, or at least less sweet, Italian dressing. Add a little extra vinegar or the juice of a lemon or lime to give the dressing more tartness. Stir in fresh herbs and spices to add your own personal touch.

Fat-free dressings and mayonnaise lose their consistency quickly once they have been mixed with other ingredients, so add them just before serving. If you expect to have leftovers, set aside part of the salad before you mix in the mayonnaise or dressing. Or you can pour off any excess liquid and then add more dressing or mayonnaise on the second day.

Cooking Times for Vegetables

When you cook lots of different kinds of vegetables together, you want them all to come out crisp and tender, not mushy. But different vegetables take different lengths of time to cook. I find it helpful to group vegetables as long cookers, medium cookers, and short cookers. Then I add them to the pot in order, so they all get cooked through and none are overcooked. Old, tough vegetables may take longer than the times given below, while very young and tender ones will cook very quickly.

Long-Cooking Vegetables
Cook 15–20 minutes or more

Potatoes	Winter squash
Onions	Turnips
Beets	Celery root
Celery	Carrots
Sweet potatoes	

Medium-Cooking Vegetables

Cook 10–15 minutes

Broccoli	Kale
Cauliflower	Kohlrabi
Brussels sprouts	Parsnips
Fennel	Lima Beans
Eggplant	Green Peppers

More Medium-Cooking Vegetables

Cook 5–10 minutes

Asparagus	Okra
Green beans	Mushrooms
Cabbage	Zucchini
Peas	

Most frozen vegetables (check package for suggested cooking time)

Quick-Cooking Vegetables

Cook less than 5 minutes

Corn	Swiss chard
Bean sprouts	Snow peas
Spinach	

About Spice Blends

Spice blends such as curry powder, chili powder, and Cajun seasoning are a great shortcut for the busy cook who wants maximum taste with minimum effort. Most supermarkets carry a variety of spice blends, or you can make your own (see pages 98–99). Use them to add infinite variety to your combinations of whole grains, vegetables, and beans.

Look for "mild" curry powder or chili powder and add the degree of heat you want with a little cayenne pepper or hot sauce such as Tabasco. If you don't like one spice blend, try another; each manufacturer has its own formula.

Recipe Symbols

🕐 A quick and easy recipe

❄ A recipe that freezes well

African Berbere Spice Blend

Berbere is the traditional Ethiopian seasoning for lentils and beans. You can use it with just about any combination of vegetables, whole grains, and legumes.

Yield: About 1/4 cup	
Calories:	12 per Tbs.
Total Fat:	1 gram
Dietary Fiber:	1 gram

    3 tablespoons sweet paprika
    2 teaspoons ground cumin
    1 teaspoon ground cinnamon
    1 teaspoon ground turmeric
    1 teaspoon ground ginger
    1 teaspoon ground coriander
    1 teaspoon ground nutmeg
    $1/2$ teaspoon ground cloves
    $1/2$ teaspoon cayenne pepper, or to taste

Mix all ingredients together in a small bowl. Store in an airtight container. ■

Garam Masala Spice Blend

Garam Masala is a mixture of warm, fragrant spices used in East Indian and Caribbean cuisine. If you don't care for curry powder, try this instead.

Yield: About 1/4 cup	
Calories:	24 per Tbs.
Total Fat:	0 grams
Dietary Fiber:	2 grams

    2 tablespoons freshly ground pepper
    2 teaspoons ground cumin
    2 teaspoons ground coriander
    2 teaspoons ground cinnamon
    1 teaspoon ground cardamom
    1 teaspoon ground nutmeg
    $1/2$ teaspoon ground cloves

Mix all ingredients together in a small bowl. Store in an airtight container. ■

Dessert Spice Blend

Yield: About 1/4 cup	
Calories:	33 per Tbs.
Total Fat:	1 gram
Dietary Fiber:	3 grams

Hot breakfast cereals and whole grain desserts can be made more delicious with a cinnamon-based spice blend. Find a good "Apple Pie Spice" or "Pumpkin Pie Spice" in your supermarket or make your own with this recipe.

>   3 tablespoons ground cinnamon
>   1 tablespoon ground nutmeg
>   1 tablespoon ground ginger
>   1 teaspoon ground cloves
>   1 teaspoon ground cardamom
>   1 teaspoon ground mace

Mix all ingredients together in a small bowl. Store in an airtight container. ■

LOW-FAT, HIGH FIBER RECIPES

• •

Harissa Sauce

Yield: About 1/4 cup	
Calories:	23 per Tbs.
Total Fat:	1 gram
Dietary Fiber:	1 gram

A little of this hot sauce goes a long way! Stir in a tiny bit while you cook, or let each person mix a little into his or her own portion of any vegetable or bean dish.

>   2 tablespoons cayenne pepper
>   1 tablespoon ground cumin
>   1 teaspoon ground caraway seeds
>   1 clove garlic
>   1/2 teaspoon salt
>   1/4 cup fat-free Italian salad dressing

Mix the spices together in a small refrigerator container. Peel the garlic clove and press it through a garlic press into the spice mixture. Stir in the salad dressing and mix well. Cover and refrigerate. ■

Summer Harira ❄

1 cup orange lentils
1 cup brown or green lentils
8 ¹/₂ cups bouillon
1 large onion, chopped
1 green bell pepper, chopped
2 stalks celery, chopped
2 cloves garlic, chopped
1 tablespoon African Berbere Spice
   Blend, or to taste (see page 98)
Pinch of cayenne pepper, or to taste
1 15-oz. can chick peas, undrained
1 15-oz. can small white beans,
   undrained

Yield: 8 to 10 servings	
Calories:	271
Total Fat:	2 grams
Dietary Fiber:	21 grams

1 cup cooked barley or other whole grains
   of your choice (see pages 68–69)
1 cup canned Italian plum
   tomatoes, chopped
¹/₂ cup chopped fresh flat-leaf
   parsley
¹/₂ cup fresh lemon juice
Lemon wedges

Cover the lentils with 8 cups of the bouillon and let them soak while you pre-pare the other ingredients. In a large pot, cook the onion, bell pepper, celery and garlic and spices in the remaining ¹/₂ cup of bouillon until softened, 5 to 10 minutes. Stir in the lentils and their soaking liquid and bring to a boil. Reduce heat and simmer until the lentils are tender, 25 to 30 minutes. Add the chick peas, white beans, barley and tomatoes; cook an additional 10 minutes. Just before serving, stir in the parsley and lemon juice. Serve with lemon wedges. ■

Irish Spring Soup ❄

6 cups onion soup made from dried or
   canned concentrate plus water
1 cup rolled oats, uncooked, or 2 cups
   cooked oat groats or other whole
   grains of your choice
   (see pages 68–69)
1 teaspoon dried oregano
Pinch of cayenne pepper, or to taste
¹/₂ pound asparagus, cut into
   1-inch pieces
¹/₄ cup chopped fresh flat-leaf parsley

Yield: 4 to 6 servings	
Calories:	156
Total Fat:	3 grams
Dietary Fiber:	5 grams

1 10-oz. bag fresh spinach, stems
   removed, leaves torn into small
   pieces, or 1 10-oz. package
   frozen spinach
Lemon wedges
Freshly ground black pepper

Combine the onion soup, oats, oregano and cayenne in a large pot and bring to a boil. Reduce heat and simmer 5 to 10 minutes. Stir in the asparagus and spinach and simmer just until the asparagus is tender, about 5 minutes. Adjust the seasonings and sprinkle with the parsley. Serve with lemon wedges and freshly ground pepper. ■

Hot and Sour Mushroom Soup

Yield: 4 servings	
Calories:	115
Total Fat:	1 gram
Dietary Fiber:	2 grams

$^1/_2$ pound cooked small shrimp
    (optional)
6 cups bouillon
1 stalk lemongrass, the bottom
    6 inches cut in $^1/_4$ inch slices
Grated rind of 1 lemon
2 cloves garlic, minced
1 teaspoon minced fresh
    ginger root
$^1/_2$ cup sliced canned bamboo shoots,
    cut into matchstick-size pieces
1 bunch green onions, thinly sliced
$^1/_4$ pound mushrooms, thinly sliced

2 tablespoons oyster sauce
2 tablespoons fresh lemon juice
2 tablespoons cornstarch
2 tablespoons mirin (rice wine)
$^1/_2$ teaspoon chili paste or hot pepper
    sauce to taste
3 to 5 steamed asparagus spears per
    serving for garnish (optional)

If using the shrimp, peel them and set aside. In a large pot, bring the bouillon, shrimp shells, lemongrass, lemon rind, garlic and ginger to a boil. Reduce heat and simmer, covered, 15 to 20 minutes. Strain to remove the solids and return the soup to the pot. Add the bamboo shoots, green onions, mushrooms, oyster sauce and lemon juice and cook 5 minutes. Mix the cornstarch and mirin into a smooth paste in a small bowl and stir into the soup. Bring the soup to a boil, stirring constantly, and cook until slightly thickened. Stir in the reserved shrimp and add chili paste to taste. Ladle into soup bowls and garnish with the asparagus spears, if using. ■

Double Mushroom-Grain Soup

Yield: 6 to 8 servings	
Calories:	133
Total Fat:	1 gram
Dietary Fiber:	5 grams

12 dried shiitake mushrooms, stems
    removed, broken in pieces
8 cups bouillon
1 large onion, chopped
2 cloves garlic, minced
2 carrots, sliced
2 stalks celery, sliced
1 small bunch broccoli, stalks sliced;
    heads broken into florets
1 cup quick-cooking oats or rolled oats
Pinch cayenne pepper, or to taste

$^1/_2$ pound fresh mushrooms, chopped
$^1/_2$ cup dry white wine or sherry
1 tablespoon Dijon mustard
$^1/_4$ cup chopped fresh flat-leaf parsley
1 cup cooked wild rice
Freshly ground black pepper to taste

Combine mushrooms and bouillon and let them soak at least 10 minutes or until soft. Add onion, garlic, carrots, celery, broccoli, oatmeal and cayenne pepper. Bring to a boil, reduce heat, and simmer, uncovered, 45 to 60 minutes, stirring occasionally. Puree with a hand blender or blender until smooth. Meanwhile, cook the fresh mushrooms in the white wine or sherry until softened, about 5 minutes. Stir the cooked mushrooms into the soup along with the mustard, parsley and wild rice, and heat through. Ladle into bowls and serve with freshly ground black pepper to taste. ■

...shroom-Barley Soup ❄

Yield: 8 to 12 servings

Calories:	233
Total Fat:	1 gram
Dietary Fiber:	8 grams

20 dried mushrooms, stems
    removed, broken in pieces
12 cups bouillon
2 onions, chopped
4 carrots, chopped
4 stalks celery, chopped
4 medium parsnips, chopped
1 cup orange lentils or yellow split peas
1 tablespoon Italian herb blend
Pinch of cayenne pepper, or to taste
1 cup barley or other whole grains of your choice (see pages 68–69)
$1/2$ cup chopped fresh flat-leaf parsley

Combine mushrooms and bouillon and let them soak at least 10 minutes, or until soft. Add the remaining ingredients except the parsley and bring to a boil. Reduce heat and simmer, uncovered, about 1 hour or until barley and vegetables are tender. When ready to serve, stir in the parsley and adjust the seasonings. If desired, you may puree the soup in a blender and return it to the pot to heat before serving. ■

Wild Rice-Pumpkin Soup ❄

Yield: 6 to 8 servings

Calories:	114
Total Fat:	1 gram
Dietary Fiber:	5 grams

3 pounds butternut or other winter
    squash or pie pumpkin (about 4 cups
    cooked)
1 onion, chopped
1 green bell pepper, chopped
3 cloves garlic, minced
8 cups bouillon
2 teaspoons Garam Masala Spice Blend
    (see page 98)

1 tablespoon oregano
Pinch of cayenne pepper, or to taste
2 cups cooked wild rice or other whole
    grains of your choice (see pages 68–69)

Puncture the squash or pumpkin skin with a knife or fork. Microwave squash or pumpkin on HIGH 3 minutes or until squash is soft enough to cut easily. Cut the squash in half and allow it to cool until you can handle it comfortably. Scoop out the seeds and discard. Either scoop the flesh from the shell, or cut the squash into chunks and pare off the peel, whichever is easier.

Cook the onion, bell pepper and garlic in $1/2$ cup of the bouillon in a large pot over medium heat until softened, about 5 minutes. Add the remaining bouillon, the cooked squash or pumpkin and seasonings to the pot, bring to a boil, reduce heat and simmer 15 to 20 minutes, stirring occasionally, or until the squash is very soft. Stir in the wild rice and heat until hot, about 5 minutes. ■

Pumpkin Soup ❄

Yield: 4 to 6 servings	
Calories:	135
Total Fat:	2 grams
Dietary Fiber:	5 grams

3 pounds butternut or other winter squash (about
   4 cups cooked) or pie pumpkin
  1 28-oz. can pumpkin puree (unsweetened)
1 large onion, chopped
4 carrots, sliced
1 teaspoon Dessert Spice Blend (see page 99)
1 teaspoon mild curry powder
8 cups bouillon
2 cups cooked oat groats or whole grains of your choice (see pages 68–69)
Hot pepper sauce (optional)

To cook squash or raw pumpkin: Puncture the skin with a knife or fork.
Microwave on HIGH 3 minutes or until squash is soft enough to cut easily. Cut
the squash in half and allow it to cool until you can handle it comfortably.
Scoop out the seeds and discard. Either scoop the flesh from the shell, or cut
the squash into chunks and pare off the peel, whichever is easier.

Place the onion, carrots, squash pieces, spices and bouillon in a large pot. (If using
canned pumpkin, add it later with the oat groats.) Bring to a boil, reduce heat,
and simmer about 20 minutes or until the squash and carrots are very tender.
Puree with a hand blender or in a blender until smooth. Stir in the oat groats and
cook, stirring frequently, 10 minutes more. Ladle soup into bowls and pass the
hot sauce if desired. ■

● ●

Speedy Chick Pea Soup ❄

Yield: 6 servings	
Calories:	183
Total Fat:	3 grams
Dietary Fiber:	11 grams

$^{1}/_{2}$ cup bulgur
4 cups bouillon
2 15-oz. cans chick peas
2 teaspoons oregano
$^{1}/_{2}$ teaspoon Harissa Sauce, or to taste
  (see page 99)
1 10-oz. bag spinach, chopped, or 1 box frozen chopped spinach
Lemon slices or wedges for garnish

Bring the bulgur and 3 cups of the bouillon to a boil. Meanwhile, place the other
cup of bouillon and 1 can of the chick peas in blender; puree until smooth. Add
them to the pot, along with the other can of chick peas, the spices and spinach.
If using frozen spinach, break up the block with a spoon. Return to boiling, then
simmer until the bulgur is soft, 5 to 10 minutes. Serve with lemon wedges. ■

Florentine Pea Soup

Yield: 6 to 8 servings	
Calories:	182
Total Fat:	1 gram
Dietary Fiber:	13 grams

1 cup split green peas
6 cups bouillon
2 onions, chopped
4 cloves garlic, minced
2 teaspoons dried oregano
Pinch of cayenne pepper, or to taste
$1/2$ cup bulgur
1 28-oz. can Italian plum tomatoes, undrained, chopped
1 pound spinach, torn into pieces
Freshly ground black pepper

Bring the split peas and bouillon to a boil in a large pot, reduce heat and simmer 20 minutes or until they are just barely tender. Add the onions, garlic, seasonings, bulgur and tomatoes and simmer until bulgur is tender, 20 to 30 minutes. Put the spinach on top of the mixture, cover the pot and simmer just until the spinach wilts, about 2 minutes. Stir and serve in bowls with ground pepper to taste. ■

Lentil-Sweet Potato Dal ❄

Yield: 4 to 6 servings	
Calories:	188
Total Fat:	0 grams
Dietary Fiber:	7 grams

1 onion, chopped
4 cloves garlic, minced
4 cups bouillon
1 cup red lentils
1 large or 2 small sweet potatoes, scrubbed
   and cut into $1/2$-inch chunks
1 tablespoon Garam Masala Spice Blend (see page 98)
Pinch of cayenne pepper, or to taste
Plain fat-free yogurt for garnish (optional)

Combine all ingredients except the yogurt in a large pot. Bring to a boil, reduce heat and simmer, uncovered, 30 to 40 minutes or until the lentils and sweet potatoes are tender. Using a hand blender or blender, puree the soup until smooth.

Ladle soup into bowls. Top each serving with a spoonful of yogurt, if desired. ■

Caribbean Lentil Soup ❄

Yield: 6 to 8 servings	
Calories:	172
Total Fat:	1 gram
Dietary Fiber:	11 grams

1 onion, chopped
1 clove garlic, minced
1 cup lentils
1 sweet potato, scrubbed and cut into
   $1/2$-inch cubes
6 cups bouillon
1 8-oz. can (1 cup) tomato sauce
1 tablespoon African Berbere Spice Mix (see page 98)
1 cup fresh or canned pineapple chunks
2 unripened bananas, cut into $1/2$-inch slices
Chopped fresh cilantro or flat-leaf parsley for garnish (optional)
Freshly ground black pepper to taste

Combine the onion, garlic, lentils, sweet potato, bouillon, tomato sauce and spice mix in a large pot. Bring to a boil, reduce heat and simmer, uncovered, 30 to 40 minutes or until the lentils and sweet potatoes are tender. Using a hand blender or a blender, process briefly to thicken , but leave it a little chunky. Stir in the pineapple and bananas. Ladle soup into bowls. Garnish with cilantro or parsley and black pepper, if desired. ■

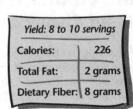

Fall Mulligatawny Soup ❄

Yield: 8 to 10 servings	
Calories:	226
Total Fat:	2 grams
Dietary Fiber:	8 grams

1 onion, chopped
2 cloves garlic, minced
1 green bell pepper, chopped
1 tablespoon fresh ginger root,
   minced
8 cups bouillon
2 parsnips, diced
2 carrots, diced
2 medium potatoes, diced
1 cup canned Italian plum
   tomatoes, chopped
1 tablespoon Garam Masala Spice
   Blend (see page 98)

Pinch of cayenne pepper, or to taste
2 apples, diced
$1/2$ cup raisins
1 15-oz. can chick peas, undrained
2 cups cooked millet or other whole
   grains of your choice
   (see pages 68–69)

Cook the onion, garlic, bell pepper and ginger in $1/2$ cup of the bouillon in a large saucepan over medium heat until softened, about 5 minutes. Add the remaining bouillon, parsnips, carrots, potatoes, tomatoes and spices, bring to a boil, reduce heat and simmer 20 to 30 minutes. Add the apples and raisins and cook 10 minutes more. Stir in the chick peas and millet and heat through. ■

Sicilian Minestrone ❄

Yield: 8 to 10 servings	
Calories:	147
Total Fat:	1 gram
Dietary Fiber:	7 grams

1 onion, chopped
2 cloves garlic, minced
1 green bell pepper, chopped
3 stalks celery, chopped
6 cups bouillon
1 29-oz. can tomato sauce
2 teaspoons dried oregano
Pinch of cayenne pepper, or to taste
2 medium potatoes, diced
1 16-oz. can cannellini or other white
beans, undrained

2 carrots, sliced
1 cup cooked whole grains such as
kamut (see pages 68–69)
$^1/_2$ cup fresh flat-leaf parsley, chopped
2 cups frozen whole-kernel corn
Freshly ground black pepper

Combine the onion, garlic, bell pepper, celery and $^1/_2$ cup of the bouillon in a large saucepan. Bring to boil, reduce heat and cook until softened, 5 to 10 minutes. Add the remaining bouillon, tomato sauce, oregano, cayenne, potatoes and carrots. Return to boiling, reduce heat and simmer 20 minutes or until the vegetables are tender. Stir in the beans, kamut, parsley and corn and simmer 5 minutes or until heated through. Serve with freshly ground pepper to taste. ■

Incredible! New England Clam Chowder ❄

Yield: 4 servings	
Calories:	105
Total Fat:	2 grams
Dietary Fiber:	4 grams

This recipe can be used to make any kind of creamy soup you like. In place of the clams, use any other seafood, or vegetables such as mushrooms, asparagus or corn. Add cubes of cooked potatoes, carrots, and any other vegetables you like, and vary the seasonings to suit your taste.

1 large onion, chopped
6 cups bouillon
1 medium cauliflower, chopped into florets
1 cup quick-cooking oats or rolled oats
1 teaspoon dried oregano
Pinch of cayenne pepper, or to taste
1 6.5-oz. can chopped clams, undrained
Freshly ground black pepper to taste
Chopped parsley or chives (optional)

Combine the onion, bouillon, cauliflower, oats and spices in a large pot and bring to a boil. Reduce heat and simmer gently 60 minutes, uncovered, stirring frequently. Allow to cool slightly. Puree the soup with a hand blender or blender until smooth and return to the pot. Stir in the clams and their juice, adjust the seasonings to your taste and reheat. Serve with freshly ground black pepper and garnish with chives or parsley if desired. ■

Spring Tonic Soup ❄

Yield: 6 to 8 servings

Calories:	150
Total Fat:	1 gram
Dietary Fiber:	7 grams

1 large Vidalia onion, chopped
2 cloves garlic, minced
2 stalks celery, chopped
8 cups bouillon
2 teaspoons dried oregano
Pinch of cayenne pepper, or
   to taste
2 cups baby carrots, cut into
   $1/_2$-inch slices
$1/_2$ pound mushrooms, sliced
2 cups cooked barley (see pages 70-72)

1 cup white wine
1 cup sugar snap peas, strings
   removed and cut into bite size
   pieces each
Freshly ground black pepper to taste

Combine the onion, garlic, celery and $1/_2$ cup of the bouillon in a medium sauce-pan and bring to a boil. Reduce heat and cook until softened, 5 to 10 minutes. Add the remaining bouillon, oregano, cayenne,, carrots, mushrooms, barley and wine. Return to a boil, reduce heat and simmer 10 to 15 minutes or until the carrots are just tender. To make a thicker soup, use a hand blender or blender to break up vegetables slightly, but do not puree (there should be lots of carrot and mushroom pieces). Stir in the snap peas and cook 3 to 5 minutes or until peas are crisp-tender. Ladle soup into bowls and serve with freshly ground pepper. ∎

Cream of Asparagus Soup ❄

Yield: 6 to 8 servings

Calories:	156
Total Fat:	2 grams
Dietary Fiber:	7 grams

2 pounds asparagus
1 large onion, chopped
2 cloves garlic, minced
2 stalks celery, sliced
2 broccoli stems, sliced (save the florets
   for another use)
6 cups bouillon
2 teaspoons dried oregano

Pinch of cayenne pepper, or to taste
1 cup rolled oats
$1/_4$ cup chopped fresh dill (optional)

Break the tough ends off the asparagus and discard. Cut the stalks into 2-inch pieces and set the tips aside. Put the asparagus stalks and the remaining ingredients except the dill in a large pot and bring to a boil. Reduce heat and simmer 45 to 60 minutes or until the vegetables are very soft. Puree with a hand blender or a blender until smooth. Return the soup to a gentle boil, stir in the asparagus tips and cook 3 to 5 minutes or until tips are crisp-tender. Stir in the chopped dill, saving a little to garnish each serving. ∎

LOW-FAT, HIGH FIBER RECIPES

Split Pea-Barley Pot ❄

Yield: 8 to 12 servings	
Calories:	284
Total Fat:	1 gram
Dietary Fiber:	18 grams

12 cups bouillon
1 pound green split peas
1 large onion, chopped
4 carrots, chopped
2 stalks celery, chopped
$^1/_2$ cup barley or other whole grains of your choice (see pages 68–69)
2 teaspoons dried oregano
Pinch of cayenne pepper, or to taste
1 tablespoon fresh lemon juice

3 cups frozen or fresh baby lima beans
1 cup loosely packed chopped fresh basil leaves
Freshly ground black pepper

Combine all ingredients except the lima beans, basil and pepper in a large pot. Bring to a boil, reduce heat and simmer, uncovered, 1 hour or until the split peas have disintegrated. Stir in the lima beans and cook 15 minutes or until beans are tender. Just before serving, stir in the basil. Ladle soup into bowls and serve with freshly ground pepper. ■

● ●

Golden Soup ❄

Yield: 8 to 10 servings	
Calories:	205
Total Fat:	1 gram
Dietary Fiber:	13 grams

1 large onion, chopped
12 cups bouillon
2 cups yellow split peas or orange lentils
1 tablespoon grated fresh ginger root
1 tablespoon Garam Masala Spice Blend (see page 98)
1 tablespoon mild chili powder
1 large sweet potato, cut into $^1/_2$-inch cubes
4 carrots, cut into $^1/_4$-inch slices, each slice halved or quartered

Juice of 2 limes
1 cup cooked oat groats or other whole grains of your choice (see pages 68–69)
Plain fat-free yogurt for garnish (optional)

Cook the onion in $^1/_2$ cup of the bouillon in a large saucepan over medium heat until softened, 5 to 10 minutes, while preparing the other ingredients. Add the remaining bouillon, split peas or lentils, seasonings, sweet potato and carrots. Bring to a boil and simmer, uncovered, about 45 minutes or until the split peas and vegetables are very tender. Stir in the lime juice; taste and adjust the seasonings. Remove about 2 cups of the vegetables with a slotted spoon and puree the rest of the soup in batches in a blender or with a hand blender until smooth. Return the reserved vegetables to the pot along with the oat groats and heat through. Ladle soup into bowls and place a dollop of yogurt in the center of each bowl, if desired. ■

Sweet Potato-Mango Soup ✻

Yield: 4 to 6 servings	
Calories:	149
Total Fat:	1 gram
Dietary Fiber:	4 grams

3 medium sweet potatoes, scrubbed or peeled
    and cut into chunks
1 large or 2 small mangoes, peeled and
    cut into chunks
1 onion, chopped
1 tablespoon minced fresh ginger root
6 cups bouillon
2 teaspoons mild curry powder
Pinch of cayenne pepper, or to taste
Chopped fresh cilantro or fresh flat-leaf parsley for garnish (optional)

Combine all ingredients except cilantro in a large pot. Bring to a boil, reduce heat and simmer, uncovered, 30 to 40 minutes or until sweet potatoes are very tender. Using a hand blender or a blender, puree the soup until smooth. Adjust the seasonings and ladle soup into bowls. Garnish with cilantro or parsley, if desired. ∎

• •

Spaghetti Squash Soup with Artichokes ✻

Yield: 6 to 8 servings	
Calories:	148
Total Fat:	2 grams
Dietary Fiber:	8 grams

1 small spaghetti squash
8 cups bouillon
2 teaspoons dried oregano
Pinch of cayenne pepper, or to taste
1 large red onion, halved lengthwise
    and thinly sliced
2 cloves garlic, minced
1 10-oz. package frozen artichoke
    hearts, cut into bite-size pieces
2 stalks celery, sliced

2 cups cooked oat groats, wild rice or
    other whole grains of your choice
    (see pages 68–69)
1 15-oz. can chick peas, undrained
1 lemon
$^1/_4$ cup chopped fresh flat-leaf parsley

To cook spaghetti squash: Puncture the skin with a knife or fork. Microwave on HIGH 3 minutes, or until squash is soft enough to cut easily. Cut the squash in half and allow it to cool until you can handle it comfortably. Scoop out the seeds and discard. Place squash halves, cut side down, in a microwave-safe dish and microwave on HIGH another 8 to 10 minutes or until squash is tender. (Squash can be baked in a conventional oven at 350°F. or 1 hour.) Allow squash to cool until you can handle it comfortably.

Meanwhile, combine the bouillon, oregano, cayenne, onion, garlic and celery and bring to a boil in a large pot. Reduce heat and simmer 5 to 10 minutes or until onion is tender.

Run a fork over the interior of the squash to separate it into spaghetti-like strands. Add these to the pot along with the artichoke hearts, cooked grains and chick peas. Return to boiling, reduce heat and simmer 15 to 20 minutes. Cut the lemon in half and squeeze the juice from one half into the soup. Stir in the parsley. Garnish with lemon slices or wedges. ∎

Broccoli Stalk Slaw

Yield: 4 to 6 servings	
Calories:	49
Total Fat:	1 gram
Dietary Fiber:	4 grams

3 broccoli stalks (reserve florets for other use
1 small red onion, diced
1 cup chopped radishes
$1/4$ cup fat-free mayonnaise
1 tablespoon Dijon mustard
2 tablespoons rice wine vinegar

Grate broccoli stalks in a food processor or with a hand grater. Combine all ingredients in a serving bowl. ∎

Mexican Slaw

Yield: 4 to 6 servings	
Calories:	132
Total Fat:	1 gram
Dietary Fiber:	8 grams

1 small head green cabbage, cored
    and shredded
2 cups frozen whole-kernel corn
1 small red onion, chopped
1 red bell pepper, chopped
$1/4$ cup chopped fresh flat-leaf parsley

Dressing
$1/4$ cup vinegar
$1/4$ cup fat-free mayonnaise
1 tablespoon Dijon mayonnaise
1 teaspoon ground cumin

Combine cabbage, corn, onion, bell pepper and parsley in a serving bowl.

Prepare the Dressing: Combine all the dressing ingredients in a small bowl. Pour dressing over the slaw and toss to combine. ∎

Potato "Egg" Salad

Yield: 4 to 6 servings

Calories:	213
Total Fat:	1 gram
Dietary Fiber:	4 grams

2 pounds red potatoes
    (about 8 medium), unpeeled
1 12-oz. container low-fat tofu
$1/4$ teaspoon turmeric
2 stalks celery, chopped
$1/4$ cup chopped red onion
$1/2$ cup fat-free mayonnaise
2 tablespoons Dijon mustard
$1/4$ cup chopped fresh flat-leaf parsley
Salt and freshly ground black pepper to taste

Add the potatoes and enough water to cover to a medium saucepan over medium heat. Bring to a boil and cook until just tender, about 20 minutes. Drain and rinse with cold water. Cut the potatoes into $1/2$-inch cubes and refrigerate until chilled, about 30 minutes.

Place the tofu and turmeric in a salad bowl and break up tofu with a fork. Stir in the chilled potatoes and the remaining ingredients. ■

Harvest Salad 🕐

Yield: 4 to 6 servings

Calories:	218
Total Fat:	2 grams
Dietary Fiber:	11 grams

2 cups cooked quinoa (see pages 70–72)
1 cup frozen whole-kernel corn, thawed
1 16-oz. can pink beans, drained and rinsed
1 tomato, chopped
1 bunch green onions, chopped
$1/4$ cup chopped fresh cilantro or flat-leaf parsley
2 tablespoons fresh lemon juice
1 teaspoon ground cumin
Hot pepper sauce to taste

Combine all ingredients except hot sauce in a serving bowl. Serve with the bottle of hot sauce on the side, so each diner can add heat to his or her taste. ■

Mango Salad with Barley and Beans ⏰

Yield: 4 to 6 servings	
Calories:	184
Total Fat:	2 grams
Dietary Fiber:	9 grams

1 small red onion, chopped
2 mangoes, peeled, pitted and chopped
1 15-oz. can black beans, drained and rinsed
2 cups cooked barley, chilled (see pages 70–72)
$1/2$ cup chopped fresh cilantro or fresh flat-leaf parsley
$1/2$ cup grapefruit juice
1 teaspoon ground cumin
1–2 jalapeño chilies, seeded and chopped (to taste)

Combine all ingredients in a serving bowl. ∎

• •

Malaysian Salad

Yield: 6 to 8 servings	
Calories:	182
Total Fat:	2 grams
Dietary Fiber:	4 grams

2 cups cooked millet or quinoa
1 small or $1/2$ large green bell pepper, chopped
1 stalk celery, chopped
1 bunch green onions, sliced thin
$1/2$ cup frozen green peas
$1/2$ cup sliced canned water chestnuts, drained
$1/2$ cup sliced canned bamboo shoots, drained
$1/2$ cup canned pineapple tidbits
$1/2$ cup golden raisins
1 orange or 2 tangerines, peeled and cut into bite-size pieces
1 cup bean sprouts
1 tablespoon toasted sesame seeds

Dressing:

$1/4$ cup rice vinegar
$1/4$ cup juice from canned or fresh pineapple
1 tablespoon minced fresh ginger root
1 clove garlic, minced
3 tablespoon soy sauce

Prepare the Dressing: Combine the dressing ingredients in a small bowl.

Combine salad ingredients in a serving bowl. Add the dressing and toss to combine. Cover and refrigerate until chilled, about 1 hour. ∎

Festive Wild Rice Salad ⏰

2 cups cooked, chilled wild rice
  (see pages 70–72)
$1/2$ red bell pepper, cut into $1/2$-inch
  diamond-shaped pieces
$1/2$ green bell pepper, cut into $1/2$-inch
  diamond-shaped pieces
$1/2$ cup dried apricots, cut into quarters
$1/2$ cup dried cranberries
1 bunch green onions, sliced
1 teaspoon mild curry powder
2 tablespoons fresh lemon juice
$1/2$ cup fat-free mayonnaise, or to taste

Yield: 6 to 8 servings	
Calories:	118
Total Fat:	0 grams
Dietary Fiber:	3 grams

Combine rice, bell peppers, apricots, and onions in a serving bowl. Stir in curry powder, lemon juice and mayonnaise. To make ahead combine all ingredients except mayonnaise, cover and refrigerate. Stir in the mayonnaise just before serving. ■

LOW-FAT, HIGH FIBER RECIPES

● ●

Spring Tabbouleh

1 cup bulgur
1 teaspoon ground cumin
1 teaspoon dried oregano
2 cloves garlic, minced
$1/2$ teaspoon ground black pepper
2 cups boiling bouillon
$1/4$ teaspoon Harissa Sauce (page 99),
  or to taste (optional)
1 bunch green onions, sliced
1 cucumber, chopped
1 16-oz. can artichokes, drained and
  cut into bite-size pieces

$1/2$ cup fresh flat-leaf parsley, chopped
2 tomatoes, chopped
$1/2$ cup fresh mint, chopped
1 teaspoon grated lemon peel
2 tablespoons fresh lemon juice
$1/4$ cup plain fat-free yogurt,
  or to taste

Yield: 4 to 6 servings	
Calories:	180
Total Fat:	1 gram
Dietary Fiber:	12 grams

Combine the bulgur, cumin, oregano, garlic and pepper in a heatproof bowl. Stir in the boiling bouillon and let sit 20 minutes or until most of the liquid is absorbed and the bulgur is soft. Drain off any excess liquid.

Add the remaining ingredients and mix to combine. ■

Minty Orange and Quinoa Salad ⏰

Yield: 4 to 6 servings

Calories:	134
Total Fat:	1 gram
Dietary Fiber:	4 grams

2 large oranges, peeled, segmented and cut
   into bite-size pieces
1 cup baby carrots, cut into matchstick-size
   pieces or sliced thin
4 stalks celery, sliced thin
2 cups cooked quinoa, millet or other whole grains of your
   choice (see pages 68–69)
$^1/_4$ cup fat-free honey mustard salad dressing
2 tablespoons fresh lemon juice, or to taste
$^1/_4$ cup chopped fresh mint
Romaine or other lettuce leaves

Combine all ingredients except the lettuce leaves in a serving bowl. Serve the salad on a bed of lettuce, or chop the lettuce and toss it with the salad before serving. ∎

Chinese Asparagus Salad

Yield: 4 to 6 servings

Calories:	173
Total Fat:	2 grams
Dietary Fiber:	9 grams

1 pound asparagus
1 red bell pepper, chopped
2 stalks celery, chopped
1 cup canned baby corn ears, drained
2 cups cooked barley, brown rice or other
   whole grains of your choice (see pages 68–69)

Dressing:

$^1/_4$ cup rice vinegar
2 cloves garlic, minced
2 tablespoons soy sauce

1 tablespoon grated fresh
   ginger root
1 teaspoon chili-garlic paste, or
   a dash of hot sauce to taste

Prepare the Dressing: Combine the dressing ingredients in a small bowl.

Break the tough ends off the asparagus and discard. Cut the stalks into 1-inch pieces. (Diagonal cuts look attractive.) Steam the asparagus over boiling water 8 minutes, or until just crisp-tender. (Or cook in boiling water 3 to 4 minutes.) Rinse the cooked asparagus in cold water and drain.

Combine the asparagus with the remaining salad ingredients in a serving bowl. Add the dressing and toss to combine. ∎

Smoked Salmon–Butter Bean Salad ⏰

Yield: 4 to 6 servings

Calories:	117
Total Fat:	1 gram
Dietary Fiber:	5 grams

$1/4$ pound smoked salmon, cut into
   bite-size pieces
1 15-oz. can butter beans (large
   limas), drained and rinsed
1 small red onion, chopped
2 stalks celery, chopped
1–2 jalapeño chilies (red if available)
   seeded and chopped (optional)
$1/2$ cup frozen green peas

$1/2$ cup fresh flat-leaf parsley, chopped
1 teaspoon dried oregano
2 tablespoons fresh lemon juice or
   2 tablespoons red wine vinegar
Fat-free Italian dressing to taste

Mix all ingredients except the Italian dressing in a serving bowl. Taste and add a little of the dressing if desired, to make the salad moist (some smoked salmon is dry, some is moist). ■

• •

Caribbean Lentil Salad

Yield: 6 to 8 servings

Calories:	111
Total Fat:	0 grams
Dietary Fiber:	5 grams

Note: This salad is supposed to be quite hot! If you make it tame, you may want to bring the bottle of hot sauce to the table so your guests can customize their own servings.

1 cup tiny green lentils
2 cloves garlic, minced
6 cups bouillon
1 small red onion, chopped
1 stalk celery, chopped
12 cherry tomatoes, halved
   or quartered
1 bunch radishes, sliced
8 tiny carrots, cut lengthwise into slivers

1–2 jalapeño chilies (red if available)
   seeded and chopped (optional)
$1/4$ cup fresh flat-leaf parsley, chopped
Juice of 1 lime
2 tablespoons red wine vinegar,
   or to taste
Hot pepper sauce to taste (optional)

Bring the lentils, garlic and bouillon to a boil in a medium saucepan. Reduce heat and simmer until the lentils are tender but not mushy, about 20 minutes. Pour the lentils into a colander in the sink, run cold water over them and let them drain.

Combine lentils with the remaining ingredients in a serving bowl. Serve at room temperature or chilled. ■

LOW-FAT, HIGH FIBER RECIPES

Sweet and Zingy Bulgur Salad

Yield: 6 to 8 servings	
Calories:	131
Total Fat:	1 gram
Dietary Fiber:	5 grams

2 cups bulgur
6 cups boiling bouillon
1 fresh pineapple, cut into bite-size pieces
    or 1 11-oz. can pineapple tidbits, drained
4 ripe peaches or nectarines, cut into $1/2$-inch pieces
1 bunch green onions, sliced
4 jalapeño chilies, seeded and minced
Juice of 2 limes
$1/4$ cup chopped fresh mint leaves
$1/4$ cup fat-free honey mustard salad dressing

Cover the bulgur with the boiling bouillon and let soak 30 minutes, or until tender. Drain off any excess liquid. Combine bulgur with the remaining ingredients in a serving bowl. ■

Sushi Salad Supreme

Yield: 4 to 6 servings	
Calories:	158
Total Fat:	3 grams
Dietary Fiber:	5 grams

$1/4$ cup rice wine vinegar
1 tablespoon soy sauce
1 teaspoon wasabi paste or to taste
2 cups cooked, chilled oat groats or other
    whole grains of your choice (see pages 68–69)
1 cup baby carrots, sliced
1 red bell pepper, chopped
1 cucumber, seeded and cut into $1/2$-inch dice
1 bunch green onions, sliced
$1/2$ pound surimi or small steamed shrimp (optional)
Romaine or Chinese cabbage leaves (optional)
1 tablespoon toasted sesame seeds

Combine the vinegar, soy sauce, wasabi and whole grains in a serving bowl. Stir in the carrots, bell pepper, cucumber, green onions and the seafood if using. Serve the salad on a bed of greens, if desired, and sprinkle with the toasted sesame seeds. ■

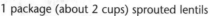

Lentil Sprouts Salad 🕐

Yield: 4 to 6 servings	
Calories:	127
Total Fat:	1 gram
Dietary Fiber:	5 grams

1 package (about 2 cups) sprouted lentils
1 ripe tomato, chopped
1 small cucumber, chopped
1 green or yellow bell pepper, chopped
2 green onions, sliced
1 cup cooked barley or other whole grains
  of your choice (see pages 68–69)
About 1/2 cup You Won't Believe It's Tofu Dressing (see page 119)
  or fat-free Italian dressing.

Combine all ingredients in a serving bowl except the dressing. Add enough of the dressing to moisten the salad. ■

Cuban Sweet Potato Salad

Yield: 4 to 6 servings	
Calories:	133
Total Fat:	3 grams
Dietary Fiber:	3 grams

4 medium sweet potatoes, cut into
  bite-size pieces
1 bunch green onions, sliced
1/2 cup pimiento-stuffed olives, sliced
About 1/4 cup fat-free mayonnaise or
  plain fat-free yogurt
1 tablespoon fresh lime juice
1 teaspoon ground cumin
1/2 teaspoon hot pepper sauce, or to taste

Steam the sweet potatoes over boiling water until just tender, about 15 minutes. Transfer sweet potatoes to a serving bowl and cool to room temperature or chill. Add the remaining ingredients and toss gently to combine. ■

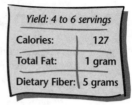

LOW-FAT, HIGH FIBER RECIPES

Barley-Bean Salad

Yield: 4 to 6 servings	
Calories:	237
Total Fat:	2 grams
Dietary Fiber:	14 grams

2 cups cooked barley or other whole grains
    of your choice (see pages 68–69)
1 15-oz. can pink or kidney beans, drained
    and rinsed
2 vine-ripened tomatoes, chopped
1 cucumber, chopped
2 stalks celery, chopped
$1/_4$ cup chopped fresh basil leaves
1 tablespoon Dijon mustard
$1/_2$ cup fat-free Italian dressing

Combine all ingredients in a serving bowl and toss to combine.
Cover and refrigerate until chilled, about 30 minutes. ∎

Southwestern Salad

Yield: 6 to 8 servings	
Calories:	162
Total Fat:	1 gram
Dietary Fiber:	6 grams

2 cups cooked brown rice, barley or other
    whole grains of your choice (see pages 68–69)
1 15-oz. can black beans, drained and rinsed
2 cups frozen whole-kernel corn, thawed
1 red bell pepper, chopped
1 small onion, chopped
$1/_4$ cup white wine vinegar, or to taste
$1/_4$ cup chopped fresh cilantro leaves
1 jalapeño chili, minced, or cayenne pepper to taste
1 teaspoon mild chili powder

Combine all ingredients in a serving bowl. For the best flavor cover and
refrigerate for at least 1 hour before serving to allow flavors to blend. ∎

Kamut Waldorf Salad ⏰

2 cups cooked kamut or other whole
    grains of your choice (see pages 68–69)
1 apple, cored and cut into bite-size pieces
1 large orange, cut into bite-size pieces
1 small fennel bulb or 2 stalks celery, cut
    into $1/_2$-inch pieces
$1/_4$ cup golden raisins
$1/_4$ cup chopped fresh flat-leaf parsley
$1/_4$ cup fat-free mayonnaise
2 tablespoons Dijon mustard
2 tablespoons lemon juice
1 teaspoon fennel seeds

Combine all ingredients in a serving bowl and toss to coat. ∎

Yield: 4 to 6 servings	
Calories:	135
Total Fat :	1 gram
Dietary Fiber:	5 grams

You Won't Believe It's Tofu Dressing ⏰

You can easily double or quadruple this recipe; it stores
well in the refrigerator up to one week. Use it in the
Lentil Sprouts Salad (see page 117) or any green salad.

2 garlic cloves, peeled, or 2 teaspoons garlic paste
1 tablespoon Dijon mustard
$1/_2$ of a 12-oz. package low-fat tofu
2 tablespoons soy sauce
2 tablespoons fresh lemon juice
1 teaspoon freshly ground black pepper

Combine all ingredients in a blender and puree until smooth. ∎

Yield: 1/2 cup	
Calories (Per 1/8 cup):	59
Total Fat:	1 gram
Dietary Fiber:	0 grams

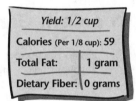

LOW-FAT, HIGH FIBER RECIPES

Extra Quick Chili ❄ ⏰

Yield: 6 to 8 servings	
Calories:	214
Total Fat:	1 gram
Dietary Fiber:	13 grams

1 10-oz. bag frozen bell pepper-onion mix
2 garlic cloves, minced
1 28-oz. can Italian plum tomatoes,
    undrained, chopped
1 teaspoon bouillon granules
1 tablespoon mild chili powder
Pinch cayenne pepper, or to taste
2 15-oz. cans kidney beans or black beans, undrained
1 teaspoon ground cumin
2 cups cooked whole grains of your choice (see pages 68–69)

Combine all ingredients in a large pot. Bring to a boil reduce heat, and simmer 5 to 10 minutes. Serve over the whole grains of your choice. ■

Two-Corn Green Chili ❄

Yield: 6 to 8 servings	
Calories:	213
Total Fat:	1 gram
Dietary Fiber:	11 grams

2 onions, chopped
4 cloves garlic, minced
1 green bell pepper, chopped
1 tablespoon mild chili powder
Pinch of cayenne pepper, or to taste
$1/2$ cup bouillon
1 cup frozen baby lima beans
1 4-oz. can chopped green chilies
$1/2$ pound fresh spinach, rinsed, stems removed, and leaves chopped or
    1 box frozen chopped spinach, thawed
1 cup frozen whole-kernel corn
2 15-oz. cans white beans, undrained
2 cups cooked polenta or other whole grains of your choice
    (see pages 68–69)
$1/4$ cup chopped fresh cilantro (optional)

Cook onions, garlic, bell pepper and seasonings in the bouillon in a large saucepan over medium heat until softened, 5 to 10 minutes. Stir in the lima beans and cook, covered, until beans are tender, 5 to 10 minutes. Add the remaining ingredients and simmer, stirring occasionally, 5 to 10 minutes or until the spinach is wilted and the chili is hot. ■

Lentil Chili ❄

Yield: 10 to 12 servings	
Calories:	231
Total Fat:	1 gram
Dietary Fiber:	12 grams

2 large onions, chopped
2 green bell peppers, chopped
4 cloves garlic, chopped
3 tablespoons mild chili powder
1 tablespoon ground cumin
1 teaspoon Dessert Spice Blend
  (see page 99)
$1/2$ teaspoon cayenne pepper,
  or to taste
5 cups bouillon
1 pound green lentils
1 cup bulgur
2 28-oz. cans Italian plum tomatoes,
  undrained, broken up

Accompaniments (optional):
  Fat-free sour cream
  Fresh salsa
  Chopped fresh cilantro
  Red, green and yellow bell
    pepper slivers
  Cooked whole grains
  Hot pepper sauce

Combine all ingredients in a large pot. Bring to a boil, reduce heat and simmer, stirring occasionally, 30 to 40 minutes or until the lentils are tender. Serve with your choice of the optional serving accompaniments. ■

Sweet Potato and Barley Chili ❄

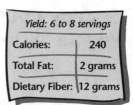

Yield: 6 to 8 servings	
Calories:	240
Total Fat:	2 grams
Dietary Fiber:	12 grams

2 onions, chopped
1 red bell pepper, chopped
6 cloves garlic, minced
2 tablespoons mild chili powder
1 tablespoon ground cumin
1 teaspoon cayenne pepper, or to taste
1 pound tomatillos, husks removed and cut into quarters, or 1 green
  bell pepper, chopped, or 1 (4-oz.) can chopped green chilies
2 large or 4 small sweet potatoes, scrubbed and cut into $1/2$-inch cubes
3 cups bouillon
1 (15-oz.) can small white beans, drained
2 cups cooked barley or other whole grain of your choice
  (see pages 68–69)

Combine the onions, bell pepper, garlic, spices, tomatillos, sweet potatoes and bouillon in a large pot. Bring to a boil, reduce heat and simmer, uncovered, 40 minutes or until the sweet potatoes are very tender.

Stir in the beans and barley and heat through. ■

Couscous on the Double

Yield: 6 to 8 servings	
Calories:	242
Total Fat:	2 grams
Dietary Fiber:	8 grams

2 cups bouillon
1 cup whole-wheat couscous
1 10-oz. bag frozen bell pepper-
   onion mix
1 10-oz. bag frozen mixed vegetables
   (such as, broccoli, carrots and
   cauliflower)
1 28-oz. can Italian plum tomatoes,
   undrained
1 15-oz. can chick peas, undrained

2 teaspoons bouillon granules
$1/2$ cup golden raisins
$1/2$ teaspoon Harissa Sauce, or to
   taste (see page 99)
Lemon wedges for garnish (optional)

Bring the bouillon to a boil in a medium saucepan. Stir in the couscous, cover and remove from heat. Let stand 5 to 10 minutes or until couscous is soft.

Combine the remaining ingredients, except the lemon wedges, in a large saucepan. Bring to a boil, reduce heat and simmer until everything is heated through.

When ready to serve, fluff the couscous with a fork. Put some couscous in each bowl, top with the vegetable mixture and garnish with the lemon wedges. ∎

Speedy Couscous and Veggie "Stir-Fry"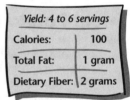

Yield: 4 to 6 servings	
Calories:	100
Total Fat:	1 gram
Dietary Fiber:	2 grams

2 cups bouillon
1 cup whole-wheat couscous
1 16-oz. bag frozen mixed stir-fry vegetables
2 tablespoons soy sauce
$1/4$ cup sherry or wine
$1/2$ teaspoon wasabi paste or pinch of cayenne pepper (optional)

Bring the bouillon to a boil in a small pot or microwave on HIGH in a microwave dish. Stir in the couscous, cover and let stand for 5 to 10 minutes or until couscous is soft. Fluff couscous with a fork.

Meanwhile, combine the remaining ingredients in a large pot. Bring to a boil, reduce heat and simmer, covered, 6 to 8 minutes or until the vegetables are crisp-tender. Stir in the couscous and serve immediately. ∎

Spring Couscous

Yield: 6 to 8 servings

Calories:	207
Total Fat:	2 grams
Dietary Fiber:	7 grams

2$^1/_2$ cups bouillon
1 cup whole wheat couscous
$^1/_2$ cup chopped canned Italian plum
   tomatoes
1 Vidalia onion, chopped
2 cloves garlic, minced
1 red, yellow or green bell pepper,
   chopped
$^1/_2$ teaspoon Harissa Sauce, plus additional for serving (see page 99)
1 cup sugar snap peas, ends and strings
   removed
$^1/_2$ cup frozen pearl onions

$^1/_2$ cup baby carrots, quartered
   lengthwise
$^1/_2$ pound fresh spinach, stems
   removed and leaves torn in
   small pieces
1 16-oz. can chick peas, drained
$^1/_2$ cup chopped fresh cilantro or fresh
   flat-leaf parsley (or some of each)

Bring 2 cups of the bouillon to a boil in a small pot. Stir in the couscous.
Remove from heat, cover and let sit 5 minutes. Stir in the chopped tomatoes
and cover until ready to serve.

Meanwhile, cook the chopped onion, garlic, bell pepper and Harissa Sauce in
the remaining $^1/_2$ cup of bouillon in a large pot over medium heat until softened, about 5 minutes. Stir in the peas, pearl onions and carrots, cover and
cook over medium heat until vegetables are just crisp-tender, about 5 minutes.
Stir in the spinach, chick peas and cilantro or parsley, cover and cook just until
the spinach is wilted, about 2 minutes. Serve over the couscous, with additional
Harissa Sauce to taste. ∎

Curried Lentils and Mushrooms ❄

Yield: 4 to 6 servings

Calories:	209
Total Fat:	0 grams
Dietary Fiber:	8 grams

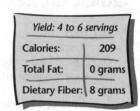

1 cup lentils
1 onion, chopped
1 carrot, chopped
6 cups bouillon
1 tablespoon chopped fresh ginger root
1 tablespoon Garam Masala Spice Blend (see page 98)
Pinch of cayenne pepper, or to taste
1 pound mushrooms, chopped
2 tablespoons fresh lemon juice or vinegar

Combine the lentils, onion, carrot, bouillon and seasonings in a large pot over
medium heat and bring to a boil. Reduce heat and simmer, uncovered, 30
minutes or until the lentils are tender and most of the liquid is absorbed. Stir
the mushrooms and lemon juice or vinegar into the lentils and cook, covered,
5 to 10 minutes or until mushrooms are softened. ∎

Three-Bean Curry ❄

Yield: 10 to 12 servings	
Calories:	223
Total Fat:	2 grams
Dietary Fiber:	12 grams

1 large onion, chopped
1 red or green bell pepper, chopped
1 cup bouillon
1 tablespoon mild curry powder
Pinch of cayenne pepper, or to taste
1 28-oz. can Italian plum tomatoes, undrained, chopped
4 small red potatoes, cut into bite-size cubes
1 15-oz. can chick peas, drained
1 15-oz. can kidney beans, drained
1 15-oz. can black beans, drained
$^1/_2$ cup chopped dried apricots
2 small zucchini, sliced
2 small yellow squash, sliced
2 cups cooked kamut or other whole grains of your choice
    (see page 68–69)

Combine the onion, bell pepper and bouillon in a large pot. Bring to a boil, reduce heat and simmer 5 to 10 minutes. Add the spices, tomatoes and potatoes and cook, covered, about 15 minutes, or until the potatoes are tender, stirring occasionally. Add the chick peas, beans, apricots, zucchini and yellow squash and cook until the zucchini is crisp-tender but still bright green, about 5 minutes. Serve over whole grains. ∎

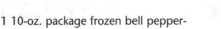

Quick Curried Chick Peas ❄ ⏱

Yield: 6 to 8 servings	
Calories:	201
Total Fat:	4 grams
Dietary Fiber:	11 grams

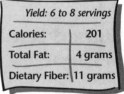

1 10-oz. package frozen bell pepper-
    onion mixture
2 (16-oz.) cans chick peas, drained
2 cups Italian plum tomatoes, undrained,
    broken up
2 teaspoons bouillon granules or 2 bouillon cubes
1 tablespoon mild curry powder
Pinch of cayenne pepper, or to taste
1 10-oz. package frozen spinach, thawed and drained
2 cups cooked oat groats, barley or other whole grain of your
    choice (see pages 68–69)

Combine all ingredients except the grains in a pot. Bring to a boil, reduce heat and simmer, stirring occasionally, 5 to 10 minutes or until vegetables are tender. Serve over whole grains. ∎

Extra-Quick Curry ❄ ⏱

Yield: 6 servings	
Calories:	231
Total Fat:	2 grams
Dietary Fiber:	13 grams

2 10-oz. bags frozen mixed vegetables such as
    onions, bell peppers, mushrooms, and broccoli;
    and beans, peas, carrots, and corn
$^1/_2$ cup bouillon
1 tablespoon mild curry powder
Pinch of cayenne pepper, or to taste
1 15-oz. can chick peas, butter beans or other beans of your choice, drained
Juice of 1 lime
1 cup plain fat-free yogurt (optional)
2 cups cooked barley or other whole grains of your choice (see pages 68–69)
Bottled mango chutney (optional)

Combine the frozen vegetables, bouillon and spices in a large pot. Bring to a
boil, reduce heat and simmer, covered, until vegetables are crisp tender, 5 to 10
minutes (check the packages for cooking times). Stir in the chick peas or beans
and the lime juice and heat through. If using the yogurt or soy milk, stir it in just
before serving the curry. Do not allow the mixture to boil after adding yogurt or
it will curdle. Serve over whole grains, with chutney on the side. ■

Moroccan Seafood Stew ❄

Yield: 8 to 10 servings	
Calories:	204
Total Fat:	3 grams
Dietary Fiber:	6 grams

1 onion, chopped
2 red or green bell peppers, chopped
2 cloves garlic, minced
1 fennel bulb or 8 stalks celery, chopped
$^1/_2$ cup water
1 28-oz. can Italian plum tomatoes,
    undrained, cut up
2 teaspoons bouillon granules
$^1/_2$ teaspoon Harissa Sauce, or to taste
    (see page 99)
$^1/_2$ pound mushrooms, quartered

$1^1/_2$ to 3 pounds seafood, cut into
    1-inch chunks (see Note below)
2 tablespoons fresh lemon juice
1 bunch cilantro, chopped
2 cups cooked barley or other whole
    grains of your choice (see pages 68–69)

Combine the onion, bell peppers, garlic, fennel or celery, tomatoes, water,
bouillon granules and Harissa Sauce in a large pot. Bring to a boil, reduce heat and
simmer 20 to 30 minutes, or until the vegetables are tender. Stir in the seafood and
mushrooms and cook until the seafood is opaque, about 5 minutes. Stir in the
lemon juice and cilantro. Serve over cooked whole grains.

Note: Seafood choices: Any combination of firm-fleshed fish and/or shellfish works
in this recipe.

Luxury version: 1 pound peeled jumbo shrimp and 1/2 pound each tuna, orange
roughy, shucked clams (12 small clams) and scallops.

Budget version: 1 pound catfish nuggets and 1 or 2 (6.5-oz.) cans chopped clams. ■

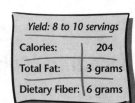

Catfish Gumbo ❄

Yield: 6 to 8 servings

Calories:	216
Total Fat:	3 grams
Dietary Fiber:	8 grams

1 large onion, chopped
4 cloves garlic, minced
1 green bell pepper, chopped
2 stalks celery, sliced
6 cups bouillon
1 28-oz. can Italian plum tomatoes,
   undrained, chopped
2 teaspoons dried oregano
$1/_8$ teaspoon cayenne pepper, or
   to taste
1 10-oz. package frozen okra, cut into
   $1/_2$-inch pieces, or 1 (10-oz.) package
   frozen green beans, or use both

1 pound catfish fillets, cut into
   1-inch pieces
1 cup frozen corn
2 cups cooked barley or other whole
   grains of your choice (see pages 68–69)
$1/_4$ cup chopped fresh flat-leaf parsley for
   garnish
Hot pepper sauce (optional)

Cook the onion, garlic, bell pepper and celery in $1/_2$ cup of the bouillon in a large saucepan over medium heat until softened, about 5 minutes. Add the remaining bouillon, tomatoes, oregano and cayenne. Bring to a boil. Reduce heat and simmer 5 to 10 minutes. Stir in the okra or green beans and simmer 5 minutes. Return the soup to a boil and stir in the catfish. Reduce heat and simmer 5 minutes or until the catfish is opaque and the vegetables are tender. Stir in the corn and heat through. Serve the gumbo over a mound of whole

Picadillo (Cuban Hash) ❄

Yield: 8 to 10 servings

Calories:	221
Total Fat:	6 grams
Dietary Fiber:	9 grams

1 onion, chopped
1 green bell pepper, chopped
1 28-oz. can Italian plum tomatoes,
   undrained, broken up
2 teaspoons bouillon granules
1 15-oz. can black beans, drained
1 cup crumbled soy or other vegetable
   burger
$1/_2$ cup pimiento-stuffed green
   olives, sliced
$1/_2$ cup golden raisins
1 tablespoon mild chili powder

2 teaspoons Dessert Spice Blend
   (see page 99)
Generous pinch of cayenne pepper,
   or to taste
2 tablespoons red wine vinegar
2 cups cooked barley or other whole
   grains of your choice (see pages 68–69)

Combine the onion, bell pepper, tomatoes and bouillon granules in a large pot. Bring to a boil, reduce heat and simmer 5 to 10 minutes. Stir in the remaining ingredients. Bring to a boil, reduce heat and simmer 15 to 20 minutes. Serve over whole grains.

Variations: Instead of the raisins, add other fruits such as chopped apples, pineapple or bananas. Or add chunks of sweet potato or winter squash (precook briefly in the microwave oven). This is also delicious served over baked sweet potatoes instead of whole grains. ■

Gabe's Famous Bean-Eggplant-Tomato Casserole —Quick Version ❄️⏱️

Yield: 8 to 10 servings	
Calories:	199
Total Fat:	1 gram
Dietary Fiber:	12 grams

1 onion, chopped
2 cloves garlic, minced
1 green bell pepper, chopped
1 28-oz. can Italian plum tomatoes, undrained, chopped
2 teaspoons bouillon granules
1 tablespoon mild chili powder
1 teaspoon dried oregano
Pinch of cayenne pepper, or to taste
1 medium eggplant, unpeeled, cut into $1/2$-inch cubes
2 15-oz. cans kidney beans, undrained
2 cups cooked barley or other whole grains of your choice (see pages 68–69)

Combine all ingredients, except barley, in a large pot. Bring to a boil, reduce heat and simmer 25 to 30 minutes, or until the eggplant is soft. Serve over barley or whole grains.

Variation: Extra-Quick Version: Substitute 1 bag frozen bell pepper-onion mix for the onions and green bell peppers. ■

• •

Quick Porotos Granados ❄️

Yield: 10 to 12 servings	
Calories:	156
Total Fat:	2 grams
Dietary Fiber:	9 grams

3 pounds butternut or other winter squash
   (about 4 cups cooked; see instructions page 103)
1 10-oz. bag frozen bell pepper-onion mix
1 28-oz. can Italian plum tomatoes, undrained, chopped
2 teaspoons dried oregano
2 15-oz. cans pinto beans or other small bean of your choice, undrained
1 cup cooked quinoa or other whole grains of your choice (see pages 68–69)
2 small yellow squash, sliced
1 cup frozen corn
3 tablespoons Pebre

Pebre:
1 tablespoon wine vinegar
2 cloves garlic, minced
$1/2$ cup chopped fresh cilantro
$1/4$ cup bouillon
2 fresh hot chilies, seeded and chopped, or to taste

Prepare Pebre: Combine all ingredients in a small bowl and let sit at least 2 hours for the flavors to blend. Use with discretion. Store any leftovers, covered, in the refrigerator. Yield: about $1/2$ cup.

Combine the cooked squash, onion-bell pepper mix, tomatoes, oregano, beans and quinoa in a large sauce pan. Bring to a boil and simmer 10 to 15 minutes. Add the yellow squash, corn and about 3 tablespoons of the Pebre or to taste and cook 5 minutes, stirring occasionally. Each diner can stir in more Pebre to his or her own taste. ■

Sweet Potato Curry with Bananas and Okra ❄

Yield: 6 to 8 servings

Calories:	250
Total Fat:	2 grams
Dietary Fiber:	9 grams

1 large onion, chopped
2 cloves garlic, minced
3 medium sweet potatoes, scrubbed or peeled and cut into 1-inch cubes
4 unripened bananas, peeled and cut in $1/2$-inch slices
1 stalk lemongrass, sliced lengthwise and crushed (optional)
3 cups bouillon
1 tablespoon mild curry powder
1 teaspoon paprika
1 teaspoon Dessert Spice Blend (see page 99) or ground cinnamon

2 cups fresh or frozen okra, whole if small or cut into $1/2$-inch slices if large
1 cup soy milk or plain fat-free yogurt
$1/4$ cup chopped fresh cilantro (optional)
2 cups cooked barley or other whole grain of your choice (see pages 68–69)

Combine the onion, garlic, sweet potatoes, bananas, lemongrass, bouillon and spices in a large pot over medium heat and bring to a boil. Reduce heat and simmer, uncovered, 30 to 40 minutes or until the sweet potatoes are tender. Remove the lemongrass.

Stir in the okra and bring to a boil. Reduce heat and simmer 10 minutes or until vegetables are tender. Add the soy milk or yogurt and heat through but do not boil. Stir in the cilantro, if desired, and serve over cooked whole grains. ■

Gallo Pinto 🕐

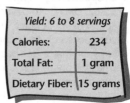

Yield: 6 to 8 servings

Calories:	234
Total Fat:	1 gram
Dietary Fiber:	15 grams

1 onion, chopped
2 cloves garlic, minced
1 red bell pepper, cut into $1/2$-inch chunks
$1/2$ cup bouillon
1 tablespoon mild chili powder
1 teaspoon mild curry powder
1 teaspoon hot pepper sauce, or to taste
2 15-oz. cans pink beans, drained
2 cups cooked barley or other whole grains of your choice (see pages 68–69)

Cook the onion, garlic and bell pepper in the bouillon in a large saucepan over medium heat until softened, about 5 minutes. Add the spices, beans and grains and cook together 5 to 10 minutes to blend the flavors. ■

Sweet and Sour Tofu

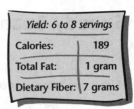

Yield: 6 to 8 servings

Calories:	189
Total Fat:	1 gram
Dietary Fiber:	7 grams

1 cup canned pineapple chunks, drained
   and juice reserved
3 tablespoons ketchup
3 tablespoons brown sugar
2 tablespoons cider vinegar
1 tablespoon soy sauce
1 tablespoon cornstarch
About $^1/_2$ cup bouillon
2 stalks celery, cut into $^1/_4$-inch
   diagonal slices
1 onion, halved lengthwise and cut into
   $^1/_4$-inch slices
1 clove garlic, minced
1 red bell pepper, cut into $^1/_2$-inch chunks

1 green bell pepper, cut into
   $^1/_2$-inch chunks
1 cup canned baby corn, cut into
   bite-size pieces
1 12-oz. package low-fat tofu, cut
   into cubes
2 cups cooked barley or other
   whole grains of your choice
   (see pages 68–69)

Make the sauce: Mix $^1/_3$ cup of the pineapple juice, ketchup, brown sugar, vinegar, soy sauce and cornstarch together in a medium bowl. Set aside.

Bring the bouillon to a boil in a large pot. Add the celery, onion, garlic and bell peppers and cook, stirring, until the vegetables are crisp-tender, about 5 minutes. Stir in the sauce mixture and cook, stirring, 1 to 2 minutes or until thickened. Add the pineapple chunks, baby corn and tofu and cook, stirring gently 2 minutes more. Serve over cooked whole grains. ■

● ●

Tofu "Fried Rice"

Yield: 6 to 8 servings

Calories:	200
Total Fat:	2 grams
Dietary Fiber:	9 grams

About $^1/_2$ cup bouillon
1 onion, chopped
1 red bell pepper, chopped
1 jalapeño chili, minced
$^1/_4$ pound mushrooms, chopped
1 tablespoon minced fresh ginger root
$^1/_2$ teaspoon turmeric
4 cups cooked barley, brown rice mix or
   oat groats (see pages 68–69)

1 (12-oz.) package low-fat tofu, cut
   into $^1/_2$-inch chunks
3 tablespoons soy sauce, or to taste
1 tablespoon toasted sesame seeds
Chopped fresh flat-leaf parsley
   for garnish

Bring the bouillon to a boil in a large pot. Add the onion, bell pepper, chili, mushrooms and ginger. Cook, stirring frequently, until softened, about 5 minutes, adding more bouillon if needed. Add the cooked whole grains, tofu, soy sauce and sesame seeds and cook over medium heat, breaking up the tofu a little so it has the consistency of scrambled eggs. Serve garnished with

Speedy Spanish "Rice" ❄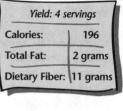

Yield: 4 servings	
Calories:	196
Total Fat:	2 grams
Dietary Fiber:	11 grams

3 cups cooked barley, brown rice or other whole
    grain of your choice (see pages 68–69)
1 cup tomato sauce
1 bunch green onions, chopped
1 teaspoon mild chili powder
$1/_2$ teaspoon ground cumin
Pinch of cayenne pepper, or to taste
$1/_2$ teaspoon dried oregano
1 cup frozen green peas
Chopped fresh cilantro or fresh flat-leaf parsley for garnish (optional)

Combine the grains, tomato sauce, onions, spices and oregano in a pot.
Bring to a boil, reduce heat and simmer 5 minutes. Stir in the peas and cook
2 to 3 minutes more or until heated through. Garnish with cilantro or parsley,
if desired. ■

Potato Goulash

Yield: 6 to 8 servings	
Calories:	216
Total Fat:	1 gram
Dietary Fiber:	8 grams

2 pounds medium red potatoes (about 8),
    cut in half lengthwise, then cut into
    $1/_4$-inch-thick slices
1 onion, chopped
2 cloves garlic, minced
2 tablespoons sweet paprika
1 teaspoon caraway seeds
1 teaspoon dried oregano
1 28-oz. can Italian plum tomatoes, undrained, broken up
2 teaspoons bouillon granules or 2 bouillon cubes
2 cups cooked barley or other whole grains of your choice
    (see pages 68–69)

Combine all ingredients except the grains in a large pot. Bring to a boil,
reduce heat and simmer, covered, 30 to 40 minutes or until the potatoes
are tender, stirring occasionally and adding water if needed. Serve over
whole grains. ■

Barbecue Beans and Barley ❄ ⏱

Yield: 8 to
Calories:
Total Fat:
Dietary Fiber: 12 grams

1 onion, chopped
2 cloves garlic, minced
1 12-oz. can light beer
$^1/_2$ cup ketchup
$^1/_2$ cup packed brown sugar
2 tablespoons Worcestershire sauce
$^1/_2$ teaspoon liquid smoke flavoring, or to taste
$^1/_2$ teaspoon Dessert Spice Blend (see page 99)
2 15-oz. cans pink beans, drained and rinsed
2 cups cooked barley or other whole grains of your choice
  (see pages 68–69)

Combine the onion, garlic, beer, ketchup, brown sugar and seasonings in a large saucepan. Bring to a boil, reduce heat and simmer, stirring occasionally, 10 minutes. Stir in the beans and barley, bring to a boil, reduce heat and simmer 10 minutes more. ■

Quinoa with Asparagus and Mushrooms

Yield: 4 to 6 servings
Calories: 152
Total Fat: 1 grams
Dietary Fiber: 6 grams

1 cup bouillon
8 dried mushrooms, stems removed, broken into small pieces
4 cloves garlic, minced
$^1/_2$ pound portobello mushrooms, cut into $^1/_2$-inch pieces
1 teaspoon dried oregano
1 pound fresh asparagus
1 red bell pepper, cut into thin strips
$^1/_2$ cup sherry
1 tablespoon cornstarch dissolved in 2 tablespoons cold water
1 tablespoon red wine vinegar
2 cups cooked quinoa (see pages 70–72)

Combine the dried mushrooms and bouillon in a large saucepan and soak for 10 minutes or until mushrooms are soft. Bring mushroom mixture to a boil, add the garlic, portobello mushrooms and oregano and simmer 5 minutes.

Meanwhile, break the tough ends off the asparagus and cut the stalks diagonally into 1-inch pieces. Add the asparagus pieces, bell pepper and sherry to the pot. Bring to a boil, reduce heat and simmer 5 to 7 minutes or until the asparagus is just crisp-tender. Stir in the cornstarch mixture and vinegar and cook, stirring, until the liquid is thickened. Serve the asparagus-mushroom mixture over the cooked quinoa and season with black pepper to taste. ■

Farmer's Paella

1 large sweet onion, chopped
3 stalks celery, chopped
3 garlic cloves, minced
$1/2$ cup bouillon
2 teaspoons dried oregano
Pinch of cayenne pepper, or to taste
1 28-oz. can Italian plum tomatoes, undrained, broken up
1 red bell pepper, cut into $1/2$ inch chunks
1 pound asparagus, cut into 1-inch pieces, tips reserved

1 16-oz. can artichoke bottoms or hearts, drained and cut into bite-size pieces
4 cups cooked barley, brown rice, or other whole grains of your choice (see pages 68–69)

Cook the onion, celery and garlic in the bouillon in a large pot over medium heat until softened, 5 to 10 minutes. Add the remaining ingredients except the asparagus tips. Bring to a boil, reduce heat and simmer, covered, 10 to 15 minutes or until the asparagus is tender. Stir in the asparagus tips and cook 3 minutes more.

Variation: This recipe makes excellent vegetable paella, but the addition of seafood makes it even more delicious. Shrimp, scallops, lobster tails, mussels, clams, chunks of white fish or surimi can be added in any combination. Stir the seafood in with the asparagus tips, cover and cook about 5 minutes or until the seafood is opaque and any shells are opened. ■

Creole Beans 'n' Greens

2 cups bouillon
1 10-oz. bag frozen bell pepper-onion mix
1 10-oz. package frozen chopped kale or spinach
$1/4$ teaspoon liquid smoke flavoring
1 teaspoon Cajun spice blend
Pinch of cayenne pepper, or to taste
2 tablespoons tomato paste
1 cup bulgur
1 15-oz. can pinto or kidney beans, drained and rinsed
4 tablespoons cider vinegar

Bring the bouillon, frozen vegetables, liquid smoke, and spices to a boil in a large pot, breaking up the vegetables with a spoon. Stir in the tomato paste and bulgur, bring to a boil, reduce heat and simmer 10 to 15 minutes or until the bulgur is soft. Stir in the beans and 2 tablespoons of the vinegar and heat through. Taste and add as much of the remaining vinegar as you like. ■

Spaghetti Squash, Thai Style

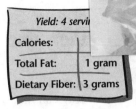

Yield: 4 servi...

Calories:	
Total Fat:	1 gram
Dietary Fiber:	3 grams

1 small spaghetti squash
$1/2$ pound medium shrimp in shells
3 tablespoons fish sauce
3 tablespoons rice vinegar
1 clove garlic, minced
1 tablespoon brown sugar
1 small hot chili, seeded and very
    thinly sliced
1 small or $1/2$ large red bell pepper, cut
    into matchstick-size pieces

1 bunch green onions, thinly sliced
1 cup bean sprouts
Chopped fresh basil or cilantro (optional)
1 tablespoon whole kasha (optional)

To cook spaghetti squash: Pierce the squash with a knife or fork Microwave on HIGH 3 to 5 minutes or until you can cut it easily. Halve and scoop out the seeds. Place the squash, cut sides down, in a microwave-safe dish and microwave on HIGH 10 minutes or until squash is tender. Let the squash sit until it is cool enough to handle. Run a fork over the interior of the squash to separate it into spaghetti-like strands and place in a serving bowl.

Meanwhile, steam the shrimp 15 minutes or boil 2 minutes. Rinse in cold water, peel and devein.

Combine the fish sauce, vinegar, garlic, brown sugar and hot chili in a small dish and mix well. Stir sauce into the spaghetti squash. Add shrimp, bell pepper, green onions, bean sprouts and basil or cilantro and toss to combine. If desired, serve with uncooked kasha sprinkled over the top as a great substitute for the classic Thai favorite, chopped peanuts. Serve at room temperature or chilled. ■

Fastest Beans and Barley ❄ ⏱

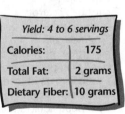

Yield: 4 to 6 servings	
Calories:	175
Total Fat:	2 grams
Dietary Fiber:	10 grams

1 15-oz. can black beans or other beans of your
    choice, undrained
2 teaspoons bouillon granules
2 cups cooked barley, brown rice or other whole
    grains (see pages 68–69)
1 tablespoon mild chili powder
$1/4$ cup chopped fresh cilantro or fresh flat-leaf parsley (optional)

Combine all ingredients in a large saucepan over medium heat. Bring to a boil, reduce heat and simmer 3 to 5 minutes. ■

Lebanese Split Peas with Spinach and Lemon ❄

Yield: 8 to 10 servings	
Calories:	254
Total Fat:	0 grams
Dietary Fiber:	5 grams

1 pound green split peas
5 cups bouillon, preferably ham flavor
1 teaspoon Harissa Sauce, or to taste (see page 99)
1 16-oz. can artichokes, cut into bite-size pieces
1 10-oz. bag fresh spinach, large stems removed and leaves chopped,
    or 1 (10-oz.) package frozen spinach, thawed and drained
2 tablespoons fresh lemon juice
2 cups cooked wild rice or other whole grains of your choice
    (see pages 68–69)

Combine the split peas and bouillon in a large saucepan over medium heat. Bring to a boil, reduce heat and simmer 45 minutes or until the peas are tender but not mushy. (Check them frequently toward the end of the cooking time.) Stir in the Harissa Sauce, artichoke hearts and spinach; cover, and cook until the spinach is wilted, 3 to 5 minutes. Stir in the lemon juice and wild rice and heat through. ■

Cassoulet ❄

Yield: 8 to 10 servings	
Calories:	267
Total Fat:	4 grams
Dietary Fiber:	10 grams

2 medium onions, chopped
6 cloves garlic, chopped
3 stalks celery, cut into $1/4$-inch slices
1 tablespoon oregano
2 cups bouillon
1 cup red wine
2 cups baby carrots
4 medium potatoes, cut into
    $1/2$-inch cubes
1 cup frozen pearl onions
1 cup Italian plum tomatoes, chopped
2 teaspoons fennel seeds
2 tablespoons Dijon mustard
$1/4$ teaspoon liquid smoke flavoring,
    or to taste
1 teaspoon minced fresh rosemary
    (optional)

Pinch of cayenne pepper to taste
1 15-oz. can white beans or pink
    beans, undrained
1 cup crumbled soy or other
    vegetable burger
Freshly ground black pepper
Chopped fresh flat-leaf parsley for
    garnish (optional)
2 cups cooked barley or other
    whole grains of your choice
    (see pages 68–69)

Cook the chopped onions, garlic, celery and oregano in $1/2$ cup of the bouillon in a large saucepan over medium heat until softened, about 5 minutes. Add the remaining bouillon, wine, carrots, potatoes, pearl onions, tomatoes and seasonings. Bring to a boil, reduce heat and simmer 15 to 20 minutes or until the carrots and potatoes are tender. Add the beans and soy burger and cook 5 to 10 minutes more. Add pepper and adjust the seasonings, garnish with chopped parsley, if desired, and serve over whole grains. ■

Stir-fry du Jour

Yield: 4 to 6 servings

Calories:	166
Total Fat:	1 gram
Dietary Fiber:	8 grams

Sauce:
1 tablespoon cornstarch
1 to 3 teaspoons sugar
$1/_2$ cup soy sauce
2 tablespoons mirin or rice wine vinegar
1 clove garlic, minced
1 tablespoon grated or minced fresh ginger
Pinch of cayenne pepper or minced fresh hot chilies, to taste

4 to 6 cups chopped, sliced or matchstick-size vegetables (choose from the following):

Mushrooms (any kind)
Onions (any kind)
Green or red bell peppers
Cabbage or Chinese cabbage
(any kind)
Carrots
Celery
Jicama

Sweet potatoes
Snow peas
Asparagus
Broccoli
Cauliflower
Fennel
Zucchini or yellow squash
Bean sprouts

Cooked whole grains of your choice (see pages 68–69)
About $1/_2$ cup bouillon

Prepare sauce: Stir the cornstarch into the liquids in a small bowl and mix until smooth. Add the other ingredients and set aside. Yield: About 6 tablespoons.

Organize vegetables according to cooking time: the harder ones take longer to cook (onions, carrots, celery) than the softer ones (beans sprouts, mushrooms, snow peas).

Have the cooked whole grains of your choice heated and ready to serve.

Heat a flat-bottomed pot or frying pan over medium-high heat and add 1 to 2 tablespoons of the bouillon. Add the longer cooking vegetables and stir-fry 3 to 5 minutes or until they start to soften, adding more bouillon as it evaporates. Continue adding the different kinds of vegetables and stir-fry until crisp-tender.

Pour $1/_4$ to $1/_2$ cup of the sauce down the side of the pan and stir to mix it into the vegetables. Cook, stirring, about 1 minute or until slightly thickened. Serve over cooked whole grains. ■

Quinoa Pilaf with Cherries

Yield: 4 to 6 servings	
Calories:	182
Total Fat:	2 grams
Dietary Fiber:	3 grams

1 onion, chopped
3 cups bouillon
2 teaspoons mild curry powder
Grated rind of 1 orange
1 cup uncooked quinoa
$1/4$ cup dried cherries
$1/4$ cup chopped fresh flat-leaf parsley, mint or cilantro
Hot pepper sauce to taste (optional)

Bring the onion, bouillon, curry powder and orange rind to a boil in a large saucepan. Stir in the quinoa and cherries, reduce heat and cook, covered, until the quinoa is tender, about 30 minutes. Stir in the parsley, mint or cilantro and hot sauce to taste. ■

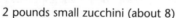

Zippy Zucchini 🕐

Yield: 4 to 6 servings	
Calories:	59
Total Fat:	1 gram
Dietary Fiber:	3 grams

2 pounds small zucchini (about 8)
3 tablespoons soy sauce
1 tablespoon Worcestershire sauce
2 tablespoons water
1 tablespoon brown sugar
1 tablespoon minced fresh ginger root
1 clove garlic, minced
Generous pinch cayenne, to taste
1 tablespoon toasted sesame seeds
2 green onions, sliced thin

Cut each zucchini in half lengthwise, then slice crosswise into $1/4$-inch slices. Place zucchini and 2 tablespoons water in a microwave-safe dish and microwave, covered, on HIGH 5 minutes or steam over boiling water about 10 minutes or until just crisp-tender. Drain.

Combine the remaining ingredients in a small bowl and stir into the zucchini. Serve warm or at room temperature. ■

LOW-FAT, HIGH FIBER RECIPES

Wild Rice with Snow Peas and Raspberries ⏰

Yield: 6 to 8 servings

Calories:	138
Total Fat:	1 gram
Dietary Fiber:	5 grams

$^1/_2$ pound fresh snow peas or 1 10-oz. package
   frozen snow peas, thawed
$^1/_2$ cup bouillon
2 teaspoons mild curry powder
1 bunch green onions, sliced
1 8-oz. can water chestnuts, drained and chopped
4 cups cooked wild rice (see pages 70–72)
1 cup fresh or frozen, thawed raspberries

Remove the tips and strings from the snow peas if using fresh . Combine the bouillon, curry powder and green onions in a pot and bring to a boil. Stir in the water chestnuts and wild rice and heat through. Add the snow peas, cover and cook 2 to 3 minutes or until just crisp-tender. Transfer the mixture to a serving dish and stir the raspberries in gently, reserving a few to garnish the top. ∎

Barley Biryani

Yield: 10 servings

Calories:	212
Total Fat:	1 gram
Dietary Fiber:	11 grams

1 sweet onion, chopped
1 green bell pepper, diced
2 carrots, diced
1 tablespoon minced fresh ginger root
2 teaspoons Garam Masala Spice Blend
   (see page 98)
$^1/_2$ cup bouillon
4 cups cooked barley or other whole grains of your choice
   (see pages 68–69)
$^1/_2$ cup golden raisins
1 15-oz. can pink beans or light red kidney beans, drained
Pinch of cayenne pepper, or to taste
1 cup frozen green peas, thawed
1 vine-ripened tomato, chopped
$^1/_4$ cup chopped fresh cilantro or flat-leaf parsley

Combine the onion, bell pepper, carrots, ginger, spice blend and bouillon in a large pot. Bring to a boil, reduce heat and simmer, covered, until the carrots are tender, about 15 minutes. Stir the cooked barley, raisins and beans into the vegetable mixture. Add cayenne to taste and heat through. Just before serving, stir in the peas, tomato and cilantro or parsley. ∎

LOW-FAT, HIGH FIBER RECIPES

Mushrooms with Grains

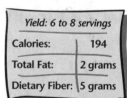

Yield: 6 to 8 servings

Calories:	195
Total Fat:	2 grams
Dietary Fiber:	7 grams

2 cups bouillon
2 cups dried mushrooms, stems removed, broken in pieces
1 onion, chopped
2 stalks celery, chopped
2 cloves garlic, minced
1 teaspoon mild chili powder
1 teaspoon dried oregano
Pinch of cayenne pepper, or to taste
2 cups cooked oat groats or other whole grains of your choice (see pages 68–69)
$1/4$ cup chopped fresh cilantro or flat-leaf parsley

Combine the mushrooms and bouillon in a large saucepan, and allow to soak at least 10 minutes or until soft. Add the onions, celery, garlic, and seasonings, bring to a boil, reduce heat and simmer 15 minutes or until most of the liquid is evaporated. Stir in the whole grains and cilantro or parsley and heat through. ■

Curried Quinoa

Yield: 6 to 8 servings

Calories:	194
Total Fat:	2 grams
Dietary Fiber:	5 grams

1 onion, chopped
3 cloves garlic, minced
2 teaspoons mild curry powder
1 tablespoon minced fresh ginger
Pinch cayenne pepper, or to taste
$2 1/2$ cups bouillon
1 cup quinoa, uncooked
$1/2$ cup golden raisins
$1/2$ cup dried apricots, cut into small pieces
2 cups frozen green peas

Cook the onion, garlic and curry powder in $1/2$ cup of the bouillon in a large saucepan over medium heat until softened, about 5 minutes. Stir in the remaining 2 cups of bouillon, the quinoa, raisins and apricots. Bring to a boil, reduce heat and simmer 15 to 20 minutes or until most of the liquid is absorbed and the quinoa is tender. Stir in the frozen peas and cook 2 to 3 minutes or until they are thawed and heated through. ■

Greek Pilaf

Yield: 8 to 10 servings

Calories:	112
Total Fat:	1 gram
Dietary Fiber:	8 grams

1 onion, chopped
$^1/_2$ cup bouillon
$^1/_2$ pound chopped mushrooms
2 cups cooked barley or other whole grains
    of your choice (see pages 68–69)
2 tablespoons tomato paste
2 teaspoons dried oregano
Pinch of cayenne pepper, or to taste
1 pound fresh spinach, rinsed, stems removed, and leaves chopped, or
    1 package frozen spinach, thawed
1 15-oz. can small white beans, drained
1 tablespoon fresh lemon juice

Optional vegetables
    8 pepperoncini peppers, stems and seeds removed,
        drained and chopped
    1 16-oz. can artichoke hearts, drained or 1 10-oz. package frozen
        artichokes, cooked, cut into bite-size pieces
    $^1/_4$ cup sliced black olives
    Freshly ground black pepper

Cook the onion in the bouillon in a large saucepan over medium heat until softened, about 5 minutes. Add the mushrooms, cover and cook until they are soft, about 5 minutes. Stir in the barley, tomato paste and seasonings and heat through. Add the spinach, cover and cook until the spinach is wilted, 3 to 5 minutes. Stir in the beans and lemon juice and any or all of the optional vegetables as desired. Cook 3 to 5 minutes more, and serve with freshly ground black pepper. ■

LOW-FAT, HIGH FIBER RECIPES

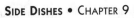

Bean-Pepper Salsa

Yield: about 2 cups	
Calories (per ¼ cup): 104	
Total Fat:	1 gram
Dietary Fiber:	5 grams

1 15-oz. can small red beans, drained and rinsed
1 15-oz. can shoepeg corn, drained
2 tablespoons hot red pepper relish, or to taste
1 bunch green onions, sliced

Mix all ingredients together in a serving bowl. Cover and refrigerate until chilled, about 30 minutes. Serve as a dip or relish. ■

Mushroom Pâté

Yield: about 2 cups.	
Calories (per ⅛ cup): 75	
Total Fat:	0 gram
Dietary Fiber:	4 grams

Serve pâté as a first course with celery sticks or your choice of veggie dippers.

6 cloves garlic
1 onion, chopped
2 stalks celery, chopped
1 pound mushrooms, cut in pieces
3 cups bouillon
1 cup red lentils
1 teaspoon dried thyme
1 teaspoon cayenne pepper, or to taste
$1/2$ cup quick-cooking rolled oats
1 envelope unflavored gelatin
$1/2$ cup cold water
1 tablespoon fresh lemon juice
Freshly ground black pepper to taste

Bring the garlic, onions, celery, mushrooms, bouillon, lentils, and thyme to a boil in a large pot. Reduce heat and simmer 20 to 30 minutes or until the lentils disintegrate. Stir in the oats and cook 5 minutes, stirring occasionally.

Meanwhile, sprinkle the gelatin on the cold water and set aside to soften, 5 to 10 minutes. Stir the softened gelatin and its soaking water, lemon juice and black pepper into lentil mixture and cook 2 to 3 minutes more. Place the mixture in a food processor and puree until smooth (or to the consistency you prefer). Pack into a mold or serving dish and chill until firm ■

LOW-FAT, HIGH FIBER RECIPES

Easy Salmon Mousse

Yield: 10 to 12 servings

Calories:	70
Total Fat:	2 grams
Dietary Fiber:	0 grams

2 envelopes unflavored gelatin
1 cup clam juice or bouillon
1 15-oz. can red salmon, undrained
1 tablespoon anchovy paste
2 tablespoons capers
1 bunch green onions, sliced
2 tablespoons fresh lemon juice
$1/_2$ teaspoon dried oregano
$1/_2$ teaspoon dried thyme
Pinch cayenne pepper, or to taste
1 cup fat-free sour cream or plain yogurt
Fresh herbs or lemon slices for garnish

Sprinkle the gelatin on the clam juice in a small saucepan and set aside to soften, 5 to 10 minutes. Heat the clam juice mixture, stirring, over low heat until gelatin dissolves. Combine with the remaining ingredients, except the sour cream or yogurt and garnish, in a food processor and blend until smooth. Stir in the yogurt or sour cream and pour into a nonstick pan or mold. Cover and refrigerate until firm, about 3 hours. Unmold and decorate as you wish. Serve as part of a buffet or as an appetizer. ■

• •

Falafel Bites

Yield: about 50

Calories (per 5 balls):	100
Total Fat:	2 grams
Dietary Fiber:	4 grams

Falafel mix is made from ground chick peas and seasonings. It's in most supermarkets in the grains section. Falafel patties are traditionally fried, but you can bake bite-size portions instead.

1 cup falafel mix
1 cup bouillon
Yogurt Dipping Sauce (see page 142)

Combine the falafel mix and the bouillon together in a bowl. Cover and refrigerate at least 60 minutes.

When ready to serve, preheat the oven or toaster oven to 400°F. Shape the mixture into about $1/_2$-inch balls. Place on a foil-covered pan or baking sheet and bake 10 to 15 minutes, or until lightly browned, dry and a little crispy on the outside. Serve with Yogurt Dipping Sauce. ■

Yogurt Dipping Sauce

This dip keeps, refrigerated, for several days, and also makes a good salad dressing.

Yield: about 1 cup.	
Calories (per ⅛ cup): **25**	
Total Fat:	0 grams
Dietary Fiber:	1 gram

> 1 cup plain fat-free yogurt
> 2 cloves garlic, minced
> ¼ cup fresh mint or cilantro leaves (optional)
> 1 cucumber, peeled, seeded and grated or finely chopped (optional)

Combine the yogurt, garlic and mint and/or cucumber, if desired. Let sit at least 30 minutes to let the flavors blend. ■

• •

Kasha-Bean "Meatballs"

You can serve these with any dipping sauce you like such as the Yogurt Dipping Sauce (see above) or use them in "spaghetti sauce and meatballs" type recipes.

Yield: about 50	
Calories (per 5 balls): **90**	
Total Fat:	1 gram
Dietary Fiber:	5 grams

> 2 cups bouillon
> 1 cup whole kasha
> 1 15-oz. can pink beans, drained and rinsed
> ½ cup cilantro or fresh flat-leaf parsley leaves
> 1 teaspoon minced ginger root
> 1 small jalapeño chili, cut into chunks
> ½ teaspoon mild curry powder
> ½ cup toasted wheat germ (optional)

Preheat the oven or toaster oven to 350°F.

Bring the bouillon to a boil in a small pot. Stir in the kasha, reduce heat and simmer, covered, until the kasha is just tender but not mushy, about 10 minutes. Drain off any excess liquid.

Meanwhile, combine the remaining ingredients, except wheat germ, in a food processor fitted with the metal blade and puree until smooth.

Transfer the bean mixture to a bowl. Combine the bean mixture and the cooked kasha. Shape into small (½-inch) balls. If you wish, roll each ball in the wheat germ to coat lightly.

Arrange the balls on a foil-covered baking sheet and bake 15 to 20 minutes or until lightly browned. Serve with toothpicks. ■

Favorite Artichoke Dip

Yield: about 3 cups.	
Calories (per 1/4 cup): 48	
Total Fat:	0 grams
Dietary Fiber:	5 grams

Serve with toasted pita wedges or sliced raw sweet potatoes.

> 1/2 pound fresh spinach, large stems removed, or 1 10-oz. package frozen spinach thawed
> 2 garlic cloves, minced
> 1 15-oz. can white beans, drained
> 1 bunch green onions, sliced
> Pinch of cayenne pepper or 1/2 teaspoon hot pepper sauce, or to taste
> 2 tablespoons fresh lemon juice
> 1 16-oz. can artichoke hearts, drained and finely chopped
> Red bell pepper rings for garnish (optional)

Wash the spinach and place it in a pot and cook over high heat until just wilted, about 2 minutes. Drain. Place the spinach and remaining ingredients, except the artichokes and garnish, in a blender or food processor and puree until smooth. Transfer the puree into a serving bowl and stir in the chopped artichoke hearts. ∎

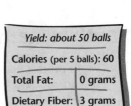

Lentil-Amaranth Canapés

Yield: about 50 balls	
Calories (per 5 balls): 60	
Total Fat:	0 grams
Dietary Fiber:	3 grams

> 2 cups bouillon
> 1/2 cup tiny green or orange lentils
> 2 cloves garlic, minced
> 2 cups cooked amaranth (see pages 70–72)
> 2 tablespoons fresh lemon juice or lime
> 1 tablespoon Dijon mustard
> 1 teaspoon mild chili powder
> Pinch of cayenne pepper, or to taste
> 1/4 cup chopped fresh flat-leaf parsley
> 1 red or yellow bell pepper, finely chopped
> Fat-free Italian salad dressing (optional)
> 2 medium zucchini, cut into 1/4-inch slices

Bring the bouillon to a boil in a medium saucepan over medium heat and stir in the lentils and garlic. Reduce heat and simmer 20 minutes or until the lentils are just tender, but not mushy. Drain the lentils and combine them with the remaining ingredients, except zucchini, in a serving bowl. Cover and refrigerate until served. If desired, moisten with a little dressing. Spoon the mixture onto zucchini slices. ∎

Caribbean Caviar

1 15-oz. can pigeon peas, drained
1 cup cooked, chilled millet, quinoa or
    amaranth (see pages 70–72)
1 Vidalia or other sweet onion, chopped
1 red or green bell pepper, chopped
2 pickled jalapeño chilies, or to taste, chopped
$1/4$ cup red wine vinegar
1 teaspoon mild chili powder
1 teaspoon mild curry powder

> Yield: about 3 cups.
>
> | Calories (per $1/4$ cup): 73 | |
> |---|---|
> | Total Fat: | 0 grams |
> | Dietary Fiber: | 4 grams |

Combine all ingredients in a serving bowl. Cover and refrigerate until chilled.
Serve as a dip or mix with salad greens for a great salad. ■

• •

Southwestern Bean Dip

$1/2$ 10-oz. bag frozen bell pepper-onion mix
$1/4$ cup bouillon
1 15-oz. can kidney beans, drained
Juice of 1 lime
2 tablespoons chopped fresh cilantro leaves
1 teaspoon mild chili powder
Pinch of cayenne pepper, or to taste
Sliced raw sweet potato or other veggie dippers of your choice

> Yield: about 2 cups.
>
> | Calories (per $1/4$ cup): 53 | |
> |---|---|
> | Total Fat: | 0 grams |
> | Dietary Fiber: | 3 grams |

Bring the onion-bell pepper mix and the bouillon to a boil in a large saucepan.
Reduce heat and simmer until soft, about 5 minutes. Combine with the
remaining ingredients, except dippers, in a blender or food processor and
puree until smooth. Serve with raw veggies. ■

Baked Peaches 🕐

4 large or 8 small ripe peaches, pitted and sliced
$^1/_4$ cup toasted wheat germ
2 tablespoons brown sugar
$^1/_4$ teaspoon Dessert Spice Blend (see page 99)
     or ground cinnamon

Yield: 4 servings	
Calories:	116
Total Fat:	1 gram
Dietary Fiber:	4 grams

Preheat the oven to 400°F

Arrange the sliced peaches in a baking dish. Mix the wheat germ, sugar and spice blend together in a small bowl and sprinkle over the peaches. Cover with foil or lid. Bake, 10 to 15 minutes or until peaches are hot. Serve warm or at room temperature.

Variation: This simple dessert works with just about any ripe fruit or combination of fruits: pears, apples, pineapple or mangoes. ■

• •

Mango-Melon Mist

1 ripe mango, peeled and cut in chunks
3 cups honeydew melon chunks
1 tablespoon fresh lime juice
$^1/_2$ cup water
1 cup cooked quinoa (see pages 70–72)
2 tablespoons brown sugar or equivalent sweetener, if needed

Yield: 4 to 6 servings	
Calories:	134
Total Fat:	1 gram
Dietary Fiber:	2 grams

Combine the mango, melon, lime juice and water in a blender and puree until smooth. Stir in the quinoa. Add the sugar or sweetener if necessary (mixture will taste less sweet when frozen).

Freeze the mixture in an ice cream freezer according to manufacturer's directions. Or pour into a shallow pan and freeze, stirring occasionally, until slushy. (If it freezes solid, cook 1 minute in a microwave oven to return it to sherbet texture.) ■

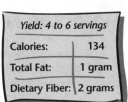

Mulled Pears

Yield: 6 to 8 servings

Calories:	184
Total Fat:	1 gram
Dietary Fiber:	6 grams

6 firm pears, cut into wedges and cored
$1/2$ cup golden raisins
1 cup red wine
1 cup water
1 teaspoon fennel seeds
$1/2$ teaspoon Dessert Spice Blend (see page 99)
$1/4$ teaspoon ground nutmeg
1 cup cooked barley or other whole grains of your choice (see pages 68–69)

Combine all ingredients except the grains in a saucepan, bring to a boil and simmer, covered, 20 minutes or until the pears are tender. Stir in the cooked grains. Serve warm or at room temperature. ■

Moroccan Fruit Pudding

Yield: 6 to 8 servings

Calories:	156
Total Fat:	0 grams
Dietary Fiber:	2 grams

4 cups soy milk or skim milk
1 teaspoon vanilla extract
$1/2$ teaspoon Dessert Spice Blend (see page 99)
$1/8$ teaspoon ground cloves
$1/4$ teaspoon salt
1 cup whole-wheat couscous
$1/4$ cup chopped dates
$1/4$ cup chopped dried apricots
$1/4$ cup dried cherries or cranberries

Heat the milk in a saucepan over medium-low heat just until hot. Stir in the vanilla, spices and salt. Stir in the couscous. Cook, stirring frequently, over low heat, 5 minutes. Add the dried fruits and cook, stirring frequently, 5 to 10 minutes or until the pudding is thick. Serve warm, at room temperature or chilled.

Variations: You can use any dried fruits of your choice or add 1–2 tablespoons of rum or your favorite liqueur; or use other spices such as mild curry powder. ■

Fruity Nuggets

Yield: 8 to 10 servings

Calories (per 5 balls): 147

| Total Fat: | 1 gram |
| Dietary Fiber: | 5 grams |

3 cups (1 pound) mixed dried fruit
Grated rind of 1 lemon
$^1/_2$ cup toasted wheat germ, plus more for rolling
$^1/_2$ teaspoon Dessert Spice Blend (see page 99)
2 tablespoons chocolate-orange liqueur (optional)

Place the fruit in the basket of an electric steamer. Fill the base with water to the lowest line. Steam the fruit 15 minutes or until soft. Process the fruit in a food processor until finely chopped. Stir in lemon rind, wheat germ, spice blend and liqueur, if using. Shape into small ($^1/_2$-inch) balls and roll in additional wheat germ.

Variations: Add festive colored sugar to the wheat germ used for rolling the balls. Use packaged mixed dried fruits or make your own combination of your favorites. ■

Clementine Sorbet

Yield: 4 servings

Calories:	74
Total Fat:	0 grams
Dietary Fiber:	3 grams

3 cups clementine, tangerine or orange segments
    (any seeds removed)
$^1/_2$ cup water
2 tablespoons Sabra liqueur
    (chocolate-orange liqueur)

Combine all ingredients in a blender or food processor and puree until smooth. Freeze in an ice cream maker according to manufacturer's instructions. Or pour into a small pan and freeze until just firm, break into chunks and whirl in a blender until softened. ■

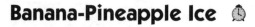

Banana-Pineapple Ice ⏰

Yield: 4 servings	
Calories:	139
Total Fat:	1 gram
Dietary Fiber:	4 grams

Whenever you have ripe (not black) bananas that you can't use up fast enough, peel them, wrap them in plastic wrap or put them in plastic freezer bags, and freeze. You can use them in fruit smoothies or this instant dessert!

> 4 frozen bananas
> 1 cup canned crushed pineapple with its juice

Process the bananas and pineapple in a blender until pureed. Pour into glasses and serve.

Variations: Needless to say, this has endless possibilities. Add some frozen strawberries or any other frozen fruit that appeals to you. Add a little liqueur—any flavor—or rum. Mix in some cooked grains before blending. ∎

Pineapple "Upside-Down Cake" Pudding

Yield: 6 servings	
Calories:	211
Total Fat:	2 grams
Dietary Fiber:	3 grams

> $^1/_2$ cup packed brown sugar
> $^1/_4$ cup water
> 1 16-oz. can pineapple chunks, drained and juice reserved
> 1 cup fat-free vanilla yogurt
> 3 cups cooked oat groats (see pages 70–72)

In a small saucepan, bring the brown sugar and water to a boil and cook over medium heat 5 minutes or until the sugar is golden brown but not burned. Slowly stir in $^1/_2$ cup of the pineapple and cook, stirring, until smooth.

Stir the yogurt into the oat groats and divide it into 6 glass dessert dishes.

Spoon pineapple mixture over oat mixture. Refrigerate until chilled, if desired. ∎

Banana "Rice" Pudding

Yield: 4 to 6 servings	
Calories:	202
Total Fat:	1 gram
Dietary Fiber:	5 grams

4 ripe bananas, sliced
2 cups cooked oat groats, brown rice or other
   whole grains of your choice (see pages 68–69)
$1/4$ cup dry sherry or rum
$1/4$ cup packed brown sugar
$1/2$ teaspoon Dessert Spice Blend (see page 99)

Combine all ingredients in a microwave-safe dish and microwave on HIGH
4 to 5 minutes or until the bananas are soft and the grain is heated through.
Mixture can also be cooked, stirring occasionally, in a saucepan over medium
heat until hot. Serve warm or at room temperature.

Variations: Add raisins, currants, chopped dried apricots or other fruits, or tiny
pieces of candied ginger, if desired. Substitute your favorite flavored liqueur for
the rum. Garnish with fresh fruits or sprinkle with a little Dessert Spice Blend
(see page 99). Leftovers are good for breakfast! ■

Two-Grain Tropical Treat

Yield: 6 to 8 servings	
Calories:	158
Total Fat:	1 gram
Dietary Fiber:	3 grams

1 16-oz. can crushed pineapple, drained and
   juice reserved
$1/2$ cup quick-cooking rolled oats
$1/4$ cup rum
$1/2$ teaspoon Dessert Spice Blend (see page 99)
$1/4$ teaspoon ground ginger
1 cup water
Pinch of salt
$1/2$ cup raisins
2 cups cooked oat groats, quinoa, or other whole grains of your choice
   (see pages 68–69)
2 kiwi fruit, peeled and sliced

Bring $1/2$ cup of the pineapple juice, the oats, rum, spice blend, ginger, water
and salt to a boil in a small saucepan. Reduce heat and simmer 5 minutes, stirring
frequently, until thick and smooth. Stir in the pineapple, raisins and cooked oat
groats and simmer, stirring occasionally, 5 to 10 minutes. Cool slightly or chill
before serving. Garnish with the kiwi slices and serve ■

Creamy Fruit Sorbet

Yield: 4 to 6 servings	
Calories:	68
Total Fat:	0 grams
Dietary Fiber:	2 grams

2 cups water
Pinch of salt
$^1/_2$ cup quick-cooking rolled oats
3 cups chopped peaches or other fresh or
    frozen fruit of your choice
2 slices candied ginger (optional), cut into small pieces
2 tablespoons sugar or 1 to 2 packets Equal or other sweetener (optional)
Extra fruit or mint leaves for garnish (optional)

Bring the water and salt to a boil in a small saucepan. Stir in the oatmeal, reduce heat and simmer until thickened, about 5 minutes. Put the fruit and candied ginger in the container of a blender or food processor. Pour in the oatmeal mixture and blend until smooth. Taste and add sweetener if desired (mixture will taste less sweet when frozen).

Freeze the mixture in an ice cream freezer according to manufacturer's directions, or pour into a shallow pan and freeze, stirring occasionally, until slushy. (If it freezes solid, cook 1 minute in a microwave oven to return it to sherbet texture.) Serve garnished with the reserved fruit or mint leaves, if desired. ■

• •

Spiced Fruit Compote

Yield: 6 servings	
Calories:	170
Total Fat:	1 gram
Dietary Fiber:	6 grams

$^1/_2$ cup dried apricots, cut into quarters
$^1/_2$ cup dried figs, cut into quarters
1 tart apple, cored and cut into bite-size pieces
1 pear, cored and cut into bite-size pieces
1 16-oz. can pineapple chunks, undrained
2 teaspoons Garam Masala Spice Blend (see page 98)
1 cup cooked barley oat groats, millet or other whole grains of your
    choice (see pages 68–69)

Cover the apricots and figs with boiling water in a medium bowl and soak about 10 minutes; then drain. Combine all of the fruits, including the juice from the canned pineapple, in a saucepan. Stir in the spice blend. Bring to a boil, reduce heat, cover and simmer, stirring occasionally, 15 to 20 minutes or until fruits are tender. Stir in the barley. Serve warm or chilled. ■

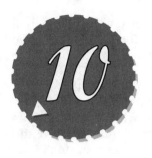

FOOD LISTS

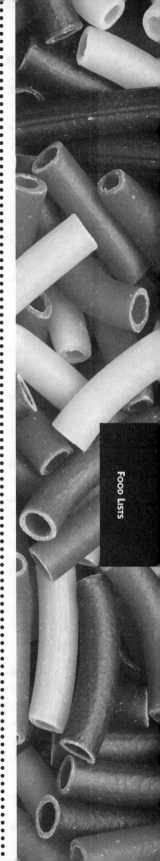

■ FOOD LIST NOTES

In assigning symbols to each food, we have relied on the information provided by the manufacturer on the package label. Products are often changed, so you may want to recheck the labels of the brands you use.

1. Foods marked ☺ are fruits, vegetables, whole grains, and beans. These are bulky foods (full of fiber and water) that fill you up without contributing a lot of calories. Eat a variety of these foods whenever you like. Generally, ☺ foods have fewer than two grams of fat and more than two grams of fiber per serving. Exceptions: oats and soybeans contain more of the "good" fats than other whole grains and beans, so products that include these ingredients may have three or more grams of fat per serving. As long as they do not contain added fats, they are ☺ foods.

2. Vegetables and fruits with a ☺ may have two or fewer grams of fiber per serving, but that is because they contain so much water that you need a huge serving size to reach a gram of fiber. All fruits and vegetables count as ☺ unless they are processed with added fats or a lot of added sugar. When you use canned fruits marked ☺, pour off the sugary juice, even if the can says "packed in natural juice" or some such term. Diabetics should always eat fruits in combination with whole grains or other foods.

3. The 👍 foods are spices, seasonings, artificial sweeteners, and other flavors that contribute fewer than 10 calories per serving. Use the ones you like whenever you wish; don't worry about the list of ingredients because the total number of calories is insignificant. However, you need to watch the serving size; a quick spritz from a can of oil spray counts as a 👍, but if you hold the button down, you'll quickly have 100 calories of fat or more.

4. A ✂ marks the foods that are low in fat but also low in fiber. They have two, one or zero grams of fat per serving and fewer than three grams of fiber. Exceptions: seafood with higher fat content is marked ✂ because the fat in fish is the "good" omega-3 fatty acids. We recommend two to three servings of seafood per week. Fish processed with added fats, such as tuna canned in oil or frozen seafood with fatty breading or sauces, are marked 💣.

5. All fat-free breads and other low-fat bakery products are marked ✂ even though they may contain whole grain flour and more than two grams of fiber, because grains ground into

flour lose their ability to suppress appetite. The whole grain versions are more nutritious, but still need to be treated with caution.

6. The 💣* foods are high in fat and usually low in fiber. Foods that contain any partially hydrogenated oils (trans fats) are marked 💣*, regardless of total fat content. All foods that contain three or more grams of fat per serving are marked 💣*. Exceptions are noted above (notes 1 & 3).

7. Breakfast cereals and other grain products receive a ☺ if the first ingredient is a whole grain or bran and there are no partially hydrogenated oils (trans fats). The ✄ applies to low-fiber cereals made from milled corn, white rice, or wheat flour. The 💣* marks cereals with added fats, which are virtually always partially hydrogenated oil (trans fats). See page 69 for more tips on picking good breakfast cereals. Watch out for trans fats in breakfast cereals; while this list was being edited, manufacturers added them to three more of our favorite brands!

8. The trans fats column will help you identify foods that contain partially hydrogenated oils, or trans fats (see pages 11–15). Food manufacturers are not required to identify trans fats on the nutrition label; you must look in the list of ingredients. Because there is no way to tell how much partially hydrogenated oil has been used in a product, we recommend that you simply avoid them whenever possible.

	Portion	Calories	Total Fat	Dietary Fiber	Trans Fat	Guide
■ BEVERAGES						
Alcoholic						
Beer, light	12 oz.	95	0	0		✂
Beer, regular	12 oz.	150	0	0		✂
California Blush, wine w/o alcohol	8 oz.	80	0	0		✂
Champagne	6 oz.	135	0	0		✂
Cordials & liqueurs	1 oz.	97	0	0		✂
Gin, 80 proof	1.5 oz.	95	0	0		✂
Gin, 86 proof	1.5 oz.	105	0	0		✂
Gin, 90 proof	1.5 oz.	110	0	0		✂
Rum, 80 proof	1.5 oz.	95	0	0		✂
Rum, 86 proof	1.5 oz.	105	0	0		✂
Rum, 90 proof	1.5 oz.	110	0	0		✂
Sherry, Medium	6 oz.	210	0	0		✂
Sparkling cider, 6.9% alcohol	6 oz.	87	0	0		✂
Vodka, 80 proof	1.5 oz.	95	0	0		✂
Vodka, 86 proof	1.5 oz.	105	0	0		✂
Vodka, 90 proof	1.5 oz.	110	0	0		✂
Whiskey, 80 proof	1.5 oz.	95	0	0		✂
Whiskey, 86 proof	1.5 oz.	105	0	0		✂
Whiskey, 90 proof	1.5 oz.	110	0	0		✂
Wine, dessert	3.5 oz.	140	0	0		✂
Wine, red	3.5 oz.	75	0	0		✂
Wine, white	3.5 oz.	80	0	0		✂
Apple						
Martinelli's, sparkling cider	8.4 oz.	150	0	0		✂
Mott's, 100%	8 oz.	110	0	0		✂
Snapple Farms	12 oz.	180	0	0		✂
White House	8 oz.	120	0	0		✂
Ziegler's, apple cider	8 oz.	120	0	0		✂
Coffee						
General Foods, Cappuccino Coolers, French vanilla	1 pkt.	60	0	0		✂
General Foods, French vanilla café	1 1/3 tbsp.	60	3	0	T	🌢
General Foods, Suisse mocha	1 1/3 tbsp.	60	2	0	T	🌢
General Foods, café Francais	1 1/3 tbsp.	60	4	0	T	🌢
General Foods, café Vienna	1 1/3 tbsp.	70	3	0	T	🌢
General Foods, hazelnut Belgian café	1 1/3 tbsp.	70	2	0	T	🌢
Maxwell House, Cafe Cappuccino, mocha	1 env.	100	3	0	T	🌢
Maxwell House, Cafe Cappuccino, mocha, decaffeinated	1 env.	100	3	0	T	🌢
Maxwell House, Cafe Cappuccino, vanilla	1 env.	90	1	0	T	🌢
Maxwell House, Cafe Cappuccino, vanilla, sugar free	1 env.	60	3	0	T	🌢
Regular, brewed	6 oz.	4	0	0		🌢
Regular, decaffeinated	6 oz.	4	0	0		🌢

☺ = *Eat as much as you want* • ✂ = *Cut Back*

	Portion	Calories	Total Fat	Dietary Fiber	Trans Fat	Guide
Regular, instant	6 oz.	4	0	0		👍
Starbucks, Frappuccino blended	12 oz.	230	3	0		🚫
Starbucks, Frappuccino, coffee	1 bottle	190	3	0		🚫
Starbucks, Frappuccino, mocha	1 bottle	190	3	0		🚫
Starbucks, Frappuccino, vanilla coffee	1 bottle	190	3	0		🚫
Starbucks, caffe Americano	12 oz.	10	0	0		👍
Starbucks, caffe latte made w/nonfat milk	12 oz.	120	1	0		✂
Starbucks, caffe latte made w/whole milk	12 oz.	210	11	0		🚫
Starbucks, caffe mocha w/nonfat mlk & crm	12 oz.	260	12	0		🚫
Starbucks, caffe mocha w/whole milk & crm	12 oz.	340	21	0		🚫
Starbucks, cappuccino made w/nonfat milk	12 oz.	80	0	0		✂
Starbucks, cappuccino made w/whole milk	12 oz.	140	7	0		🚫
Starbucks, drip	12 oz.	10	0	0		👍

Diet/Supplement/Sport

	Portion	Calories	Total Fat	Dietary Fiber	Trans Fat	Guide
All Sport Body Quencher, all flavors	8 oz.	70	0	0		✂
Boost, chocolate	1 can	240	4	0		🚫
Boost, strawberry	1 can	240	4	0		🚫
Boost, vanilla	1 can	240	4	0		🚫
Boost Plus, chocolate	1 can	360	14	1		🚫
Ensure, Light, French vanilla	1 can	200	3	0		🚫
Ensure, Light, strawberry swirl	1 can	200	3	0		🚫
Ensure, chocolate	1 can	250	6	0		🚫
Ensure, strawberry	1 can	250	6	0		🚫
Ensure, vanilla	1 can	250	6	0		🚫
Ensure, w/Fiber, chocolate	1 can	250	6	4		🚫
Ensure, w/Fiber, vanilla	1 can	250	6	4		🚫
Gatorade, all flavors	8 oz.	50	0	0		✂
Nestlé, Sweet Success, chocolate mocha supreme	1 can	200	3	3		🚫
Nestlé, Sweet Success, creamy vanilla delight	1 can	200	3	3		🚫
Nestlé, Sweet Success, dark chocolate fudge	1 can	200	3	3		🚫
Nestlé, Sweet Success, strawberries & cream	1 can	200	3	3		🚫
Powerade, mountain blast	8 oz.	70	0	0		✂
Slim-Fast, Jump Start Program, chocolate	1 pkt.	150	2	5		🚫
Slim-Fast, Jump Start Program, vanilla	1 pkt.	150	1	5		🚫
Slim-Fast, Ultra, French vanilla	1 can	220	3	5	T	🚫
Slim-Fast, Ultra, chocolate royale	1 can	220	3	5	T	🚫
Slim-Fast, Ultra, milk chocolate	1 can	220	3	5	T	🚫
Slim-Fast, Ultra, orange pineapple	1 can	220	2	5		🚫
Slim-Fast, Ultra, orange strawberry banana	1 can	220	2	5		🚫
Slim-Fast, Ultra, strawberry	1 can	220	3	5	T	🚫
Sustacal, vanilla	1 can	240	6	0	T	🚫
Sustacal Plus, chocolate	1 can	240	6	0	T	🚫
Sustacal Plus, vanilla	1 can	360	14	0		🚫

Frozen Concentrate

	Portion	Calories	Total Fat	Dietary Fiber	Trans Fat	Guide
Dole, tropical fruit	1/4 cup	160	0	0		✂
Five-Alive	2 oz.	110	0	0		✂

🚫 = Avoid • 👍 = Add for flavor

	Portion	Calories	Total Fat	Dietary Fiber	Trans Fat	Guide
Just Pik't, orange	2 oz.	120	0	0		✂
Minute Maid, apple	2 oz.	110	0	0		✂
Minute Maid, citrus punch	2 oz.	120	0	0		✂
Minute Maid, fruit punch	2 oz.	120	0	0		✂
Minute Maid, lemonade	2 oz.	110	0	0		✂
Minute Maid, orange, original	2 oz.	110	0	0		✂
Seneca, Granny Smith apple	2 oz.	110	0	0		✂
Tropicana Twister, orange peach	$1/4$ cup	120	0	0		✂
Welch's, 100% Grape	2 oz.	160	0	0		✂
Welch's, apple grape raspberry	2 oz.	140	0	0		✂
Welch's, cranberry	2 oz.	140	0	0		✂
Welch's, cranberry raspberry	2 oz.	150	0	0		✂
Welch's, cranberry raspberry, lite	2 oz.	50	0	0		✂
Welch's, orange pineapple apple	2 oz.	140	0	0		✂
Welch's, passionfruit	2 oz.	140	0	0		✂
Welch's, strawberry breeze	2 oz.	130	0	0		✂
Welch's, white grape	2 oz.	140	0	0		✂
Welch's, white grape peach	2 oz.	150	0	0		✂

Lemonade

	Portion	Calories	Total Fat	Dietary Fiber	Trans Fat	Guide
Arizona, pink	8 oz.	110	0	0		✂
Minute Maid, pink	8 oz.	110	0	0		✂
Newman's Own, old fashioned	1 cup	110	0	0		✂
Snapple	8 oz.	100	0	0		✂

Mixes

	Portion	Calories	Total Fat	Dietary Fiber	Trans Fat	Guide
Carnation, malted milk	3 tbsp.	90	2	0		✂
Country Time, Lem'n Berry Sippers, strawberry lemonade	8 oz.	90	0	0		✂
Country Time, Lem'n Berry Sippers, wild berry lemonade	$1/8$ cap	90	0	0		✂
Crystal Light, raspberry ice	8 oz.	5	0	0		👍
Lipton Iced Tea, decaffeinated lemon, sugar sweet	$1 2/3$ tbsp.	90	0	0		✂
Nestle Quik, chocolate	2 tbsp.	90	1	1		✂
Nestle Quik, strawberry	2 tbsp.	90	0	0		✂
Ovaltine	1 env.	110	2	0		✂
Ovaltine, chocolate malt	4 tbsp.	80	0	0		✂
Swiss Miss, French vanilla	1 env.	120	3	0	T	●
Swiss Miss, chocolate sensation	1 env.	150	4	1	T	●
Swiss Miss, fat free	1 env.	50	0	1		✂
Swiss Miss, lite	1 env.	80	1	2	T	●
Swiss Miss, milk chocolate	1 env.	120	3	1	T	●
Swiss Miss, milk chocolate w/marshmallows	1 env.	120	3	1	T	●
Swiss Miss, rich chocolate	1 env.	110	2	1	T	●
Tang	2 tbsp.	90	0	0		✂
Weight Watchers, Smart Options, hot cocoa	1 env.	70	0	1		✂
Weight Watchers, shake, chocolate fudge, low fat	1 pkg.	80	1	2		✂

☺ = Eat as much as you want • ✂ = Cut Back

	Portion	Calories	Total Fat	Dietary Fiber	Trans Fat	Guide
Nectar						
Goya, de guanabana	12 oz.	230	0	1		✂
Goya, de tamarindo	12 oz.	240	0	1		✂
Goya, guava	12 oz.	240	0	2		✂
Goya, pear	12 oz.	240	0	2		✂
Goya, mango	12 oz.	230	0	2		✂
Libby's, apricot	8 oz.	140	0	0		✂
Libby's, pear	8 oz.	150	0	0		✂
Orange						
Donald Duck, pure	8 oz.	120	0	0		✂
Five-Alive, citrus	8 oz.	120	0	0		✂
Minute Maid, premium country style	8 oz.	110	0	0		✂
Minute Maid, premium original	8 oz.	110	0	0		✂
Minute Maid, premium original calcium	8 oz.	120	0	0		✂
Snapple Farms, orange grove	12 oz.	170	0	0		✂
Sunkist, pulp free	8 oz.	110	0	0		✂
Sunny Delight, citrus	8 oz.	130	0	0		✂
Tropicana, pure premium calcium	8 oz.	110	0	0		✂
Tropicana, pure premium original	8 oz.	110	0	0		✂
Tropicana, pure premium tangerine orange	8 oz.	110	0	0		✂
Other						
Arizona, pina colada	8 oz.	140	1	0		✂
Chiquita, kiwi strawberry	8 oz.	120	0	0		✂
Crystal Bay, cherry	8 oz.	90	0	0		✂
Crystal Bay, strawberry	8 oz.	90	0	0		✂
Dole, country raspberry	8 oz.	140	0	0		✂
Dole, cranberry apple	8 oz.	120	0	0		✂
Dole, orange-peach-mango	8 oz.	120	0	0		✂
Dole, pine-orange banana	8 oz.	120	0	0		✂
Dole, pineapple orange	8 oz.	120	0	0		✂
Dole, tropical fruit	8 oz.	160	0	0		✂
Edge 2 O, caffeinated	8 oz.	0	0	0		👍
Fruitopia, fruit integration	8 oz.	110	0	0		✂
Fruitopia, strawberry passion awareness	8 oz.	110	0	0		✂
Fruitopia, the great grape beyond	8 oz.	120	0	0		✂
Fruitopia, tremendously tangerine	8 oz.	110	0	0		✂
Goya, coconut milk	1 tbsp.	50	5	0		💧
Hi-C, blue cooler	8 oz.	120	0	0		✂
Hi-C, boppin' berry	8 oz.	120	0	0		✂
Hi-C, ecto-cooler	8 oz.	120	0	0		✂
Kame, coconut milk lite	1/4 cup	35	3	0		💧
Mistic, black cherry	8 oz.	100	0	0		✂
Mistic, kiwi strawberry	8 oz.	120	0	0		✂
Mondo	8 oz.	110	0	0		✂
Nantucket Nectars, orange mango	8 oz.	130	0	0		✂

💧 = *Avoid* • 👍 = *Add for flavor*

	Portion	Calories	Total Fat	Dietary Fiber	Trans Fat	Guide
Nantucket Nectars, pineapple orange guava	8 oz.	120	0	0		✄
Ocean Spray, cranapple	8 oz.	160	0	0		✄
Ocean Spray, cranraspberry	8 oz.	140	0	0		✄
Ocean Spray, cranstrawberry	8 oz.	140	0	0		✄
Ocean Spray, island guava	8 oz.	130	0	0		✄
Ocean Spray, mango mango	8 oz.	130	0	0		✄
Ocean Spray, paradise passion	8 oz.	130	0	0		✄
Ocean Spray, ruby red & mango	8 oz.	130	0	0		✄
Snapple, apple cherry	8 oz.	120	0	0		✄
Snapple, kiwi strawberry cocktail	8 oz.	110	0	0		✄
Snapple, mango madness	8 oz.	110	0	0		✄
Snapple, strawberry	8 oz.	120	0	0		✄
Snapple Farms, cranberry apple	12 oz.	200	0	0		✄
Snapple Farms, dixie peach	12 oz.	170	0	0		✄
Tropicana Twister, apple berry pear	8 oz.	140	0	0		✄
Tropicana Twister, apple raspberry blackberry	8 oz.	130	0	0		✄
Tropicana Twister, orange cranberry	8 oz.	130	0	0		✄
Tropicana Twister, orange peach	8 oz.	120	0	0		✄
Tropicana Twister, orange strawberry banana	8 oz.	130	0	0		✄
Tropicana Twister, pink grapefruit cocktail	8 oz.	120	0	0		✄
Tropicana Twister, strawberry orange peach	8 oz.	130	0	0		✄

Punch

	Portion	Calories	Total Fat	Dietary Fiber	Trans Fat	Guide
Hawaiian Punch, fruit juicy red	8 oz.	120	0	0		✄
Mistic, fruit	8 oz.	120	0	0		✄
Snapple, fruit	8 oz.	110	0	0		✄
Tropicana, fruit	8 oz.	130	0	0		✄

Soda

	Portion	Calories	Total Fat	Dietary Fiber	Trans Fat	Guide
7-Up	8 oz.	110	0	0		✄
7-Up, Cherry	8 oz.	100	0	0		✄
7-Up, Diet	8 oz.	0	0	0		👍
7-Up, Diet Cherry	8 oz.	0	0	0		👍
A & W Root beer	8 oz.	110	0	0		✄
Barq's, Old Tyme root beer	8 oz.	110	0	0		✄
Canada Dry, cherry ginger ale	8 oz.	100	0	0		✄
Canada Dry, club	8 oz.	0	0	0		👍
Canada Dry, cranberry ginger ale	8 oz.	0	0	0		👍
Canada Dry, diet ginger ale	8 oz.	0	0	0		👍
Canada Dry, ginger ale	8 oz.	80	0	0		✄
Canada Dry, lemon ginger ale	8 oz.	90	0	0		✄
Citra	8 oz.	90	0	0		✄
Coca-Cola, Caffeine Free	8 oz.	100	0	0		✄
Coca-Cola, Classic	8 oz.	100	0	0		✄
Coke, Caffeine Free Diet	8 oz.	0	0	0		👍
Coke, Cherry	8 oz.	100	0	0		✄
Coke, Diet	8 oz.	0	0	0		👍
Diet Rite Cola	8 oz.	0	0	0		👍
Dr. Pepper	8 oz.	100	0	0		✄

☺ = Eat as much as you want • ✄ = Cut Back

	Portion	Calories	Total Fat	Dietary Fiber	Trans Fat	Guide
Dr. Pepper, Diet	8 oz.	0	0	0		👍
Fresca	8 oz.	0	0	0		👍
IBC, diet root beer	12 oz.	0	0	0		👍
IBC, root beer	12 oz.	180	0	0		✂
Minute Maid, orange	8 oz.	120	0	0		✂
Mountain Dew	8 oz.	110	0	0		✂
Mountain Dew, diet	8 oz.	0	0	0		👍
Old Tyme, cream soda	8 oz.	110	0	0		✂
Old Tyme, root beer	8 oz.	110	0	0		✂
Orange Crush	8 oz.	120	0	0		✂
Orangina	1 bottle	120	1	0		✂
Orangina, light	1 bottle	20	0	0		✂
Pepsi	8 oz.	100	0	0		✂
Pepsi, Caffeine Free	8 oz.	100	0	0		✂
Pepsi, Diet	8 oz.	0	0	0		👍
Pepsi, Wild Cherry	8 oz.	110	0	0		✂
RC Cola	8 oz.	100	0	0		✂
Schweppes, club	8 oz.	0	0	0		👍
Schweppes, diet tonic water	8 oz.	0	0	0		👍
Seagram's, ginger ale	8 oz.	100	0	0		✂
Slice, fruit punch	8 oz.	120	0	0		✂
Slice, lemon lime	8 oz.	100	0	0		✂
Slice, mandarin orange	8 oz.	130	0	0		✂
Sprite	8 oz.	100	0	0		✂
Sprite, Diet	8 oz.	0	0	0		👍
Squirt	8 oz.	100	0	0		✂
Squirt, Diet	8 oz.	0	0	0		👍
Sunkist, orange	8 oz.	130	0	0		✂
Surge	8 oz.	120	0	0		✂
Tab	8 oz.	0	0	0		👍

Soy/Tofu

	Portion	Calories	Total Fat	Dietary Fiber	Trans Fat	Guide
Pro Soya, So Nice, chocolate	1 cup	110	4	0		✂
Pro Soya, So Nice, soy	1 cup	70	3	0		✂
Pro Soya, So Nice, vanilla	1 cup	90	3	0		✂
Rice Dream, organic brown rice	8 oz.	120	2	0		✂
Silk, dairyless soy	1 cup	80	3	0		✂
Vitasoy, creamy original	8 oz.	160	7	1		🛢
Vitasoy, rich cocoa	8.45 oz.	220	6	1		🛢

Tea & Iced Tea

	Portion	Calories	Total Fat	Dietary Fiber	Trans Fat	Guide
Arizona, ginseng	8 oz.	60	0	0		✂
Arizona, green w/ginseng & honey	8 oz.	70	0	0		✂
Arizona, herbal w/honey	8 oz.	70	0	0		✂
Bigelow, all flavors	8 oz.	0	0	0		👍
Celestial Seasonings, all flavors	8 oz.	0	0	0		👍
Crystal Light Teas, iced tea	8 oz.	5	0	0		👍
Lipton, brisk lemon	8 oz.	80	0	0		✂
Lipton, sugar sweetened	8 oz.	80	0	0		✂

🛢 = Avoid • 👍 = Add for flavor

	Portion	Calories	Total Fat	Dietary Fiber	Trans Fat	Guide
Lipton, unsweetened, no lemon	8 oz.	0	0	0		👍
Nestea	8 oz.	90	0	0		✂
Nestea, cool	8 oz.	80	0	0		✂
Snapple	8 oz.	100	0	0		✂
Snapple, Diet	8 oz.	0	0	0		👍
Snapple, ginseng	8 oz.	80	0	0		✂
Twinings, all flavors	8 oz.	0	0	0		👍

Vegetable

	Portion	Calories	Total Fat	Dietary Fiber	Trans Fat	Guide
Beefamato, tomato cocktail	8 oz.	80	0	1		✂
Campbell's, Healthy Request	8 oz.	50	0	1		✂
Campbell's, tomato	8 oz.	50	0	1		✂
Carrot juice	12 oz.	120	1	1		✂
Clamato, tomato cocktail	8 oz.	60	0	1		✂
Looza, tomato cocktail	8 oz.	35	0	0		✂
V-8, Healthy Request	8 oz.	50	0	1		✂
V-8, Splash, berry blend	8 oz.	110	0	0		✂
V-8, Splash, strawberry kiwi	8 oz.	110	0	0		✂
V-8, Splash, tropical blend	8 oz.	120	0	0		✂
V-8, low sodium	8 oz.	50	0	2		✂
V-8, picante mild flavor	8 oz.	50	0	1		✂
V-8, spicy hot	8 oz.	50	0	1		✂
V-8, vegetable	8 oz.	50	0	1		✂

■ BREAKFAST FOODS & CEREALS

Breakfast Foods, Cereal Bar

	Portion	Calories	Total Fat	Dietary Fiber	Trans Fat	Guide
Entenmann's, Multi-Grain, real chocolate chip, chewy	1 bar	140	3	1	T	🌢
Entenmann's, Multi-Grain, real strawberry	1 bar	140	3	0	T	🌢
Hostess, Fruit and Grain, apple	1 bar	120	2	1	T	🌢
Hostess, Fruit and Grain, raspberry	1 bar	120	2	1	T	🌢
Kellogg's, Nutri-Grain, blueberry	1 bar	140	3	1		🌢
Kellogg's, Nutri-Grain, raspberry	1 bar	140	3	1		🌢
Kellogg's, Nutri-Grain, strawberry	1 bar	140	3	1		🌢
Quaker, Fruit n' Oatmeal, apple cinnamon	1 bar	140	3	1	T	🌢
Quaker, Fruit n' Oatmeal, blueberry	1 bar	140	3	1	T	🌢
Quaker, Fruit n' Oatmeal, strawberry	1 bar	140	3	1	T	🌢
SnackWell's, Fruit n' Grain, blueberry	1 bar	120	0	1		✂
SnackWell's, Fruit n' Grain, cherry	1 bar	130	3	0	T	🌢
SnackWell's, Fruit n' Grain, mixed berry	1 bar	130	3	0	T	🌢
SnackWell's, Fruit n' Grain, raspberry	1 bar	120	0	1		✂
SnackWell's, apple cinnamon, fat free	1 bar	120	0	1		✂

Breakfast Foods, Donut

	Portion	Calories	Total Fat	Dietary Fiber	Trans Fat	Guide
Entenmann's, Light, fantastic fudge	1 donut	210	9	1	T	🌢
Entenmann's, Rich frosted popems	4 pieces	280	20	1	T	🌢
Entenmann's, cinnamon	1 donut	310	19	0	T	🌢

☺ = Eat as much as you want • ✂ = Cut Back

FOOD LISTS

	Portion	Calories	Total Fat	Dietary Fiber	Trans Fat	Guide
Entenmann's, crumb topped	1 donut	420	22	1	T	🩸
Entenmann's, frostee powdered popettes	4 popettes	270	16	0	T	🩸
Entenmann's, glazed popems	4 pieces	210	10	0	T	🩸
Entenmann's, rich frosted donut	1 donut	400	27	1	T	🩸
Hostess, Frosted donettes	3 donettes	230	14	0	T	🩸
Hostess, cinnamon donettes	4 donettes	250	11	1	T	🩸
Hostess, donut bites & glazed donut holes	4 holes	250	15	0	T	🩸
Hostess, frosted	1 donut	330	17	1	T	🩸
Hostess, glazed & raised	1 donut	150	8	0	T	🩸
Hostess, plain	1 donut	150	8	0	T	🩸
Hostess, powdered	1 donut	230	11	0	T	🩸
Hostess, powdered donettes	4 donettes	250	11	1	T	🩸
Krispy Kreme, cinnamon	1 donut	210	11	0	T	🩸
Krispy Kreme, fudge iced glazed	1 donut	210	9	2	T	🩸
Krispy Kreme, original	1 donut	200	11	2	T	🩸
Krispy Kreme, plain	1 donut	200	11	0	T	🩸
Krispy Kreme, powdered sugar	1 donut	220	11	0	T	🩸
Tastykake, rich frosted mini donuts	4 donuts	240	14	2	T	🩸

Breakfast Foods, Donut, Dunkin' Donuts

	Portion	Calories	Total Fat	Dietary Fiber	Trans Fat	Guide
Bagel, plain	1 serv.	200	1	0	n.a.	✂
Cake donut, chocolate	1 serv.	210	14	1	n.a.	🩸
Cake donut, chocolate glazed	1 serv.	250	14	1	n.a.	🩸
Cake donut, cinnamon	1 serv.	300	19	1	n.a.	🩸
Cake donut, powdered	1 serv.	310	19	1	n.a.	🩸
Cake donut, whole wheat glazed	1 serv.	230	11	2	n.a.	🩸
Croissant, almond	1 serv.	360	21	2	n.a.	🩸
Croissant, chocolate	1 serv.	370	23	1	n.a.	🩸
Croissant, plain	1 serv.	270	17	0	n.a.	🩸
Cruller, glazed	1 serv.	340	14	2	n.a.	🩸
Muffin, banana nut	1 serv.	340	12	2	n.a.	🩸
Muffin, blueberry	1 serv.	310	10	2	n.a.	🩸
Muffin, chocolate chip	1 serv.	400	16	2	n.a.	🩸
Muffin, lowfat, banana	1 serv.	240	2	1	n.a.	✂
Muffin, lowfat, blueberry	1 serv.	230	2	1	n.a.	✂
Muffin, lowfat, bran	1 serv.	260	2	4	n.a.	✂
Yeast donut, Bavarian kreme	1 serv.	250	11	1	n.a.	🩸
Yeast donut, Boston kreme	1 serv.	270	11	1	n.a.	🩸
Yeast donut, apple n' spice	1 serv.	230	10	1	n.a.	🩸
Yeast donut, chocolate kreme	1 serv.	320	16	1	n.a.	🩸
Yeast donut, glazed	1 serv.	160	7	1	n.a.	🩸
Yeast donut, jelly filled	1 serv.	240	10	1	n.a.	🩸

Breakfast Foods, Drinks

	Portion	Calories	Total Fat	Dietary Fiber	Trans Fat	Guide
Carnation, Instant Breakfast, French vanilla	1 env.	70	1	1		✂
Carnation, Instant Breakfast, classic chocolate malt	1 env.	70	1	1		✂
Carnation, Instant Breakfast, creamy milk chocolate	1 env.	70	1	1		✂
Carnation, Instant Breakfast, strawberry cream	1 env.	70	1	1		✂

🩸 = *Avoid* • 💧 = *Add for flavor*

FOOD LISTS • CHAPTER 10   161

	Portion	Calories	Total Fat	Dietary Fiber	Trans Fat	Guide
Carnation, InstantBreakfast, cafe mocha	1 env.	70	1	1		✄

Breakfast Foods, French Toast, Frozen

	Portion	Calories	Total Fat	Dietary Fiber	Trans Fat	Guide
Aunt Jemima, cinnamon	2 slices	240	7	2	T	🌢
Aunt Jemima, homestyle plain	2 slices	240	7	2	T	🌢

Breakfast Foods, Frozen Entree

	Portion	Calories	Total Fat	Dietary Fiber	Trans Fat	Guide
Morningstar Farms, breakfast links	2 links	60	3	2		🌢
Morningstar Farms, breakfast patties	1 pattie	70	3	2		🌢
Morningstar Farms, breakfast strips	2 strips	60	5	0		🌢
Swanson, Great Starts, French toast w/sge	1 pkg.	410	26	3	T	🌢
Swanson, Great Starts, breakfast burrito, bacon	1 pkg.	250	11	1	T	🌢
Swanson, Great Starts, breakfast burrito, sausage	1 pkg.	240	12	1	T	🌢
Swanson, Great Starts, budget, 6 slvr dlr pncke w/sge	1 pkg.	340	18	1	T	🌢
Swanson, Great Starts, budget, scrmbld egg & pncke	1 pkg.	250	14	1	T	🌢
Swanson, Great Starts, cinn swrl French tst w/sge	1 pkg.	440	28	2	T	🌢
Swanson, Great Starts, egg, can bacon & cheese mffn	1 pkg.	290	15	2	T	🌢
Swanson, Great Starts, french toast strips w/syrup	1 pkg.	320	10	2	T	🌢
Swanson, Great Starts, pancakes w/bacon	1 pkg.	400	20	1		🌢
Swanson, Great Starts, pancakes w/sausage	1 pkg.	490	25	3	T	🌢
Swanson, Great Starts, sausage, egg & cheese bsct	1 pkg.	460	28	3	T	🌢
Swanson, Great Starts, scrambled eggs & bacon w/home fries	1 serv.	290	19	1	T	🌢

Breakfast Foods, Pancake, Frozen

	Portion	Calories	Total Fat	Dietary Fiber	Trans Fat	Guide
Hungry Jack, Microwave, blueberry	3 pancakes	240	4	1	T	🌢
Hungry Jack, Microwave, buttermilk	3 pancakes	270	5	1	T	🌢
Hungry Jack, Microwave, original	3 pancakes	270	5	1	T	🌢
Kellogg's, Eggo, buttermilk	3 pancakes	270	8	1	T	🌢

Breakfast Foods, Pancake, Mix

	Portion	Calories	Total Fat	Dietary Fiber	Trans Fat	Guide
Arrowhead Mills, multi-grain	1/4 cup	120	1	3		☺
Aunt Jemima, buttermilk, complete	1/3 cup	160	2	1	T	🌢
Aunt Jemima, buttermilk, reduced calorie	1/3 cup	140	2	5	T	🌢
Aunt Jemima, original	1/3 cup	160	1	1		✄
Bisquick, Shake and Pour	1/2 cup	200	4	0	T	🌢
Bisquick, buttermilk	1/2 cup	200	3	1	T	🌢
Hungry Jack, buttermilk complete	1/3 cup	160	2	0	T	🌢
Hungry Jack, extra light & fluffy	1/3 cup	160	2	0	T	🌢
Hungry Jack, original	1/3 cup	150	2	0	T	🌢
Mrs. Butterworth's, country breakfast	1/3 cup	160	2	0	T	🌢

☺ = Eat as much as you want • ✄ = Cut Back

	Portion	Calories	Total Fat	Dietary Fiber	Trans Fat	Guide

Breakfast Foods, Pastry

	Portion	Calories	Total Fat	Dietary Fiber	Trans Fat	Guide
Entenmann's, apple strudel	1/4 strudel	310	14	2	T	🖤
Entenmann's, cheese danish twist	1/8 danish	230	12	0	T	🖤
Entenmann's, cheese topped bun	1 bun	300	15	1	T	🖤
Entenmann's, cherry cheese danish	1/8 danish	190	9	0	T	🖤
Entenmann's, cinnamon filbert ring	1/5 danish	260	16	1	T	🖤
Entenmann's, cinnamon swirl bun	1 bun	300	13	1	T	🖤
Entenmann's, light, cherry cheese pastry	1/9 danish	130	0	1		✂
Entenmann's, light, cinnamon apple twist	1/8 danish	140	0	1		✂
Entenmann's, light, lemon twist	1/8 danish	130	0	1		✂
Entenmann's, light, raspberry twist	1/8 danish	140	0	1		✂
Entenmann's, pecan danish ring	1/6 danish	250	15	1	T	🖤
Entenmann's, pineapple cheese strudel	1/4 strudel	370	20	0	T	🖤
Entenmann's, raspberry danish twist	1/8 danish	220	11	0	T	🖤
Entenmann's, walnut danish ring	1/6 danish	240	15	1	T	🖤
Hostess, iced honey bun	1 bun	420	25	1	T	🖤
Kellogg's Pop-Tarts, frosted blueberry	1 pastry	200	5	1	T	🖤
Kellogg's Pop-Tarts, frosted cherry	1 pastry	200	5	1	T	🖤
Kellogg's Pop-Tarts, low fat, apple cinnamon	1 pastry	190	3	1	T	🖤
Kellogg's Pop-Tarts, low fat, frosted chocolate fudge	1 pastry	190	3	2	T	🖤
Kellogg's Pop-Tarts, low fat, blueberry	1 pastry	190	3	1	T	🖤
Kellogg's Pop-Tarts, low fat, frosted brown sugar cinnamon	1 pastry	210	7	1	T	🖤
Kellogg's Pop-Tarts, s'mores	1 pastry	200	6	1	T	🖤
Kellogg's Pop-Tarts, strawberry	1 pastry	200	5	1	T	🖤
Kellogg's Pop-Tarts, wild berry	1 pastry	210	5	1	T	🖤
Kellogg's Pop-Tarts, wild watermelon	1 pastry	210	5	1	T	🖤
Krispy Kreme, honey bun	1 bun	410	24	1	T	🖤

Breakfast Foods, Pastry, Frozen

	Portion	Calories	Total Fat	Dietary Fiber	Trans Fat	Guide
Pepperidge Farm, turnover, apple	1 turnover	290	15	2	T	🖤
Pillsbury Toaster Strudel, apple	1 pastry	200	9	0	T	🖤
Pillsbury Toaster Strudel, cherry	1 pastry	190	8	0	T	🖤
Pillsbury Toaster Strudel, cream cheese & blueberry	1 pastry	200	10	0	T	🖤
Pillsbury Toaster Strudel, cream cheese & strawberry	1 pastry	200	10	0	T	🖤
Pillsbury Toaster Strudel, raspberry	1 pastry	190	8	0	T	🖤
Pillsbury Toaster Strudel, strawberry	1 pastry	200	9	0	T	🖤
Pillsbury Toaster Strudel, wildberry	1 pastry	190	8	0	T	🖤

Breakfast Foods, Syrup

	Portion	Calories	Total Fat	Dietary Fiber	Trans Fat	Guide
Aunt Jemima, butter lite	1/4 cup	100	0	0		✂
Aunt Jemima, butter rich	1/4 cup	210	0	0		✂
Aunt Jemima, lite	1/4 cup	100	0	0		✂
Aunt Jemima, original rich maple	1/4 cup	210	0	0		✂
Cozy Cottage, sugar free, low calorie	1/4 cup	35	0	0		✂
Hungry Jack, butter maple	1/4 cup	210	0	0		✂

🖤 = Avoid • 💧 = Add for flavor

	Portion	Calories	Total Fat	Dietary Fiber	Trans Fat	Guide
Hungry Jack, lite, microwave ready	1/4 cup	100	0	0		✂
King	2 tbsp.	125	0	0		✂
Log Cabin	1/4 cup	200	0	0		✂
Log Cabin Lite, reduced calorie	1/4 cup	100	0	0		✂
Maple Grove Farms, pure maple	1/4 cup	200	0	0		✂
Mrs. Butterworth's, lite	1/4 cup	100	0	0		✂
Mrs. Butterworth's, original	1/4 cup	230	0	0		✂
Smucker's, natural blueberry	1/4 cup	210	0	0		✂

Breakfast Foods, Waffle, Frozen

	Portion	Calories	Total Fat	Dietary Fiber	Trans Fat	Guide
Aunt Jemima, blueberry	2 waffles	190	6	1	T	🌢
Aunt Jemima, buttermilk	2 waffles	200	6	1	T	🌢
Aunt Jemima, homestyle	2 waffles	200	6	1	T	🌢
Hungry Jack, blueberry	2 waffles	210	7	0	T	🌢
Hungry Jack, buttermilk	2 waffles	190	6	0	T	🌢
Hungry Jack, homestyle	2 waffles	180	6	0	T	🌢
Hungry Jack, mini, cinnamon toast	3 (st of 4) wffls	270	8	0	T	🌢
Hungry Jack, mini, funfetti	3 (st of 4) wffls	260	8	1	T	🌢
Kellogg's, Eggo, Nutri-Grain, made w/whole wheat	2 waffles	190	6	4	T	🌢
Kellogg's, Eggo, Nutri-Grain, multi-grain	2 waffles	180	6	6	T	🌢
Kellogg's, Eggo, Special K, fat free	2 waffles	120	0	1		✂
Kellogg's, Eggo, apple cinnamon	2 waffles	220	8	1	T	🌢
Kellogg's, Eggo, banana bread	2 waffles	200	7	2	T	🌢
Kellogg's, Eggo, blueberry	2 waffles	220	9	1	T	🌢
Kellogg's, Eggo, buttermilk	2 waffles	220	8	1	T	🌢
Kellogg's, Eggo, cinnamon toast	3 (st of 4) wffls	290	10	2	T	🌢
Kellogg's, Eggo, golden oat, made w/oat bran	2 waffles	150	3	3	T	🌢
Kellogg's, Eggo, homestyle	2 waffles	220	8	1	T	🌢
Kellogg's, Eggo, homestyle minis	3 (st of 4) wffls	260	9	2	T	🌢
Kellogg's, Eggo, homestyle, low fat	2 waffles	180	3	1	T	🌢
Kellogg's, Eggo, strawberry	2 waffles	220	8	1	T	🌢

Cereals, Cold

	Portion	Calories	Total Fat	Dietary Fiber	Trans Fat	Guide
Barbara's, Puffins, crunchy corn	3/4 cup	90	1	5		☺
Barbara's, Shredded Wheat	2 biscuits	140	1	5		☺
Barbara's, multi-grain shredded spoonfuls, low fat	3/4 cup	120	2	4		☺
Familia, Muesli	1/2 cup	210	3	5		☺
General Mills, Basic 4	1 cup	200	3	3	T	🌢
General Mills, Cheerios	1 cup	110	2	3		☺
General Mills, Cheerios, apple cinnamon	3/4 cup	120	2	1	T	🌢
General Mills, Cheerios, frosted	1 cup	120	1	1		✂
General Mills, Cheerios, honey nut	1 cup	120	2	2		✂
General Mills, Cheerios, multi-grain plus	1 cup	110	1	3	T	🌢
General Mills, Cheerios, team	1 cup	120	1	1		✂
General Mills, Chex, corn	1 cup	110	0	0		✂
General Mills, Chex, multi-bran	1 cup	200	2	7		☺
General Mills, Chex, rice	1 1/4 cups	120	0	0		✂

☺ = Eat as much as you want   •   ✂ = Cut Back

	Portion	Calories	Total Fat	Dietary Fiber	Trans Fat	Guide
General Mills, Chex, wheat	1 cup	180	1	5		☺
General Mills, Cinnamon Grahams	3/4 cup	120	2	1	T	☻
General Mills, Cinnamon Toast Crunch	3/4 cup	130	4	1	T	☻
General Mills, Clusters, honey nut	1 cup	210	3	3		✂
General Mills, Cocoa Puffs	1 cup	120	1	0	T	☻
General Mills, Cookie Crisp, chocolate chip	1 cup	120	2	0	T	☻
General Mills, Count Chocula	1 cup	120	1	0	T	☻
General Mills, Fiber One	1/2 cup	60	1	13		☺
General Mills, French Toast Crunch	3/4 cup	120	1	0	T	☻
General Mills, Golden Grahams	3/4 cup	120	1	1	T	☻
General Mills, Kix	1 1/3 cups	120	1	1		✂
General Mills, Kix, berry berry	3/4 cup	120	2	0	T	☻
General Mills, Lucky Charms	1 cup	120	1	1		✂
General Mills, Oatmeal Crisp, almond	1 cup	220	5	4		☺
General Mills, Oatmeal Crisp, apple cinnamon	1 cup	210	2	4		☺
General Mills, Oatmeal Crisp, raisin	1 cup	210	3	4		☺
General Mills, Raisin Nut Bran	3/4 cup	200	4	5	T	☻
General Mills, Reese's Peanut Butter Puffs	3/4 cup	130	3	0	T	☻
General Mills, Total, corn flakes	1 1/3 cups	110	0	0		✂
General Mills, Total, raisin bran	1 cup	180	1	5		☺
General Mills, Total, whole grain	3/4 cup	110	1	3		☺
General Mills, Trix w/wildberry	1 cup	120	2	1	T	☻
General Mills, Wheaties	1 cup	110	1	3	T	☻
General Mills, Wheaties, crispy 'n raisins	1 cup	190	1	4		☺
General Mills, Wheaties, honey frosted	3/4 cup	110	0	0		✂
Health Valley, Fiber7 flakes	3/4 cup	100	0	4		☺
Health Valley, oat bran flakes	3/4 cup	100	0	4		☺
Health Valley, oat bran flakes w/raisins	3/4 cup	110	0	4		☺
Health Valley, organic bran w/raisins	3/4 cup	160	0	6		☺
Health Valley, organic healthy fiber multigrain flake	3/4 cup	100	0	4		☺
Health Valley, raisin bran flakes	1 1/4 cups	190	0	6		☺
Kasha medley	1/2 cup	100	1	2		☺
Kellogg's, All-Bran, bran buds	1/3 cup	80	1	13		☺
Kellogg's, All-Bran, extra fiber	1/2 cup	50	1	13		☺
Kellogg's, All-Bran, original	1/2 cup	80	1	10		☺
Kellogg's, Apple Jacks	1 cup	120	0	1		✂
Kellogg's, Breakfast Mates, corn flakes	3/4 cup	80	0	1		✂
Kellogg's, Breakfast Mates, frosted flakes	3/4 cup	110	0	1		✂
Kellogg's, Breakfast Mates, milk	1 carton	60	3	0		☻
Kellogg's, Cocoa Frosted Flakes	3/4 cup	120	0	0	T	☻
Kellogg's, Cocoa Krispies	3/4 cup	120	1	0	T	☻
Kellogg's, Complete Oat Bran Flakes	3/4 cup	110	1	4		☺
Kellogg's, Complete Wheat Bran Flakes	3/4 cup	90	1	5		☺
Kellogg's, Corn Flakes	1 cup	100	0	1		✂
Kellogg's, Corn Flakes, honey crunch	3/4 cup	110	1	1		✂
Kellogg's, Corn Pops	1 cup	120	0	0		✂
Kellogg's, Cracklin' Oat Bran	3/4 cup	190	6	6	T	☻
Kellogg's, Crispix	1 cup	110	0	1		✂

☻ = Avoid • ☙ = Add for flavor

	Portion	Calories	Total Fat	Dietary Fiber	Trans Fat	Guide
Kellogg's, Froot Loops	1 cup	120	1	1	T	💣
Kellogg's, Frosted Flakes	3/4 cup	120	0	1		✂
Kellogg's, Granola w/out raisins, low fat	1/2 cup	190	3	3	T	💣
Kellogg's, Granola w/raisins, low fat	2/3 cup	220	3	3	T	💣
Kellogg's, Healthy Choice, almond crunch w/raisins	1 cup	210	2	5	T	💣
Kellogg's, Healthy Choice, low fat granola w/raisins	1/2 cup	190	3	3	T	💣
Kellogg's, Healthy Choice, toasted brown sugar squares	1 cup	190	1	5		☺
Kellogg's, Just Right, crunchy nugget	1 cup	210	2	3	T	💣
Kellogg's, Just Right, fruit & nut	1 cup	220	2	3		☺
Kellogg's, Mini-Wheats, frosted	5 biscuits	180	1	5		☺
Kellogg's, Mini-Wheats, frosted, bite size	1 cup	200	1	6		☺
Kellogg's, Mini-Wheats, raisin squares	3/4 cup	180	1	5		☺
Kellogg's, Mini-Wheats, strawberry squares	3/4 cup	170	1	5	T	💣
Kellogg's, Mueslix	2/3 cup	200	3	4	T	💣
Kellogg's, Nutri-Grain, almond raisin	1 1/4 cups	180	3	3		✂
Kellogg's, Nutri-Grain, golden wheat	3/4 cup	100	1	3		☺
Kellogg's, Product 19	1 cup	100	0	1		✂
Kellogg's, Raisin Bran	1 cup	200	2	8		☺
Kellogg's, Rice Krispies	1 cup	120	0	0		✂
Kellogg's, Rice Krispies, razzle dazzle	3/4 cup	110	0	0		✂
Kellogg's, Smacks	3/4 cup	100	1	1	T	💣
Kellogg's, Smart Start	1 cup	180	1	2		✂
Kellogg's, Special K	1 cup	110	0	1		✂
Oat bran	1/3 cup	150	3	7		☺
Post, 100% Bran	1/3 cup	80	1	7		☺
Post, Alpha-Bits, frosted	1 cup	130	2	1	T	💣
Post, Alpha-Bits, marshamallow	1 cup	120	1	0	T	💣
Post, Bran Flakes	3/4 cup	100	1	5		☺
Post, Cocoa Pebbles	3/4 cup	120	1	0	T	💣
Post, Fruit & Fibre, dates, raisins, walnuts	1 cup	210	3	5	T	💣
Post, Fruit & Fibre, peaches, raisins, almonds	1 cup	210	3	5	T	💣
Post, Fruity Pebbles	3/4 cup	110	1	0	T	💣
Post, Golden Crisp	3/4 cup	110	0	0	T	💣
Post, Grape-nuts	1/2 cup	200	1	5		☺
Post, Grape-nuts flakes	3/4 cup	100	1	3	T	💣
Post, Honey Bunches of Oats, almond	3/4 cup	130	3	1	T	💣
Post, Honey Bunches of Oats, honey-roasted	3/4 cup	120	2	1	T	💣
Post, Honey-Comb	1 1/3 cups	110	1	1		✂
Post, Morning Traditions, banana nut crunch	1 cup	250	6	4	T	💣
Post, Morning Traditions, blueberry morning	1 1/4 cups	210	3	2	T	💣
Post, Morning Traditions, cranberry almond crunch	1 cup	220	3	3	T	💣
Post, Morning Traditions, great grains, crnchy pcn	2/3 cup	220	6	4	T	💣
Post, Morning Traditions, great grains, rsn, dt, pc	2/3 cup	210	5	4	T	💣
Post, Oreo O's	3/4 cup	110	3	1	T	💣

☺ = Eat as much as you want • ✂ = Cut Back

	Portion	Calories	Total Fat	Dietary Fiber	Trans Fat	Guide
Post, Raisin Bran, whole grain wheat	1 cup	190	1	8		☺
Post, Shredded Wheat	2 biscuits	160	1	5		☺
Post, Shredded Wheat 'n bran	1 1/4 cups	200	1	8		☺
Post, Shredded Wheat, frosted	1 cup	190	1	5		☺
Post, Shredded Wheat, honey nut, bite size	1 cup	200	2	4	T	♠
Post, Shredded Wheat, spoon size	1 cup	170	1	5		☺
Post, Waffle Crisp	1 cup	130	3	0	T	♠
Puffed kashi	1 cup	70	0	2		☺
Quaker, 100% Natural, granola w/raisins, low fat	2/3 cup	210	3	3	T	♠
Quaker, 100% Natural, granola, oats, honey & raisins	1/2 cup	230	9	3	T	♠
Quaker, Apple Zaps	1 cup	120	1	1	T	♠
Quaker, Cap'n Crunch	3/4 cup	110	2	1	T	♠
Quaker, Cap'n Crunch's, crunch berries	3/4 cup	100	2	1	T	♠
Quaker, Cap'n Crunch's, oops! all berries	1 cup	130	2	1	T	♠
Quaker, Cap'n Crunch's, peanut butter crunch	3/4 cup	110	3	1	T	♠
Quaker, Cocoa Blasts	1 cup	130	1	1	T	♠
Quaker, Life	3/4 cup	120	2	2		✂
Quaker, Life, cinnamon	3/4 cup	120	1	2		✂
Quaker, Oat Bran	1 1/4 cups	210	3	6		☺
Quaker, Oatmeal Squares	1 cup	220	3	4		☺
Quaker, Puffed Rice	1 cup	50	0	0		✂
Quaker, Puffed Wheat	1 1/4 cups	50	0	1		☺
Quaker, Sweet Crunch	1 cup	110	2	1	T	♠
Quaker, Toasted Oatmeal	1 cup	190	3	3	T	♠
Quaker, Toasted Oatmeal, honey nut	1 cup	190	3	3	T	♠
Toasted wheat bran	1/4 cup	30	1	7		☺

Cereals, Hot

	Portion	Calories	Total Fat	Dietary Fiber	Trans Fat	Guide
Fantastic Foods, Hearty grains	1 pkg.	260	3	4		☺
Fantastic Foods, apple cinnamon oatmeal	1 pkg.	170	2	4		☺
Fantastic Foods, maple raisin three grain	1 pkg.	190	2	5		☺
Farina	3 tbsp.	120	0	0		✂
Matzo	1/4 cup	110	0	1		✂
Nabisco, Cream of Rice	1/4 cup	170	0	0		✂
Nabisco, Cream of Wheat (all cking times)	3 tbsp.	120	0	1		✂
Nabisco, Cream of Wheat, instant	1 pkt.	100	0	1		✂
Nabisco, Cream of Wheat, instant, brown sugar cinnamon	1 pkt.	130	0	1		✂
Nabisco, Cream of Wheat, multigrain, apple cranberry c	1 pkt.	140	1	3		☺
Nabisco, Cream of Wheat, multigrain, banana nut bread	1 pkt.	150	2	3		☺
Nabisco, Cream of Wheat, multigrain, blueberry muffin	1 pkt.	140	1	2	T	♠
Nabisco, Cream of Wheat, multigrain, cinnamon raisin	1 pkt.	150	1	3		☺
Quaker, Instant Oatmeal, apple & cinnamon	1 pkt.	130	2	3		☺
Quaker, Instant Oatmeal, maple & brown sugar	1 pkt.	160	2	3		☺

♠ = *Avoid* • ♨ = *Add for flavor*

	Portion	Calories	Total Fat	Dietary Fiber	Trans Fat	Guide
Quaker, Instant Oatmeal, raisins & spice	1 pkt.	150	2	3		☺
Quaker, Instant Oatmeal, regular	1 pkt.	100	2	3		☺
Quaker, Oats, old fashioned	1/2 cup dry	150	3	4		☺
Quaker, Oats, quick-1 minute	1/2 cup dry	150	3	4		☺
Quaker, Quick'n Hearty, microwave, appl spc	1 pkt.	170	2	3		☺
Quaker, Quick'n Hearty, microwave, brwn sgr cnnmn	1 pkt.	160	2	3		☺
Quaker, Quick'n Hearty, microwave, honey bran	1 pkt.	150	2	3		☺
Quaker, Quick'n Hearty microwave, regular,	1 pkt.	110	2	2		☺
Quaker, bran, unprocessed	1/3 cup	35	1	8		☺
Quaker, grits, instant original	1 pkt.	100	0	1		✂
Quaker, grits, old fashioned	1/4 cup	140	1	2		✂
Quaker, grits, quick	1/4 cup	130	1	2		✂
Quaker, multi grain	1/2 cup	130	1	5		☺
Quaker, oat bran	1/2 cup	150	3	6		☺
Wheat germ	2 tbsp.	50	1	2		☺
Wheatena	1/3 cup	150	1	5		☺

■ CONDIMENTS & SAUCES

Condiments, Bacon Bits

	Portion	Calories	Total Fat	Dietary Fiber	Trans Fat	Guide
Betty Crocker, Bac-Os	1 1/2 tbsp.	30	1	0	T	💧
Hormel, real bacon pieces	1 tbsp.	25	2	0		💧
McCormick, bac'n pieces	1 1/2 tbsp.	30	2	0	T	💧

Condiments, Capers

	Portion	Calories	Total Fat	Dietary Fiber	Trans Fat	Guide
Capers, non pareille	20 capers	2	0	0		👍

Condiments, Clam Juice

	Portion	Calories	Total Fat	Dietary Fiber	Trans Fat	Guide
Doxsee	1 tbsp.	0	0	0		👍
Progresso, white clam	1/2 cup	150	10	0		💧

Condiments, Cooking Wine

	Portion	Calories	Total Fat	Dietary Fiber	Trans Fat	Guide
Holland House, red	2 tbsp.	20	0	0		✂
Holland House, sherry	2 tbsp.	45	0	0		✂
Holland House, white	2 tbsp.	20	0	0		✂
Pineapple Chinese flavored	3 tbsp.	15	0	0		✂

Condiments, Dips

	Portion	Calories	Total Fat	Dietary Fiber	Trans Fat	Guide
Athenos, Mediterranean Spreads, hummus, original	2 tbsp.	50	4	1		💧
Athenos, Mediterranean Spreads, hummus, roasted garlic	2 tbsp.	50	3	1		💧
Athenos, Mediterranean Spreads, hummus, roasted red pepper	2 tbsp.	50	4	1		💧
Athenos, Mediterranean Spreads, hummus, spicy three pepper	2 tbsp.	50	4	1		💧
Bearitos, vegetarian bean, fat free	2 tbsp.	25	0	1		👍
Bearitos, vegetarian black bean, fat free	2 tbsp.	25	0	1		👍

☺ = Eat as much as you want • ✂ = Cut Back

	Portion	Calories	Total Fat	Dietary Fiber	Trans Fat	Guide
Breakstone's, Chesapeake clam	2 tbsp.	50	4	0		🌢
Deans', French onion, no fat	2 tbsp.	30	0	0		✂
Deans', guacamole	2 tbsp.	80	8	0		🌢
Deans', ranch	2 tbsp.	60	5	0		🌢
Fantastic Foods, hummus	2 tbsp.	60	2	2		✂
Frito Lay, bean	2 tbsp.	40	1	1	T	🌢
Frito Lay, chili cheese dip	2 tbsp.	45	3	0	T	🌢
Frito Lay, jalapeno cheddar cheese dip	2 tbsp.	50	4	0	T	🌢
Guacamole	2 tbsp.	60	5	0		🌢
Heluva Good, French onion	2 tbsp.	50	5	0		🌢
Heluva Good, French onion, fat free	2 tbsp.	25	0	0		✂
Heluva Good, bacon horseradish	2 tbsp.	60	5	0		🌢
Heluva Good, classic ranch	2 tbsp.	60	5	0		🌢
Kraft, French onion	2 tbsp.	45	4	0		🌢
Old El Paso, black bean dip	2 tbsp.	25	0	1		☺
Old El Paso, cheese 'n salsa dip	2 tbsp.	40	3	0	T	🌢
Old El Paso, jalapeño bean dip	2 tbsp.	30	1	2		☺
Tribe of Two Sheiks, hummus	2 tbsp.	50	3	1		🌢
Tribe of Two Sheiks, hummus w/cracked chili peppers	2 tbsp.	50	3	1		🌢
Tribe of Two Sheiks, hummus w/forty spices	2 tbsp.	50	3	1		🌢
Tribe of Two Sheiks, hummus w/roasted garlic	2 tbsp.	50	3	1		🌢
Tribe of Two Sheiks, hummus w/roasted red peppers	2 tbsp.	50	3	1		🌢
Tribe of Two Sheiks, hummus, dill	2 tbsp.	50	3	1		🌢
Walden Farms, onion, fat free	2 tbsp.	20	0	0		✂
Walden Farms, roasted pepper, fat free	2 tbsp.	30	0	1		✂

Condiments, Mayonnaise

	Portion	Calories	Total Fat	Dietary Fiber	Trans Fat	Guide
Hellmann's, light	1 tbsp.	50	5	0		🌢
Hellmann's, low fat	1 tbsp.	25	1	0		✂
Hellmann's, real	1 tbsp.	100	11	0		🌢
Kraft, Miracle Whip	1 tbsp.	70	7	0		🌢
Kraft, Miracle Whip free	1 tbsp.	15	0	0		✂
Kraft, Miracle Whip light	1 tbsp.	35	3	0		🌢
Kraft, mayo fat free	1 tbsp.	10	0	0		💧
Kraft, mayo light	1 tbsp.	50	5	0		🌢
Kraft, mayo real	1 tbsp.	100	11	0		🌢
Kraft, mayo real squeeze	1 tbsp.	100	11	0		🌢
Smart Beat, fat free	1 tbsp.	10	0	0		💧
Weight Watchers, light	1 tbsp.	25	2	0		✂

Condiments, Mustard

	Portion	Calories	Total Fat	Dietary Fiber	Trans Fat	Guide
French's, classic yellow	1 tbsp.	0	0	0		💧
French's, hearty deli	1 tbsp.	5	0	0		💧
Grey Poupon, honey	1 tbsp.	10	0	0		💧
Grey Poupon, w/white wine	1 tbsp.	5	0	0		💧
Gulden's, spicy brown	1 tbsp.	0	0	0		💧
Healthy Farms, honey orange	1 tbsp.	15	0	0		✂

🌢 = Avoid • 💧 = Add for flavor

	Portion	Calories	Total Fat	Dietary Fiber	Trans Fat	Guide
Condiments, Olives						
Almond stuffed	2 olives	25	3	0		🫒
Garlic stuffed	2 olives	20	2	0		✂
Jalapeño stuffed	2 olives	25	2	0		✂
Onion stuffed	2 olives	20	2	0		✂
Pimiento stuffed	2 olives	20	2	0		✂
Stuffed Spanish	5 olives	25	2	0		✂
Sun of Italy, Spanish olives	2 olives	10	1	1		✂
Condiments, Pickles						
Claussen, Kosher dill halves	$1/2$ pickle	5	0	0		👍
Claussen, Kosher dill mini	1 pickle	5	0	0		👍
Claussen, Kosher dill spears	1 spear	5	0	0		👍
Claussen, Kosher dill spear slices for burgers	1 slice	5	0	0		👍
Claussen, Sandwich Slices, bread 'n butter	2 slices	25	0	0		✂
Mt. Olive, Kosher dill cocktail midgets	3 pickles	5	0	0		👍
Mt. Olive, Kosher dill strips	1 strip	0	0	0		👍
Mt. Olive, bread & butter	6 chips	25	0	0		✂
Mt. Olive, salad sweet cubes	1 tbsp.	20	0	0		✂
Mt. Olive, sour	1 pickle	0	0	0		👍
Mt. Olive, sweet gherkins	1 pickle	35	0	0		✂
Okra pickles	2 pieces	10	0	0		👍
Vlasic, Bread & butter chips	3 chips	25	0	0		✂
Vlasic, Bread & butter reduced sodium	3 chips	25	0	0		✂
Vlasic, Kosher dill baby whole pickles	1 pickle	5	0	0		👍
Vlasic, Kosher dill reduced sodium	$3/4$ spear	5	0	0		👍
Vlasic, Kosher dill spears	$3/4$ spear	5	0	0		👍
Vlasic, Original Sandwich Stackers, bread & butter	2 slices	25	0	0		✂
Vlasic, Original Sandwich Stackers, hearty garlic	2 slices	5	0	0		👍
Vlasic, Original Sandwich Stackers, kosher dill	2 slices	5	0	0		👍
Vlasic, Original Sandwich Stackers, zesty dill	2 slices	5	0	0		👍
Vlasic, Snack'mms, bread & butter	3 pickles	35	0	0		✂
Vlasic, Snack'mms, kosher dill	2 pickles	5	0	0		👍
Vlasic, bread & butter spears	$3/4$ spear	25	0	0		✂
Vlasic, cauliflower, hot & spicy	$1/4$ cup	5	0	0		👍
Vlasic, sweet gherkins	3 pickles	35	0	0		✂
Vlasic, sweet midgets	3 pickles	35	0	0		✂
Vlasic, sweet salad cubes	1 tbsp.	20	0	0		✂
Vlasic, zesty bread & butter chips	3 chips	40	0	0		✂
Vlasic, zesty dill spears	3/4 spear	5	0	0		👍
Watermelon rind, sweet pickled	2 tbsp.	70	0	0		✂
Condiments, Relish						
Heinz, hamburger relish	1 tbsp.	10	0	0		👍
Mt. Olive, sweet relish	1 tbsp.	20	0	0		✂
Vlasic, dill relish	1 tbsp.	5	0	0		👍
Vlasic, hot dog relish	1 tbsp.	20	0	0		👍
Vlasic, sweet relish	1 tbsp.	15	0	0		✂

☺ = Eat as much as you want • ✂ = Cut Back

	Portion	Calories	Total Fat	Dietary Fiber	Trans Fat	Guide
Condiments, Vinegar						
Balsamic	1 tbsp.	5	0	0		🖐
Heinz	1/2 oz.	2	0	0		🖐
Heinz, apple cider	1/2 oz.	2	0	0		🖐
Kame, rice wine vinegar	1 tbsp.	0	0	0		🖐
Pompeian, red wine	1 tbsp.	2	0	0		🖐
Regina, light, wine	1 tbsp.	0	0	0		🖐
Rice	1 tbsp.	20	0	0		✂
White House, apple cider	1 tbsp.	0	0	0		🖐
Sauces, Asian						
Chun King, soy sauce	1 tbsp.	10	0	0		🖐
Dai Day, duck sauce	2 tbsp.	80	0	0		✂
Dai Day, sweet & sour duck sauce	2 tbsp.	80	0	0		✂
Dynasty, plum sauce	2 tbsp.	70	0	0		✂
Dynasty, sweet & hot mustard	1 tsp.	10	0	0		🖐
Ebara, stir fry sauce	16 g.	10	0	0		💧
Emperor's, stir fry sauce	1/4 cup	110	6	0		💧
House of Tsang, sweet & sour stir fry sauce	1 tbsp.	35	0	0		✂
Kame, hoisin sauce	2 tbsp.	70	0	0		✂
Kame, soy sauce, dark	1 tbsp.	10	0	0		🖐
Kikkoman, soy sauce	1 tbsp.	10	0	0		🖐
Kikkoman, stir fry sauce	1 tbsp.	15	0	0		✂
Kikkoman, sweet & sour sauce	2 tbsp.	35	0	0		✂
Kikkoman, teriyaki, base & glaze	2 tbsp.	50	0	0		✂
Kikkoman, teriyaki, marinade & sauce	1 tbsp.	15	0	0		✂
Kikkoman, teriyaki, roasted garlic	1 tbsp.	25	0	0		✂
La Choy, soy sauce	1 tbsp.	10	0	0		🖐
La Choy, soy sauce, lite	1 tbsp.	15	0	0		✂
La Choy, sweet & sour sauce	2 tbsp.	60	0	0		✂
Lawry's, teriyaki sauce	1 tbsp.	20	0	0		✂
San-j, Szechuan hot & spice sauce	1 tsp.	5	0	0		🖐
San-j, Thai peanut	2 tbsp.	70	3	1		💧
San-j, soy sauce, tamari	1 tbsp.	15	0	0		✂
World Harbors, Maui Mountain, sweet'n sour, Hawaiian style	2 tbsp.	60	0	0		✂
World Harbors, Maui Mountain, teriyaki, Hawaiian style	2 tbsp.	70	0	0		✂
Sauces, Clam						
Sun of Italy, red	1/2 cup	120	5	0		💧
Sun of Italy, white	1/2 cup	110	6	0		💧
Sauces, Dry Mix						
Knorr, Classic Sauces, bernaise	1 tsp.	10	0	0		🖐
Knorr, Classic Sauces, hollandaise	1 tsp.	10	0	0	T	💧
Knorr, Pasta Sauces, 4 cheese toscana	2 tbsp.	70	4	0	T	💧
Knorr, Pasta Sauces, creamy pesto	1 tbsp.	30	1	0	T	💧
Knorr, Pasta Sauces, garlic herb	2 tbsp.	70	4	0	T	💧

💧 = Avoid • 🖐 = Add for flavor

	Portion	Calories	Total Fat	Dietary Fiber	Trans Fat	Guide
Knorr, Pasta Sauces, parma rosa	2 tbsp.	60	3	0	T	🌢
Knorr, Pasta Sauces, red bell pepper pesto	1 tbsp.	30	1	0	T	🌢
Knorr, Pasta Sauces, sun dried tomato pesto	1 1/2 tbsp.	45	1	1	T	🌢
McCormick, 3 cheese chicken sauce blend	1 tbsp. dry mix	45	3	0		🌢
McCormick, chicken Dijon sauce blend	1 2/3 tbsp.	40	2	0		✂
McCormick, Grill Mates, mesquite marinade	2 tsp. dry	15	0	0	T	🌢
McCormick, Grill Mates, zesty herb marinade	2 tsp. dry	10	0	0		👍
McCormick, alfredo pasta sauce blend	2 tbsp.	60	2	0		✂
McCormick, bernaise sauce blend	1 tsp. dry	10	0	0		👍
McCormick, chicken teriyaki sauce blend	1 1/3 tbsp. dry	40	1	0	T	🌢
McCormick, green peppercorn sauce blend	2 tsp. dry	20	0	0		✂
McCormick, hollandaise sauce blend	2 tsp. dry	15	0	0		✂
McCormick, lemon herb chicken sauce blend	1 tbsp. dry mix	30	0	0		✂
McCormick, spaghetti sauce	1 tsp. dry	25	0	0		✂

Sauces, Gravy

	Portion	Calories	Total Fat	Dietary Fiber	Trans Fat	Guide
Franco-American, slow roast beef	1/4 cup	25	1	0		✂
Franco-American, slow roast chicken	1/4 cup	25	1	0		✂
Heinz, Homestyle, classic chicken	1/4 cup	25	1	0	T	🌢
Heinz, Homestyle, rich mushroom	1/4 cup	20	1	0		✂
Heinz, Homestyle, roasted turkey	1/4 cup	30	2	0	T	🌢
Heinz, Homestyle, savory beef	1/4 cup	25	1	0	T	🌢
Heinz, Homestyle, zesty onion	1/4 cup	25	1	0		✂
Heinz, fat free, beef	1/4 cup	10	0	0		👍
Heinz, fat free, chicken	1/4 cup	15	0	0		✂
Heinz, fat free, turkey	1/4 cup	15	0	0		✂

Sauces, Gravy Mix

	Portion	Calories	Total Fat	Dietary Fiber	Trans Fat	Guide
Butterball, turkey	2 tsp.	15	0	0	T	🌢
Knorr, Gravy Classics, aujus	1 tsp.	10	0	0	T	🌢
Knorr, Gravy Classics, roasted chicken	1 tbsp.	30	1	0		✂
Knorr, Gravy Classics, roasted turkey	1 tbsp.	25	1	0		✂
Knorr, classic brown	2 tsp.	20	1	0	T	🌢
McCormick, brown	1 tsp. dry	20	1	0		✂
McCormick, chicken	2 tsp. dry	20	0	0		✂
McCormick, country	1 1/3 tbsp.	45	2	0	T	🌢
McCormick, mushroom	1 tsp. dry	20	1	0		✂
McCormick, onion	1/4 pkg.	20	1	0		✂
McCormick, pork	1 tsp. dry	20	0	0		✂
McCormick, turkey	2 tsp. dry	20	0	0		✂
Pillsbury, Hungry Jack, biscuit gravy mix	1 tbsp.	40	2	0	T	🌢

Sauces, Marinade

	Portion	Calories	Total Fat	Dietary Fiber	Trans Fat	Guide
Lawry's, herb & garlic	1 tbsp.	10	0	0		👍
Lawry's, lemon pepper	1 tbsp.	10	0	0		👍
Lawry's, mesquite	1 tbsp.	5	0	0		👍
Lawry's, teriyaki	1 tbsp.	25	0	0		✂
McCormick, Golden Dipt, cajun style	1 tbsp.	60	5	0		🌢

☺ = Eat as much as you want • ✂ = Cut Back

	Portion	Calories	Total Fat	Dietary Fiber	Trans Fat	Guide
McCormick, Golden Dipt, ginger teriyaki	1 tbsp.	60	3	0		🫗
McCormick, Golden Dipt, lemon herb	1 tbsp.	80	8	0		🫗
World Harbors, Acadia, lemon pepper & garlic	2 tbsp.	35	0	0		✂

Sauces, Mexican

Old El Paso, enchilada sauce	$1/4$ cup	30	2	0		✂
Old El Paso, taco sauce	1 tbsp.	5	0	0		👍
Taco Bell, hot sauce	1 tsp.	0	0	0		👍
Taco Bell, taco sauce, medium	2 tbsp.	15	0	0		✂

Sauces, Other

Del Monte, sloppy joe	$1/4$ cup	50	0	0		✂
French's, worcestershire	1 tbsp.	0	0	0		👍
Hunt's, sloppy joe, classic recipe	$1/2$ cup	70	1	2		✂
Kraft, free, horseradish	1 tbsp.	20	2	0		✂
Lea & Perrins, Worcestershire	1 tbsp.	5	0	0	T	🫗
Manwich, sloppy joe	$1/4$ cup	45	0	0		✂
McCormick, Golden Dipt, honey soy, fat free	1 tbsp.	30	0	0		✂
McCormick, Golden Dipt, lemon butter dill	2 tbsp.	120	10	0		🫗
McCormick, Golden Dipt, sun-dried tomato & basil	2 tbsp.	25	1	0		✂
McCormick, mesquite, fat free	1 tbsp.	10	0	0		👍
World Harbors, Blue Mountain, jerk, Jamaican style	2 tbsp.	70	0	0		✂

Sauces, Pasta

Barilla, marinara	$1/2$ cup	80	4	3		🫗
Barilla, tomato & basil	$1/2$ cup	70	2	3		✂
Classico, pecorino romano & herb	$1/2$ cup	80	3	2		🫗
Classico, roasted garlic	$1/2$ cup	60	2	2		🫗
Classico, spicy red pepper	$1/2$ cup	60	3	2		🫗
Classico, tomato & basil	$1/2$ cup	50	1	2		✂
Five Brothers, French tomato basil	$1/2$ cup	60	2	3		✂
Five Brothers, alfredo w/mushroom	$1/2$ cup	160	12	0		🫗
Five Brothers, alfredo, creamy	$1/2$ cup	200	18	0		🫗
Five Brothers, alfredo, tomato	$1/2$ cup	140	8	2		🫗
Five Brothers, creamy pesto	$1/2$ cup	200	18	0		🫗
Five Brothers, grilled summer vegetable	$1/2$ cup	80	5	3		🫗
Five Brothers, marinara & burgundy wine	$1/2$ cup	80	3	3		🫗
Healthy Choice, garlic & herb	$1/2$ cup	50	0	2		☺
Healthy Choice, super chunky tomato, mushroom & garlic	$1/2$ cup	45	0	2		☺
Healthy Choice, traditional	$1/2$ cup	50	0	2		☺
Hunt's, tomato sauce	$1/2$ cup	30	0	1		☺
Newman's Own, garlic & peppers	$1/2$ cup	70	3	4		🫗
Newman's Own, sockarooni spaghetti	$1/2$ cup	60	2	3		✂
Prego, 3 cheese	$1/2$ cup	100	2	3		✂
Prego, diced onion & garlic	$1/2$ cup	110	3	3		🫗
Prego, extra chunky garden combination	$1/2$ cup	90	1	3		☺

🫗 = *Avoid* • 👍 = *Add for flavor*

	Portion	Calories	Total Fat	Dietary Fiber	Trans Fat	Guide
Prego, mushroom parmesan	1/2 cup	120	4	3		🔴
Prego, tomato & basil	1/2 cup	110	3	3		🔴
Prego, tomato parmesan	1/2 cup	120	3	3		🔴
Prego, traditional	1/2 cup	140	5	2		🔴
Ragu, Chunky Garden Style, mushroom & green peppers	1/2 cup	110	4	3		🔴
Ragu, Chunky Garden Style, roasted red pepper & onions	1/2 cup	110	4	2		🔴
Ragu, Chunky Garden Style, super vegetable primavera	1/2 cup	110	4	4		🔴
Ragu, Chunky Garden Style, tomato, garlic & onion	1/2 cup	120	4	3		🔴
Ragu, LIght, tomato & basil	1/2 cup	50	0	2		☺
Ragu, cheese creations	1/2 cup	220	20	0		🔴
Ragu, hearty, 7 herb tomato	1/2 cup	110	3	3		🔴
Ragu, hearty, parmesan & romano	1/2 cup	120	4	3		🔴
Ragu, hearty, sauteed onion & garlic	1/2 cup	120	4	4		🔴
Ragu, hearty, spicy red pepper	1/2 cup	110	2	3		✂
Ragu, light, chunky mushroom & garlic	1/2 cup	70	0	3		☺
Ragu, meat	1/2 cup	80	4	3		🔴
Ragu, mushroom	1/2 cup	80	3	3		🔴
Ragu, spicy cheddar & tomato	1/2 cup	100	4	0		🔴
Ragu, traditional	1/2 cup	80	3	3		🔴

Sauces, Pasta, Refrigerated

	Portion	Calories	Total Fat	Dietary Fiber	Trans Fat	Guide
Contadina, alfredo	1/4 cup	180	16	0		🔴
Contadina, alfredo, light	1/4 cup	80	5	0		🔴
Contadina, alfredo, mushroom	1/4 cup	100	7	1		🔴
Contadina, garden vegetable	1/2 cup	40	0	2		☺
Contadina, marinara	1/2 cup	80	4	2		🔴
Contadina, pesto w/basil	1/4 cup	290	24	3		🔴
Contadina, pesto w/basil, reduced fat	1/4 cup	230	18	2		🔴
DiGiorno, alfredo	1/4 cup	180	18	0		🔴
Monterey Pasta Company, sundried tomato cream	1/2 cup	160	11	1		🔴
Trio's, tomato	1/2 cup	100	7	0		🔴

Sauces, Pizza

	Portion	Calories	Total Fat	Dietary Fiber	Trans Fat	Guide
Contadina	1/4 cup	25	1	1		✂
Contadina, squeeze	1/4 cup	35	2	1		✂
Donpepino	1/4 cup	45	3	1		🔴
Ragu	1/4 cup	30	1	1		✂
Ragu, pizza quick traditional	1/4 cup	40	2	1		✂

Sauces, Salsa

	Portion	Calories	Total Fat	Dietary Fiber	Trans Fat	Guide
Chi-Chi's, Chunky Restaurante Salsa, mild	2 tbsp.	10	0	0		👍
Chi-Chi's, salsa, con queso	2 tbsp.	90	7	0	T	🔴
Enrico's, salsa	2 tbsp.	15	0	0		✂
Goya, hot sauce, salsa picante	1 tsp.	0	0	0		👍
Newman's Own, salsa, mild	2 tbsp.	10	0	0		👍

☺ = Eat as much as you want • ✂ = Cut Back

	Portion	Calories	Total Fat	Dietary Fiber	Trans Fat	Guide
Old El Paso, salsa, hot	2 tbsp.	10	0	0		👍
Pace, picante sauce, mild	2 tbsp.	10	0	0		👍
Pace, Thick & Chunky Salsa, cilantro	2 tbsp.	10	0	0		👍
Taco Bell, salsa, con queso, mild	2 tbsp.	40	3	0		💧
Tostitos, salsa	2 tbsp.	15	0	1		✂
Tostitos, salsa, con queso	2 tbsp.	40	2	0		✂

Sauces, Seafood

	Portion	Calories	Total Fat	Dietary Fiber	Trans Fat	Guide
Hellmann's, tartar	2 tbsp.	80	7	0		💧
Ken's, cocktail	2 tbsp.	30	1	1		✂
Ken's, tartar	2 tbsp.	170	19	0		💧
Kraft, free, tartar	2 tbsp.	25	0	0		✂
McCormick, Golden Dipt, tartar, fat free	2 tbsp.	35	0	0		✂
Old Bay, cocktail	1/4 cup	110	1	1		✂
Phillips, cocktail	1/4 cup	70	1	1		✂
Phillips, tartar	2 tbsp.	140	15	0		💧

Sauces, Steak

	Portion	Calories	Total Fat	Dietary Fiber	Trans Fat	Guide
A-1, Bold & Spicy Steak	1 tbsp.	20	0	0		✂
A-1, steak	1 tbsp.	15	0	0		✂
Heinz, 57 steak	1 tbsp.	15	0	0		✂
Lea & Perrins, steak	1 tbsp.	25	0	0		✂
Newman's Own, steak	1 tbsp.	20	1	0		✂

■ DAIRY PRODUCTS

Cheese

	Portion	Calories	Total Fat	Dietary Fiber	Trans Fat	Guide
Alpine Lace, cheddar, fat free	1/6 bar	45	0	0		✂
Apetina, feta	1 oz.	80	7	0		💧
Athenos, feta, crumbled basil & tomato	1 oz.	80	6	0		💧
Athenos, feta, crumbled mild	1 oz.	80	6	0		💧
Athenos, feta, crumbled reduced fat	1 oz.	60	4	0		💧
Athenos, feta, traditional	1 oz.	80	6	0		💧
Babybel, semi-soft part skim	1 oz.	90	7	0		💧
Belmont, goat	1 oz.	70	6	0		💧
Boursin, spice gournay w/garlic	2 tbsp.	120	13	0		💧
Breakstone's, Temptee whipped	2 tbsp.	80	8	0		💧
Cabot, cheddar, Vermont	1 oz.	110	9	0		💧
Cabot, cheddar, light	1 oz.	70	5	0		💧
Cabot, pepper jack, Vermont	1 oz.	110	9	0		💧
Cheddar, Wisconsin sharp	1 oz.	110	9	0		💧
Cheese log	2 tbsp.	110	9	0		💧
Country Castle, limburger	1 oz.	90	12	0		💧
Country Line, cheddar, mild	1 oz.	110	9	0		💧
Country Line, colby	1 oz.	110	9	0		💧
Country Line, mozzarella, string	1 piece	80	6	0		💧
Cracker Barrel, cheddar, 2%	1 oz.	90	6	0		💧
Cracker Barrel, cheddar, Vermont sharp white	1 oz.	110	9	0		💧

💧 = Avoid • 👍 = Add for flavor

	Portion	Calories	Total Fat	Dietary Fiber	Trans Fat	Guide
Cracker Barrel, cheddar, extra sharp	1 oz.	90	6	0		🩸
Cracker Barrel, cheddar, sharp white	1 oz.	120	10	0		🩸
Cracker Barrel, cheddar, whipped sharp	2 tbsp.	80	8	0		🩸
Double-H, cheese ball	2 tbsp.	100	7	1		🩸
Havarti	1 oz.	120	7	0		🩸
Havarti, cream	1 oz.	130	11	0		🩸
Healthy Choice, mozzarella, low fat	1 cube	60	2	0		✂
Healthy Choice, string, mozzarella	1 piece	50	2	0		✂
Heluva Good, Monterey jack	1 oz.	110	9	0		🩸
Heluva Good, cheddar, sharp	1 oz.	110	9	0		🩸
Ile de France, brie, double cream	1 oz.	110	9	0		🩸
Ile de France, camembert	1 oz.	110	9	0		🩸
King's Choice, gouda, smoked	1 oz.	90	8	0		🩸
Kraft, Monterey jack, 2% milk	1 oz.	80	6	0		🩸
Land O Lakes, Monterey jack	1 oz.	110	8	0		🩸
Land O Lakes, cheddar, extra sharp	1 oz.	110	9	0		🩸
Land O Lakes, cheddar, mild	1 oz.	110	9	0		🩸
Land O Lakes, cheddar, sharp	1 oz.	110	9	0		🩸
May-bud, edam	1 oz.	100	8	0		🩸
Monterey Jack	1 oz.	100	8	0		🩸
Papillon, brie, herb	1 oz.	100	9	0		🩸
Polly-O, string	1 stick	80	6	0		🩸
Port Salut, semi-soft	1 oz.	91	7	0		🩸
Provolone	1 oz.	100	8	0		🩸
Rosenborg, blue, extra creamy in oil	1 oz.	180	19	0		🩸
Saga, soft-ripened	1 oz.	120	12	0		🩸
Saladena, goat, crumbles	1/4 cup	80	6	0		🩸
Sorrento, Deli Style, ricotta, low fat	1/4 cup	70	3	0		🩸
Sorrento, Deli Style, ricotta, part skim	1/4 cup	100	6	0		🩸
Sorrento, Deli Style, ricotta, whole milk	1/4 cup	110	8	0		🩸
Sorrento, mozzarella, part skim	1 oz.	80	5	0		🩸
Sorrento, ricotta, fat free	1/4 cup	60	0	0		✂
Stella, romano	1 oz.	100	8	0		🩸
Swiss, natural	1 oz.	100	8	0		🩸
Treasure Cave, blue	1 oz.	110	9	0		🩸
Treasure Cave, blue, crumbled	1 oz.	110	9	0		🩸
Weight Watchers, cheddar, mild	1 oz.	80	5	0		🩸
Wispride, cheddar, port wine	2 tbsp.	90	7	0		🩸
Wispride, cheddar, sharp	2 tbsp.	90	7	0		🩸

Cheese, Cream

	Portion	Calories	Total Fat	Dietary Fiber	Trans Fat	Guide
Healthy Choice, fat free, non fat	2 tbsp.	25	0	0		✂
Kraft, Philadelphia	2 tbsp.	100	10	0		🩸
Kraft, Philadelphia, 1/3 less fat	1 oz.	70	6	0		🩸
Kraft, Philadelphia, free	1 oz.	30	0	0		✂
Kraft, Philadelphia, light	2 tbsp.	70	5	0		🩸
Kraft, Philadelphia, neufchatel, 1/3 less fat	1 oz.	70	6	0		🩸
Kraft, Philadelphia, whipped	2 tbsp.	70	7	0		🩸
Kraft, Philly Flavors, apple cinnamon	2 tbsp.	100	8	0		🩸
Kraft, Philly Flavors, chive & onion	2 tbsp.	110	10	0		🩸

☺ = Eat as much as you want • ✂ = Cut Back

	Portion	Calories	Total Fat	Dietary Fiber	Trans Fat	Guide
Kraft, Philly Flavors, garden vegetable	2 tbsp.	110	10	0		☁
Kraft, Philly Flavors, honeynut	2 tbsp.	110	9	0		☁
Kraft, Philly Flavors, pineapple	2 tbsp.	100	9	0		☁
Kraft, Philly Flavors, salmon	2 tbsp.	100	9	0		☁
Vita, smoked salmon	2 tbsp.	100	9	0		☁

Cheese, Grated

	Portion	Calories	Total Fat	Dietary Fiber	Trans Fat	Guide
Kraft, Parm Plus!, zesty red pepper	2 tsp.	15	0	0		✂
Kraft, mozzarella, Free	2 tsp.	15	0	0		✂
Kraft, parmesan, 100%	2 tsp.	20	2	0		✂
Kraft, romano, sharp	2 tsp.	20	2	0		✂
Suprema, parmesan	1 tbsp.	25	2	0		✂

Cheese, Sauce

	Portion	Calories	Total Fat	Dietary Fiber	Trans Fat	Guide
Campbell's, cheddar cheese	1/2 cup	130	8	1	T	☁
Chef Garcia, nacho	2 tbsp.	20	1	0		✂
Kaukauna, nacho, medium	2 tbsp.	90	7	0		☁
Kaukauna, nacho, mild	2 tbsp.	90	7	0		☁
Pablo's, jalapeño	2 tbsp.	150	9	0		☁

Cheese, Shredded

	Portion	Calories	Total Fat	Dietary Fiber	Trans Fat	Guide
Healthy Choice, mozzarella, garlic lovers	1/4 cup	50	2	1		✂
Healthy Choice, mozzarella, low fat	1/4 cup	50	2	0		✂
Healthy Choice, pizza cheese, low fat	1/4 cup	50	2	0		✂
Kraft, cheddar, sharp	1/4 cup	110	9	0		☁
Kraft, cheddar, sharp 2% milk, reduced fat	1/4 cup	90	6	0		☁
Kraft, mozzarella, 2% milk	1/4 cup	70	5	0		☁
Sargento, mozzarella	1/4 cup	80	6	0		☁
Sargento, mozzarella, light, low fat	1/4 cup	70	4	0		☁
Sorrento, 6 cheese	1/4 cup	90	7	0		☁
Sorrento, Monterey jack, fancy	1/4 cup	110	9	0		☁
Sorrento, cheddar, fancy mild	1/4 cup	110	9	0		☁
Sorrento, double cheese	1/4 cup	90	6	0		☁
Sorrento, mozzarella, whole milk	1/4 cup	90	6	0		☁
Sorrento, nacho & taco	1/4 cup	110	9	0		☁
Sorrento, pizza, 3 cheese blend	1/4 cup	100	7	0		☁

Cheese, Sliced

	Portion	Calories	Total Fat	Dietary Fiber	Trans Fat	Guide
Alpine Lace, fat free	1 slice	30	0	0		✂
Alpine Lace, swiss, reduced fat	1 slice	110	8	0		☁
Borden, American, the big	1 slice	80	6	0		☁
Borden, fat free	1 slice	30	0	0		✂
Borden, low fat, sharp	1 slice	30	1	0		✂
Cooper, CV sharp	1 slice	80	7	0		☁
Double-H, munster	1 oz.	100	8	0		☁
Emmen Taler, Swiss	1 oz.	120	9	0		☁
Healthy Choice, American singles	1 slice	40	1	0		✂
Kraft, American, deluxe	1 slice	70	6	0		☁
Kraft, Free Singles, American	1 slice	30	0	0		✂

☁ = Avoid • ☁ = Add for flavor

	Portion	Calories	Total Fat	Dietary Fiber	Trans Fat	Guide
Kraft, Free Singles, sharp cheddar	1 slice	35	0	0		✄
Kraft, Singles, American	1 slice	60	5	0		🌢
Kraft, Singles, American, 2% milk	1 slice	50	3	0		🌢
Kraft, Singles, mild Mexican style	1 slice	70	5	0		🌢
Kraft, Swiss	1 slice	150	12	0		🌢
Kraft, Swiss, 2% milk	1 slice	130	9	0		🌢
Kraft, Swiss, deli thin	1 slice	90	7	0		🌢
Kraft, Velveeta	1 slice	70	5	0		🌢
Kraft, cheddar, mild	1 slice	110	9	0		🌢
Land O Lakes, American singles	1 slice	70	5	0		🌢
Sargento, Jarlsberg	1 slice	120	9	0		🌢
Sargento, Monterey jack	1 slice	100	9	0		🌢
Smart Beat, fat free	1 slice	25	0	0		✄

Cheese, Spread

	Portion	Calories	Total Fat	Dietary Fiber	Trans Fat	Guide
Alouette, French onion melange	2 tbsp.	80	7	0		🌢
Alouette, garlic et herbes classique	2 tbsp.	70	7	0		🌢
Alouette, garlic et herbes, light	2 tbsp.	50	4	0		🌢
Alouette, spring vegetable jardin, light	2 tbsp.	50	4	0		🌢
Kraft, Cheez Whiz	2 tbsp.	90	7	0		🌢
Kraft, Cheez Whiz, jalapeño	2 tbsp.	100	8	0		🌢
Kraft, Cheez Whiz, light	2 tbsp.	80	3	0		🌢
Kraft, Olive & pimento	2 tbsp.	70	6	0		🌢
Kraft, Velveeta	1 oz.	90	6	0		🌢
Kraft, bacon	2 tbsp.	90	5	0		🌢
Kraft, old English	2 tbsp.	90	8	0		🌢
Kraft, pimento	2 tbsp.	80	6	0		🌢
Montrachet, goat, cracked peppercorn	2 tbsp.	40	3	0		🌢
Prices, pimiento	2 tbsp.	80	7	0		🌢
Rondele, black pepper	2 tbsp.	90	9	0		🌢
Rondele, garden vegetable	2 tbsp.	90	9	0		🌢
Rondele, garlic & herbs	2 tbsp.	100	9	0		🌢
Rondele, garlic & herbs, lite	2 tbsp.	60	4	0		🌢

Cheese, Squeeze

	Portion	Calories	Total Fat	Dietary Fiber	Trans Fat	Guide
Kraft, Cheez Whiz, cheezin 'n squeezin	2 tbsp.	100	8	0	T	🌢
Nabisco, Easy Cheese, American	2 tbsp.	100	7	0		🌢
Nabisco, Easy Cheese, cheddar	2 tbsp.	100	7	0		🌢
Nabisco, Easy Cheese, sharp cheddar	2 tbsp.	100	7	0		🌢
Old Fashioned Foods, cheddar, sharp	2 tbsp.	70	5	0		🌢

Egg

	Portion	Calories	Total Fat	Dietary Fiber	Trans Fat	Guide
Chicken, Fresh, extra large	1 egg	90	6	0		🌢
Chicken, Fresh, large	1 egg	80	5	0		🌢
Chicken, Fresh, medium	1 egg	70	4	0		🌢
Chicken, Fresh, small	1 egg	60	4	0		🌢
Chicken, Fresh, white only	1 egg	17	0	0		✄
Chicken, Fresh, yolk only	1 egg	59	5	0		🌢
Chicken, fried w/butter	1 egg	91	7	0		🌢

☺ = *Eat as much as you want* • ✄ = *Cut Back*

	Portion	Calories	Total Fat	Dietary Fiber	Trans Fat	Guide
Chicken, poached in salt water	1 egg	74	5	0		🌢
Chicken, scrambled w/milk in butter	1 egg	110	8	0		🌢
Chicken, soft cooked	1 egg	80	5	0		🌢
Duck, Fresh, whole	1 egg	130	10	0		🌢
Goose, Fresh, whole	1 egg	267	19	0		🌢
Quail, Fresh, whole	1 egg	14	1	0		✂
Turkey, Fresh, whole	1 egg	135	9	0		🌢

Egg Substitute

	Portion	Calories	Total Fat	Dietary Fiber	Trans Fat	Guide
Fleischmann's, Egg Beaters	$1/4$ cup	30	0	0		✂
Healthy Choice, cholesterol free	$1/4$ cup	30	0	0		✂
Morningstar Farms, Better'n Eggs	$1/4$ cup	20	0	0		✂
Morningstar Farms, Scramblers	$1/4$ cup	35	0	0		✂
Papetti Foods, Better'n Eggs	$1/4$ cup	30	0	0		✂
Second Nature, Eggs, fat free	$1/4$ cup	30	0	0		✂

Ice Cream

	Portion	Calories	Total Fat	Dietary Fiber	Trans Fat	Guide
Ben & Jerry's, New York super fudge chunk	$1/2$ cup	290	20	2		🌢
Ben & Jerry's, cherry Garcia	$1/2$ cup	240	16	0		🌢
Ben & Jerry's, chocolate chip cookie dough	$1/2$ cup	270	17	0	T	🌢
Ben & Jerry's, chocolate fudge brownie	$1/2$ cup	260	13	2	T	🌢
Ben & Jerry's, chunky monkey	$1/2$ cup	280	19	1		🌢
Ben & Jerry's, coconut almond fudge chip	$1/2$ cup	310	22	2		🌢
Ben & Jerry's, coffee w/heath toffee crunch	$1/2$ cup	280	19	0	T	🌢
Ben & Jerry's, cool Britannia	$1/2$ cup	260	15	0	T	🌢
Ben & Jerry's, low fat, blackberry cobbler	$1/2$ cup	180	3	0		🌢
Ben & Jerry's, low fat, sweet cream & cookies	$1/2$ cup	170	3	0		🌢
Ben & Jerry's, mint chocolate cookie	$1/2$ cup	260	17	1	T	🌢
Ben & Jerry's, peanut butter & jelly	$1/2$ cup	280	16	0		🌢
Ben & Jerry's, peanut butter cup	$1/2$ cup	370	26	2	T	🌢
Ben & Jerry's, totally nuts	$1/2$ cup	310	21	0		🌢
Ben & Jerry's, vanilla caramel fudge	$1/2$ cup	280	17	1		🌢
Ben & Jerry's, wavy gravy	$1/2$ cup	330	24	2		🌢
Ben & Jerry's, world's best vanilla	$1/2$ cup	250	17	0		🌢
Breyers, butter pecan	$1/2$ cup	180	12	0		🌢
Breyers, caramel & cream, homemade	$1/2$ cup	160	8	0	T	🌢
Breyers, chocolate chip cookie dough	$1/2$ cup	180	10	0		🌢
Breyers, mint chocolate chip	$1/2$ cup	170	10	0		🌢
Breyers, mint chocolate chip, light	$1/2$ cup	140	5	0		🌢
Breyers, mint chocolate chip, no sugar added	$1/2$ cup	100	5	0		🌢
Breyers, peanut butter w/fudge swirls	$1/2$ cup	180	9	0		🌢
Breyers, strawberry, natural	$1/2$ cup	130	7	0		🌢
Breyers, vanilla & chocolate	$1/2$ cup	150	9	0		🌢
Breyers, vanilla chocolate strawberry	$1/2$ cup	150	8	0		🌢
Breyers, vanilla, French	$1/2$ cup	160	10	0		🌢
Breyers, vanilla, cherry	$1/2$ cup	150	8	0		🌢
Breyers, vanilla, fat free	$1/2$ cup	90	0	0		✂
Breyers, vanilla, homemade	$1/2$ cup	150	8	0		🌢
Breyers, vanilla, light	$1/2$ cup	130	5	0		🌢

🌢 = Avoid • 🌢 = Add for flavor

	Portion	Calories	Total Fat	Dietary Fiber	Trans Fat	Guide
Breyers, vanilla, natural	1/2 cup	150	9	0		🌢
Breyers, vanilla, no sugar added	1/2 cup	90	5	0		🌢
Edy's, Nestlé Toll House coffee jar	1/2 cup	180	9	0	T	🌢
Edy's, butter pecan, light, no sugar added	1/2 cup	110	5	0		🌢
Edy's, cherry chocolate chip	1/2 cup	150	8	0		🌢
Edy's, chocolate fudge mousse	1/2 cup	110	3	0		🌢
Edy's, chocolate fudge sundae	1/2 cup	170	9	0	T	🌢
Edy's, cookie dough	1/2 cup	170	9	0	T	🌢
Edy's, fat free, black cherry vanilla swrl	1/2 cup	100	0	0		✂
Edy's, fat free, caramel praline crunch	1/2 cup	120	0	0		✂
Edy's, fat free, chocolate brownie chunk	1/2 cup	130	0	1		✂
Edy's, fat free, chocolate fudge	1/2 cup	120	0	1		✂
Edy's, fat free, chocolate peanut butter chunk	1/2 cup	120	0	1		✂
Edy's, fat free, cookie chunk	1/2 cup	120	0	0		✂
Edy's, fat free, no sugar added, brwn sndae	1/2 cup	110	0	0	T	🌢
Edy's, fat free, no sugar added, choc fudge	1/2 cup	100	0	1		✂
Edy's, fat free, no sugar added, rspbry vnlla swrl	1/2 cup	90	0	0		✂
Edy's, fat free, no sugar added, vanilla	1/2 cup	90	0	0		✂
Edy's, fat free, no sugar added, vnlla choc swrl	1/2 cup	90	0	0		✂
Edy's, rocky road	1/2 cup	170	10	1		🌢
Edy's, vanilla, French	1/2 cup	160	10	0		🌢
Edy's, vanilla, homemade	1/2 cup	140	7	0		🌢
Edy's, vanilla, light	1/2 cup	100	3	0		🌢
Healthy Choice, cappuccino chocolate chunk	1/2 cup	120	2	1		✂
Healthy Choice, cookie creme de mint, fat free	1/2 cup	130	2	0		✂
Healthy Choice, cookies & cream	1/2 cup	120	2	0		✂
Healthy Choice, mint chocolate chip	1/2 cup	120	2	0		✂
Healthy Choice, praline & caramel	1/2 cup	130	2	0		✂
Healthy Choice, praline caramel cluster, low fat	1/2 cup	130	2	0		✂
Healthy Choice, rocky road	1/2 cup	140	2	0		✂
Healthy Choice, turtle fudge cake, low fat	1/2 cup	130	2	2	T	🌢
Häagen-Dazs, butter pecan	1/2 cup	310	23	0		🌢
Häagen-Dazs, chocolate	1/2 cup	270	18	1		🌢
Häagen-Dazs, coffee	1/2 cup	270	18	0		🌢
Häagen-Dazs, dulce de leche caramel	1/2 cup	290	17	0		🌢
Häagen-Dazs, macadamia brittle	1/2 cup	300	20	0		🌢
Häagen-Dazs, mint chip	1/2 cup	290	19	0		🌢
Häagen-Dazs, rum raisin	1/2 cup	270	17	0		🌢
Häagen-Dazs, strawberry	1/2 cup	250	16	0		🌢
Häagen-Dazs, strawberry, low fat	1/2 cup	150	2	0		✂
Häagen-Dazs, vanilla	1/2 cup	270	18	0		🌢
Häagen-Dazs, vanilla fudge	1/2 cup	290	18	0		🌢
Häagen-Dazs, vanilla, cherry	1/2 cup	240	15	0		🌢
Häagen-Dazs, vanilla, low fat	1/2 cup	170	3	0		🌢
Kemps, fat free, caramel praline crunch	1/2 cup	120	1	0		✂
Kemps, fat free, cookies 'n cream	1/2 cup	110	0	0		✂
Lactaid, vanilla, 70% lactose reduced	1/2 cup	160	9	0		🌢
Newman's Own, milk chocolate mud bath	1/2 cup	190	10	1		🌢
Newman's Own, obscene vanilla bean	1/2 cup	170	10	0		🌢

☺ = *Eat as much as you want* • ✂ = *Cut Back*

	Portion	Calories	Total Fat	Dietary Fiber	Trans Fat	Guide
Newman's Own, pistol packin' praline pecan	1/2 cup	200	11	0		🌢
Starbucks, caffe almond fudge	1/2 cup	250	13	1	T	🌢
Starbucks, chocolate chocolate fudge	1/2 cup	290	17	2		🌢
Starbucks, java chip	1/2 cup	250	13	0		🌢
Starbucks, low fat, latte	1/2 cup	170	3	0		🌢
Starbucks, low fat, mocha mambo	1/2 cup	170	3	0		🌢

Ice Cream, Bar

	Portion	Calories	Total Fat	Dietary Fiber	Trans Fat	Guide
Dove, dark dark chocolate	1 bar	260	17	0		🌢
Dove, french vanilla, bite size	5 bars	330	21	0		🌢
Dove, milk chocolate w/almonds	1 bar	280	19	1		🌢
Dove, milk chocolate w/vanilla	1 bar	260	17	0		🌢
Eskimo Pie, vanilla	1 bar	120	8	0		🌢
Good Humor, chocolate eclair	1 bar	170	9	1	T	🌢
Good Humor, premium ice cream bar	1 bar	190	12	0	T	🌢
Good Humor, strawberry shortcake	1 bar	160	7	0	T	🌢
Good Humor, toasted almond	1 bar	180	8	0	T	🌢
Häagen-Dazs, reduced fat, vanilla & milk chocolate	1 bar	230	13	0		🌢
Häagen-Dazs, mint dark chocolate	1 bar	290	20	1		🌢
Häagen-Dazs, reduced fat, vanilla caramel	1 bar	240	13	0		🌢
Häagen-Dazs, strawberry & white chocolate	1 bar	270	19	0		🌢
Häagen-Dazs, vanilla & almond	1 bar	320	23	1		🌢
Klondike, choco taco	1 bar	310	17	1	T	🌢
Klondike, krispy krunch	1 piece	300	19	0		🌢
Klondike, neapolitan	1 piece	280	19	0		🌢
Klondike, original	1 piece	290	20	0		🌢
Nestlé Crunch, reduced fat	1 bar	150	9	0		🌢
Nestlé Crunch, vanilla	1 bar	200	14	0	T	🌢
Snickers	1 bar	180	11	0		🌢
Starbucks, Frappuccino coffee low fat	1 bar	110	2	0		✂
Starbucks, Frappuccino coffee mocha	1 bar	120	2	0		✂
Starbucks, caffe almond roast	1 bar	280	18	1		🌢
Weight Watchers, Smart Ones, chocolate mousse	1 bar	40	1	1		✂
Weight Watchers, chocolate treat	1 bar	100	1	1		✂
Yoo-hoo, fudge bars	1 bar	70	0	0		✂

Ice Cream, Baskin Robbins

	Portion	Calories	Total Fat	Dietary Fiber	Trans Fat	Guide
Blast, cappuccino w/whipped cream	8 oz.	160	7	0	n.a.	🌢
Blast, chocolate w/whipped cream	8 oz.	250	7	0	n.a.	🌢
Blast, mocha cappy w/whipped cream	8 oz.	180	6	0	n.a.	🌢
Ice Cream, Regular Deluxe, chocolate	1/2 cup	150	9	0	n.a.	🌢
Ice Cream, Regular Deluxe, chocolate chip cookie dough	1/2 cup	170	9	0	n.a.	🌢
Ice Cream, Regular Deluxe, cookies 'n cream	1/2 cup	170	11	0	n.a.	🌢
Ice Cream, Regular Deluxe, jamoca	1/2 cup	140	9	0	n.a.	🌢
Ice Cream, Regular Deluxe, mint chocolate chip	1/2 cup	150	10	0	n.a.	🌢

🌢 = Avoid • 💧 = Add for flavor

	Portion	Calories	Total Fat	Dietary Fiber	Trans Fat	Guide
Ice Cream, Regular Deluxe, old fashion butter pecan	1/2 cup	160	11	0	n.a.	🌢
Ice Cream, Regular Deluxe, vanilla	$^1/_2$ cup	140	8	0	n.a.	🌢
Ice Cream, Regular Deluxe, very berry strawberry	1/2 cup	130	7	0	n.a.	🌢
Ice Cream, non fat, chocolate van twist	$^1/_2$ cup	100	0	0	n.a.	✂
Ice Cream, non fat, espresso 'n cream	$^1/_2$ cup	100	3	1	n.a.	🌢
Ice Cream, non fat, jamoca swirl	$^1/_2$ cup	110	0	0	n.a.	✂
Sherbet, orange	$^1/_2$ cup	120	2	0	n.a.	✂
Sherbet, rainbow	$^1/_2$ cup	120	2	0	n.a.	✂
Smoothies, aloha berry banana	8 oz.	180	0	1	n.a.	✂
Smoothies, sunset orange	8 oz.	150	0	2	n.a.	✂
Smoothies, tropical tango	8 oz.	190	0	1	n.a.	✂

Ice Cream, Cone

	Portion	Calories	Total Fat	Dietary Fiber	Trans Fat	Guide
Joy, cake	1 cup	20	0	0	T	🌢
Joy, sugar	1 cone	50	0	0	T	🌢
Keebler	1 cup	15	0	0	T	🌢
Keebler, fudge dipped	1 cone	35	2	0	T	🌢
Keebler, sugar	1 cone	50	2	0	T	🌢
Keebler, waffle bowl	1 bowl	50	1	0	T	🌢
Keebler, waffle cone	1 cone	50	1	0	T	🌢
Nabisco, Comet cups	1 cup	20	0	0	T	🌢
Nabisco, Comet rainbow cups	1 cup	20	0	0	T	🌢
Nabisco, Comet sugar cones	1 cone	60	0	0	T	🌢
Nabisco, Oreo chocolate cone	1 cone	50	1	0	T	🌢

Ice Cream, Dessert Cone

	Portion	Calories	Total Fat	Dietary Fiber	Trans Fat	Guide
Edy's, sundae cones, vanilla fudge	1 cone	240	11	1		🌢
Good Humor, premium sundae cone	1 cone	290	14	1	T	🌢
Nestle, Drumstick, supreme, triple chocolate	1 cone	260	13	2	T	🌢
Nestle, Drumstick, vanilla, reduced fat	1 cone	300	14	2	T	🌢
Snickers, Ice cream cones	1 cone	290	15	1	T	🌢

Ice Cream, Frozen Dessert

	Portion	Calories	Total Fat	Dietary Fiber	Trans Fat	Guide
Breyers, Viennetta	1 slice	190	11	0		🌢
Derring, Spumoni	1 slice	280	11	0		🌢
Nestlé, Bon Bons	8 pieces	350	25	0	T	🌢
Weight Watchers, Smart Ones, chocolate chip cookie dough sundae	1 dessert	190	5	1	T	🌢
Weight Watchers, Smart Ones, strawberry parfait royale	1 parfait	180	2	0		✂

Ice Cream, Fruit Bar

	Portion	Calories	Total Fat	Dietary Fiber	Trans Fat	Guide
Dole, Fruit 'n ice juice, strawberry	1 bar	70	0	0		✂
Dole, Fruit juice, sugar free	1 bar	25	0	0		✂
Edy's, strawberry	1 bar	90	0	0		✂
Minute Maid, Fruit Juicee, all flavors	1 bar	60	0	0		✂
Starburst, fruit juice, all flavors	1 bar	20	0	0		✂

☺ = Eat as much as you want • ✂ = Cut Back

	Portion	Calories	Total Fat	Dietary Fiber	Trans Fat	Guide
Tropicana, fruit juice, all flavors	1 bar	45	0	0		✂
Tropicana, orange cream	1 bar	70	1	0		✂
Welch's, fruit juice	1 bar	45	0	0		✂
Welch's, fruit juice, no sugar added, all flavors	1 bar	25	0	0		✂

Ice Cream, Ices

	Portion	Calories	Total Fat	Dietary Fiber	Trans Fat	Guide
Lemon chill	1 cup	130	0	0		✂
Luigi's, Italian ice, lemon, real	1 cup	110	0	0		✂
Mama Tish's, Italian ice, no sugar added, all flavors	4 oz.	70	0	0		✂
Mama Tish's, Italian ice, raspberry, premium	4 oz.	100	0	0		✂

Ice Cream, Pops

	Portion	Calories	Total Fat	Dietary Fiber	Trans Fat	Guide
Creamsicle, fat free	1 piece	60	0	0		✂
Flavor Ice	1 pop	30	0	0		✂
Fudgsicle, sugar free	1 piece	40	1	0		✂
Lifesavers, flavor pops, all flavors	1 bar	40	0	0		✂
Nestlé, Cool Creations, tiger tails	1 pop	60	0	0		✂
Nestlé, Push-Up, all flavors	1 tube	100	2	0		✂
Popsicle, Big Stick, all flavors	1 piece	60	0	0		✂
Popsicle, Tingle Twister	1 piece	45	0	0		✂
Popsicle, fantastic fruity	1 piece	60	0	0		✂
Popsicle, original, orange, grape & chrry	1 piece	45	0	0		✂
Popsicle, sugar free, all flavors	1 piece	15	0	0		✂

Ice Cream, Sandwich

	Portion	Calories	Total Fat	Dietary Fiber	Trans Fat	Guide
Betty Crocker, Healthy Temptations, snack sandwiches, low fat	1 sandwich	80	2	0	T	◓
Eskimo Pie, no sugar added	1 sandwich	160	4	0	T	◓
Klondike, Big Bear, ice cream cookie	1 sandwich	290	13	1	T	◓
Klondike, Big Bear, neapolitan	1 sandwich	200	7	0	T	◓
Klondike, Big Bear, premium	1 sandwich	200	7	0	T	◓
Mr. Cookie Face, chocolate vanilla swirl, low fat	1 sandwich	130	2	0		✂
Weight Watchers, vanilla	1 sandwich	150	3	1	T	◓

Ice Cream, Sherbet

	Portion	Calories	Total Fat	Dietary Fiber	Trans Fat	Guide
Lemon	1/2 cup	110	2	0		✂
Orange	1/2 cup	100	2	0		✂
Pineapple	1/2 cup	100	1	2		✂
Raspberry	1/2 cup	110	2	0		✂

Ice Cream, Sorbet

	Portion	Calories	Total Fat	Dietary Fiber	Trans Fat	Guide
Ben & Jerry's, Doonesberry, fat free	1/2 cup	130	0	0		✂
Ben & Jerry's, lemon swirl, fat free	1/2 cup	120	0	0		✂
Ben & Jerry's, purple passionfruit, fat free	1/2 cup	120	0	0		✂
Cascadian Farm Organic, orange	1/2 cup	120	3	0		◓
Cascadian Farm Organic, raspberry	1/2 cup	80	0	2		✂
Edy's, whole Fruit, peach	1/2 cup	130	0	1		✂
Edy's, whole Fruit, raspberry	1/2 cup	130	0	1		✂

◓ = Avoid • ◔ = Add for flavor

	Portion	Calories	Total Fat	Dietary Fiber	Trans Fat	Guide
Häagen-Dazs, chocolate	1/2 cup	120	0	2		✂
Häagen-Dazs, raspberry	1/2 cup	120	0	2		✂
Häagen-Dazs, vanilla	1/2 cup	120	0	0		✂
Häagen-Dazs, zesty lemon	1/2 cup	120	0	0		✂
Real Fruit Chunky, Georgia peach	1/2 cup	110	0	0		✂
Real Fruit Chunky, mountain strawberry	1/2 cup	100	0	0		✂
Real Fruit Chunky, wild berries	1/2 cup	110	0	0		✂

Milk

	Portion	Calories	Total Fat	Dietary Fiber	Trans Fat	Guide
Borden, egg nog	1/2 cup	160	9	0		💧
Buttermilk, cultured, fat free	8 oz.	80	0	0		✂
Buttermilk, lowfat 1%	1 cup	110	3	0		💧
Dairy Ease 100, 2% reduced fat, lactose free	1 cup	130	5	0		💧
Hershey's, chocolate, fat free	8 oz.	150	0	0		✂
Horizon Organic	1 cup	150	8	0		💧
Horizon Organic, 2% reduced fat	1 cup	120	5	0		💧
Lactaid 100, 100% lactose reduced, fat free	1 cup	90	0	0		✂
Lactaid 70, 70% lactose reduced	1 cup	110	3	0		💧
Milk, 2%	8 oz.	120	5	0		💧
Milk, Vitamin A & D, 1% milkfat	1 cup	100	3	0		💧
Milk, chocolate, 2% reduced fat	8 oz.	190	5	1		💧
Milk, fat free	8 oz.	80	0	0		✂
Milk, lowfat, 1% milkfat	1 cup	110	3	0		💧
Milk, whole	8 oz.	150	8	0		💧
Nestle Quik, chocolate	1 cup	230	8	1		💧
Parmalat, long life whole milk vitamin D	1 cup	160	8	0		💧
Vitamite, 2% fat, non-dairy lactose free	1 cup	110	5	0		💧
Yoo-Hoo, chocolate drink	8 oz.	130	1	0		✂

Milk Products, Cottage Cheese

	Portion	Calories	Total Fat	Dietary Fiber	Trans Fat	Guide
Axelrod, lowfat	1/2 cup	90	2	0		✂
Axelrod, lowfat, no salt, 1% milkfat	1/2 cup	90	1	0		✂
Axelrod, lowfat, pineapple	1/2 cup	120	2	0		✂
Axelrod, nonfat	1/2 cup	90	0	0		✂
Axelrod, w/added pineapple	1/2 cup	90	0	0		✂
Breakstone's, 2% milkfat, low fat	1/2 cup	90	3	0		💧
Breakstone's, 4% milkfat	1/2 cup	120	5	0		💧
Breakstone's, free	1/2 cup	80	0	0		✂
Cottage cheese, low fat, 1%	1/2 cup	80	1	0		✂
Cottage cheese, w/pineapple	1/2 cup	130	4	0		💧
Lactaid 70, low fat	1/2 cup	80	1	0		✂
Light 'n Lively, free	1/2 cup	80	0	0		✂
Light n' Lively	1/2 cup	80	2	0		✂

Milk Products, Cream

	Portion	Calories	Total Fat	Dietary Fiber	Trans Fat	Guide
Half & half	2 tbsp.	40	3	0		💧
Heavy whipping	1 tbsp.	50	5	0		💧
Land O Lakes, Gourmet, fat free	2 tbsp.	20	0	0		✂
Land O Lakes, Gourmet, half & half	2 tbsp.	40	4	0		💧

☺ = Eat as much as you want • ✂ = Cut Back

	Portion	Calories	Total Fat	Dietary Fiber	Trans Fat	Guide
Sweetened baker's cream	1 tbsp.	60	5	0		♠
Table	1 tbsp.	30	3	0		♠
Whipping	1 tbsp.	45	5	0		♠

Milk Products, Creamer, Dry

	Portion	Calories	Total Fat	Dietary Fiber	Trans Fat	Guide
Carnation, Coffee-mate	1 tsp.	10	1	0	T	♠
Carnation, Coffee-mate fat free	1 tsp.	10	0	0	T	♠
Carnation, Coffee-mate lite	1 tbsp.	10	1	0	T	♠
Carnation, Coffee-mate, French vanilla	1 tbsp.	40	2	0	T	♠
Carnation, Coffee-mate, French vanilla, fat free	1 tbsp.	25	0	0	T	♠
Carnation, Coffee-mate, Swiss chocolate	1 1/3 tbsp.	50	1	0	T	♠
Carnation, Coffee-mate, amaretto	1 1/3 tbsp.	60	3	0	T	♠
Carnation, Coffee-mate, hazelnut	1 tbsp.	40	2	0	T	♠
Carnation, Coffee-mate, hazelnut, fat free	1 tbsp.	25	0	0	T	♠
Creamer	1 tsp.	10	1	0	T	♠
Creamer, fat free	1 tsp.	10	0	0	T	♠
Creamer, light	1 tsp.	10	0	0	T	♠

Milk Products, Creamer, Refrigerated

	Portion	Calories	Total Fat	Dietary Fiber	Trans Fat	Guide
Carnation, Coffee-mate	1 tbsp.	20	1	0	T	♠
Carnation, Coffee-mate fat free, lactose & chol. free	1 tbsp.	10	0	0	T	♠
Carnation, Coffee-mate lactose & chol. free	1 tbsp.	20	1	0	T	♠
Carnation, Coffee-mate lite, lactose & chol. free	1 tbsp.	10	1	0	T	♠
Carnation, Coffee-mate, French vanilla	1 tbsp.	40	2	0	T	♠
Carnation, Coffee-mate, French vanilla, fat free	1 tbsp.	25	0	0	T	♠
Carnation, Coffee-mate, hazelnut	1 tbsp.	40	2	0	T	♠
Carnation, Coffee-mate, vanilla nut	1 tbsp.	40	2	0	T	♠
Creamer	1 tbsp.	20	2	0	T	♠
Creamer, light	1 tbsp.	10	1	0	T	♠
International Delight, French vanilla, fat free	1 tbsp.	30	0	0	T	♠
International Delight, Irish cream	1 tbsp.	35	2	0	T	♠
International Delight, Irish cream, fat free	1 tbsp.	30	0	0	T	♠
International Delight, Swiss chocolate	1 tbsp.	40	2	0	T	♠
International Delight, amaretto	1 tbsp.	35	2	0	T	♠
International Delight, amaretto, fat free	1 tbsp.	30	0	0	T	♠
International Delight, cafe de Mexico	1 tbsp.	40	2	0	T	♠
International Delight, cinnamon hazelnut	1 tbsp.	35	2	0	T	♠
International Delight, cinnamon hazelnut, fat free	1 tbsp.	30	0	0	T	♠
International Delight, southern butter pecan	1 tbsp.	35	2	0	T	♠
International Delight, vanilla toffee caramel	1 tbsp.	35	2	0	T	♠
Rich's, Coffee Rich	1 tbsp.	20	2	0	T	♠
Rich's, Farm Rich	1 tbsp.	20	2	0	T	♠
Rich's, Farm Rich fat free	1 tbsp.	10	0	0	T	♠

Milk Products, Sour Cream

	Portion	Calories	Total Fat	Dietary Fiber	Trans Fat	Guide
Axelrod	2 tbsp.	60	5	0		♠
Axelrod, light	2 tbsp.	40	3	0		♠

♠ = Avoid • ♭ = Add for flavor

	Portion	Calories	Total Fat	Dietary Fiber	Trans Fat	Guide
Axelrod, nonfat	2 tbsp.	20	0	0		✂
Breakstone's	2 tbsp.	60	5	0		●
Breakstone's, free, fat free	2 tbsp.	35	0	0		✂
Breakstone's, free, reduced fat	2 tbsp.	45	4	0		●
Land O Lakes, light	2 tbsp.	40	2	0		✂
Land O Lakes, no fat	2 tbsp.	30	0	0		✂
Land O Lakes, regular	2 tbsp.	60	6	0		●
Naturally Yours, fat free	2 tbsp.	20	0	0		✂

Milk, Condensed

	Portion	Calories	Total Fat	Dietary Fiber	Trans Fat	Guide
Borden, Eagle, creamy chocolate	2 tbsp.	120	3	0		●
Borden, Eagle, sweetened	2 tbsp.	130	3	0		●
Borden, Eagle, sweetened, fat free	2 tbsp.	110	0	0		✂
Carnation, sweetened	2 tbsp.	130	3	0		●
Condensed milk	2 tbsp.	130	3	0		●

Milk, Evaporated

	Portion	Calories	Total Fat	Dietary Fiber	Trans Fat	Guide
Carnation	2 tbsp.	40	2	0		✂
Carnation, fat free	2 tbsp.	25	0	0		✂
Evaporated milk	2 tbsp.	40	2	0		✂
Evaporated milk, fat free	2 tbsp.	25	0	0		✂
Pet	2 tbsp.	40	2	0		✂

Milk, Powdered

	Portion	Calories	Total Fat	Dietary Fiber	Trans Fat	Guide
Carnation, dry milk, non fat	$1/3$ cup dry	80	0	0		✂
Dry milk, non fat	$1/3$ cup	80	0	0		✂
Saco, cultured buttermilk blend	4 tbsp.	80	0	0		✂

Yogurt

	Portion	Calories	Total Fat	Dietary Fiber	Trans Fat	Guide
Breyers, Black cherry	1 container	230	2	0		✂
Breyers, Blueberry	8 oz.	220	2	0		✂
Breyers, Light Fat Free, apple pie a la mode	1 container	130	0	0		✂
Breyers, Light Fat Free, black cherry jubilee	1 container	130	0	0		✂
Breyers, Light Fat Free, blueberries 'n cream	1 container	130	0	0		✂
Breyers, Light Fat Free, cherry vanilla cream	8 oz.	130	0	0		✂
Breyers, Light Fat Free, classic strawberry	1 container	130	0	0		✂
Breyers, Light Fat Free, key lime pie	8 oz.	130	0	0		✂
Breyers, Light Fat Free, lemon chiffon	1 container	130	0	0		✂
Breyers, Light Fat Free, peaches 'n cream	1 container	130	0	0		✂
Breyers, Light Fat Free, raspberries 'n cream	8 oz.	130	0	0		✂
Breyers, Light Fat Free, strawberry chscake	1 container	130	0	0		✂
Breyers, Mixed berry	1 container	220	2	0		✂
Breyers, Peach	1 container	230	2	0		✂
Breyers, Peach a la mode	1 container	280	3	0		●
Breyers, Pineapple	1 container	230	2	0		✂
Breyers, Raspberry a la mode	1 container	280	3	0		●
Breyers, Red raspberry	1 container	220	2	0		✂
Breyers, Smooth & Creamy, black cherry parfait	8 oz.	240	2	0		✂

☺ = Eat as much as you want • ✂ = Cut Back

FOOD LISTS

	Portion	Calories	Total Fat	Dietary Fiber	Trans Fat	Guide
Breyers, Smooth & Creamy, classic strawberry	1 container	230	2	0		✂
Breyers, Smooth & Creamy, peaches 'n cream	8 oz.	230	2	0		✂
Breyers, Smooth & Creamy, raspberries 'n cream	8 oz.	230	2	0		✂
Breyers, Smooth & Creamy, strawbrry banana splt	1 container	240	2	0		✂
Breyers, Strawberry	1 container	220	2	0		✂
Breyers, Strawberry a la mode	1 container	280	3	0		●
Breyers, Strawberry banana	1 container	230	2	0		✂
Colombo, Classic Fat Free, cherry	8 oz.	200	0	0		✂
Colombo, Classic Fat Free, peach	8 oz.	200	0	0		✂
Colombo, Classic Fat Free, raspberry	8 oz.	200	0	0		✂
Colombo, Classic Fat Free, strawberry	8 oz.	200	0	0		✂
Dannon, Blended Fat Free, all flavors	1 container	110	0	0		✂
Dannon, Chunky Fruit Fat Free, blueberry	6 oz.	160	0	0		✂
Dannon, Chunky Fruit Fat Free, cherry vanilla	6 oz.	160	0	0		✂
Dannon, Chunky Fruit Fat Free, strawberry banana	6 oz.	160	0	0		✂
Dannon, Danimals, blueberry	4 oz.	130	1	0		✂
Dannon, Danimals, cherry	4 oz.	130	1	0		✂
Dannon, Danimals, vanilla	4 oz.	120	1	0		✂
Dannon, Double Delights, caramel praline	1 container	220	1	0		✂
Dannon, Double Delights, cherry cheesecake	1 container	170	1	0		✂
Dannon, Double Delights, chocolate cheesecake	1 container	220	1	0		✂
Dannon, Double Delights, chocolate eclair	1 container	220	1	0		✂
Dannon, Double Delights, lemon meringue pie	1 container	190	1	0		✂
Dannon, Double Delights, strawberry cheesecake	1 container	170	1	0		✂
Dannon, Light, blueberry	8 oz.	100	0	0		✂
Dannon, Light, cherry vanilla	8 oz.	100	0	0		✂
Dannon, Light, cookies 'n cream	8 oz.	130	0	0		✂
Dannon, Light, lemon blueberry cobbler	8 oz.	140	0	0		✂
Dannon, Light, peach	8 oz.	100	0	0		✂
Dannon, Light, raspberry	8 oz.	100	0	0		✂
Dannon, Light, strawberry banana	8 oz.	100	0	0		✂
Dannon, Light, strawberry kiwi	8 oz.	100	0	0		✂
Dannon, Sprinkl'ins w/magic crystals	1 container	110	1	0		✂
Dannon, blueberry	8 oz.	240	3	0		●
Dannon, cherry	8 oz.	240	3	0		●
Dannon, fat free, plain	8 oz.	110	0	0		✂
Dannon, raspberry	8 oz.	240	3	0		●
Dannon, strawberry	8 oz.	230	3	0		●
Dannon, strawberry banana	8 oz.	230	3	0		●
Horizon Organic, non fat, blueberry	3/4 cup	120	0	1		✂
Horizon Organic, non fat, raspberry	3/4 cup	110	0	0		✂
Horizon Organic, non fat, strawberry	3/4 cup	110	0	0		✂
Horizon Organic, plain	3/4 cup	80	0	0		✂
La Yogurt, peach	6 oz.	170	2	0		✂
La Yogurt, raspberry	6 oz.	170	2	0		✂

● = Avoid • ◌ = Add for flavor

	Portion	Calories	Total Fat	Dietary Fiber	Trans Fat	Guide
La Yogurt, strawberry	6 oz.	170	2	0		✂
La Yogurt, strawberry banana	6 oz.	170	2	0		✂
La Yogurt, white chocolate almond	6 oz.	170	3	0		⬤
SnackWell's, double chocolate	³/₄ cup	190	0	0		✂
SnackWell's, milk chocolate	³/₄ cup	160	0	0		✂
SnackWell's, milk chocolate almond	³/₄ cup	160	0	1		✂
SnackWell's, milk chocolate caramel nut	³/₄ cup	160	0	1		✂
SnackWell's, milk chocolate cheesecake	3/4 cup	160	0	1		✂
Stonyfield Farm, French vanilla	8 oz.	160	0	0		✂
Stonyfield Farm, Lotsa lemon	8 oz.	160	0	0		✂
Stonyfield Farm, apricot mango	8 oz.	160	0	0		✂
Stonyfield Farm, fat free, blueberry	8 oz.	160	0	0		✂
Stonyfield Farm, fat free, strawberry fields	8 oz.	160	0	0		✂
Yoplait, Custard Style, adventure pack	1 container	120	2	0		✂
Yoplait, Custard Style, banana	6 oz.	190	3	0		⬤
Yoplait, Custard Style, blueberries & cream	6 oz.	190	4	0		⬤
Yoplait, Custard Style, key lime pie	6 oz.	190	4	0		⬤
Yoplait, Custard Style, vanilla	6 oz.	190	3	0		⬤
Yoplait, Light Fat Free, harvest peach	6 oz.	90	0	0		✂
Yoplait, Light Fat Free, strawberry	6 oz.	90	0	0		✂
Yoplait, Trix	1 container	130	2	0		✂

Yogurt, Frozen

	Portion	Calories	Total Fat	Dietary Fiber	Trans Fat	Guide
Ben & Jerry's, coffee almond fudge	¹/₂ cup	180	5	1		⬤
Ben & Jerry's, low fat, brownie	¹/₂ cup	180	2	2	T	⬤
Ben & Jerry's, low fat, cherry Garcia	¹/₂ cup	170	3	0		⬤
Ben & Jerry's, vanilla w/Heath toffee crunch	¹/₂ cup	210	6	0	T	⬤
Breyers, vanilla, chocolate, strawberry	¹/₂ cup	120	3	0		⬤
Breyers, vanilla, natural	¹/₂ cup	120	3	0		⬤
Cascadian Farm Organic, apple streudel	¹/₂ cup	130	3	0		⬤
Cascadian Farm Organic, harvest berry	¹/₂ cup	120	2	1		✂
Colombo, non fat, strawberry	¹/₂ cup	110	0	0		✂
Dannon, Fat Free Light, cappuccino	¹/₂ cup	80	0	0		✂
Dannon, Fat Free Light, chocolate	¹/₂ cup	80	0	0		✂
Dannon, Fat Free Light, vanilla	¹/₂ cup	80	0	0		✂
Dannon, Light n' Crunchy, triple chocolate	¹/₂ cup	110	1	0		✂
Edy's, Heath toffee crunch	¹/₂ cup	120	4	0	T	⬤
Edy's, cherry chocolate chunk	¹/₂ cup	110	3	0		⬤
Edy's, chocolate brownie chunk	¹/₂ cup	120	4	1		⬤
Edy's, cookies 'n cream	¹/₂ cup	110	3	0	T	⬤
Edy's, fat free, black cherry vanilla swirl	¹/₂ cup	90	0	0		✂
Edy's, fat free, caramel praline crunch	¹/₂ cup	100	0	0		✂
Edy's, fat free, chocolate silk mousse	¹/₂ cup	90	0	1		✂
Edy's, fat free, coffee fudge sundae	¹/₂ cup	100	0	0		✂
Edy's, fat free, vanilla	¹/₂ cup	90	0	0		✂
Edy's, fat free, vanilla chocolate swirl	¹/₂ cup	80	0	1		✂
Edy's, vanilla	¹/₂ cup	100	3	0		⬤
Häagen-Dazs, vanilla fudge	¹/₂ cup	160	0	0		✂
Häagen-Dazs, vanilla raspberry swirl	¹/₂ cup	130	0	0		✂

☺ = Eat as much as you want • ✂ = Cut Back

	Portion	Calories	Total Fat	Dietary Fiber	Trans Fat	Guide
Kemps, fat free, chocolate	$^1/_2$ cup	100	0	0		✂
Kemps, fat free, neapolitan	$^1/_2$ cup	100	0	0		✂
Kemps, fat free, peach	$^1/_2$ cup	90	0	0		✂
Kemps, fat free, vanilla	$^1/_2$ cup	100	0	0		✂
Kemps, pralines 'n caramel	$^1/_2$ cup	150	4	0		🌢

■ DESSERTS, TOPPINGS & BAKING INGREDIENTS

Baking Ingredients, Baking Mix

Betty Crocker, Bisquick	$^1/_3$ cup	170	6	0	T	🌢
Betty Crocker, Bisquick, reduced fat	$^1/_3$ cup	150	3	0	T	🌢
Gold Medal, Wondra flour	$^1/_4$ cup	100	0	0		✂
Jiffy	$^1/_4$ cup	130	5	1	T	🌢

Baking Ingredients, Baking Powder

Calumet, double acting	$^1/_4$ tsp.	0	0	0		👆

Baking Ingredients, Baking Soda

Arm & Hammer	$^1/_8$ tsp.	0	0	0		👆

Baking Ingredients, Chocolate, Baking

Baker's, German's sweet chocolate	2 squares	60	4	0		🌢
Baker's, semi-sweet chocolate	$^1/_2$ square	70	5	1		🌢
Baker's, unsweetened squares	$^1/_2$ square	70	7	2		🌢
Baker's, white chocolate, premium	$^1/_2$ square	80	5	0		🌢
Hershey's, unsweetened	$^1/_2$ bar	90	7	2		🌢
Nestlé, Toll House, premier white	$^1/_2$ oz.	80	5	0	T	🌢
Nestlé, Toll House, semi-sweet	$^1/_2$ oz.	70	4	2		🌢
Nestlé, Toll House, unsweetened	$^1/_2$ oz.	80	7	3		🌢

Baking Ingredients, Chocolate, Chip/Morsel

Ghirardelli, semi-sweet chocolate	1 $^1/_3$ tbsp.	70	4	1		🌢
Heath, Bits' o Brickle	1 tbsp.	80	5	0	T	🌢
Hershey's, milk chocolate chips	1 tbsp.	80	5	0		🌢
Hershey's, mini-kisses	11 pieces	80	5	0		🌢
Hershey's, reduced fat, baking chips semi-sweet chocolate	1 tbsp.	60	4	0		🌢
M & M's, milk chocolate mini	$^1/_2$ oz.	70	4	0		🌢
Nestlé, Toll House, butterscotch morsels	1 tbsp.	80	4	0	T	🌢
Nestlé, Toll House, milk chocolate morsels	1 tbsp.	70	4	0		🌢
Nestlé, Toll House, premier white morsels	1 tbsp.	80	4	0	T	🌢
Nestlé, Toll House, semi-sweet choc, mega	1 tbsp.	70	4	2		🌢
Reese's, peanut butter chips	1 tbsp.	80	4	0	T	🌢

Baking Ingredients, Cocoa

Hershey's, European-style Dutch	1 tbsp.	20	1	1		✂
Hershey's, cocoa	1 tbsp.	20	1	1		✂

🌢 = Avoid • 👆 = Add for flavor

	Portion	Calories	Total Fat	Dietary Fiber	Trans Fat	Guide
Baking Ingredients, Coconut Flake						
Baker's, Angel Flake	2 tbsp.	70	5	1		🌢
Baking Ingredients, Corn Starch						
Argo	1 tbsp.	30	0	0		✂
Cream, pure	1 tbsp.	40	0	0		✂
Baking Ingredients, Corn Syrup						
Karo, dark	2 tbsp.	120	0	0		✂
Karo, light	2 tbsp.	120	0	0		✂
King	2 tbsp.	125	0	0		✂
Baking Ingredients, Crumbs						
Cracker Meal, cracker crumbs	$1/4$ cup	110	0	1		✂
Nabisco, Honey Maid, graham cracker crumbs	$2 1/2$ tbsp.	70	2	0	T	🌢
Salerno, graham cracker crumbs	3 tbsp.	80	2	0	T	🌢
Sunshine, graham cracker crumbs	3 tbsp.	80	2	0	T	🌢
Baking Ingredients, Filling						
Gourmet Award, almond paste	2 oz.	298	10	4		🌢
Gourmet Award, marzipan	2 oz.	298	10	4		🌢
Solo, almond	2 tbsp.	120	3	2		🌢
Solo, poppyseed	2 tbsp.	140	4	3		🌢
Solo, prune plum, lekvar	2 tbsp.	80	0	2		✂
Baking Ingredients, Marshmallow Creme						
Jet-Puffed	2 tbsp.	40	0	0		✂
Baking Ingredients, Pie Crust						
Betty Crocker, Mix	$1/8$ crust	110	8	0	T	🌢
Jiffy, Mix	$1/4$ cup	180	10	0	T	🌢
Keebler, Ready Crust, Hershey's chocolate	$1/8$ crust	110	5	0	T	🌢
Keebler, Ready Crust, graham cracker	$1/10$ crust	130	6	0	T	🌢
Keebler, Ready Crust, graham cracker, reduced fat	$1/8$ crust	100	3	0	T	🌢
Keebler, Ready Crust, shortbread	$1/8$ crust	100	5	0	T	🌢
Nabisco, Oreo crust	$1/6$ crust	140	7	1	T	🌢
Pillsbury, pie shell, deep dish, frozen	$1/8$ crust	90	5	0	T	🌢
Pillsbury, refrigerated dough	$1/8$ crust	120	7	0	T	🌢
Baking Ingredients, Yeast						
Redstar, active dry	$1/4$ tsp.	0	0	0		☺
Desserts, Brownie						
Entenmann's, Light, fudge brownies	$1/10$ strip	110	0	1		✂
Entenmann's, Ultimate fudge brownies	1 brownie	220	13	2		🌢
Hostess, Brownie Bites	3 pieces	170	9	1	T	🌢
Little Debbie, Brownie Lights	1 brownie	190	3	1	T	🌢

☺ = Eat as much as you want • ✂ = Cut Back

	Portion	Calories	Total Fat	Dietary Fiber	Trans Fat	Guide
Little Debbie, Fudge Brownies	1 brownie	270	13	0	T	🌢
SnackWell's, Fudge Brownies	1 brownie	130	2	1	T	🌢

Desserts, Brownie Mix

	Portion	Calories	Total Fat	Dietary Fiber	Trans Fat	Guide
Betty Crocker, Stir'n Bake	$1/6$ pkg.	220	8	1	T	🌢
Betty Crocker, Sweet Rewards, fudge brownie	$1/18$ pkg.	130	3	1	T	🌢
Betty Crocker, Sweet Rewards, supreme, reduced fat	$1/20$ pkg.	120	1	0	T	🌢
Betty Crocker, chocolate chunk supreme	$1/20$ pkg.	130	3	0	T	🌢
Betty Crocker, dark chocolate supreme	$1/20$ pkg.	120	2	0	T	🌢
Betty Crocker, original supreme	$1/20$ pkg.	120	2	0	T	🌢
Duncan Hines, Chocolate Lovers, chewy fudge	$1/20$ pkg.	120	2	1	T	🌢
Duncan Hines, Chocolate Lovers, double fudge	$1/20$ pkg.	140	4	0	T	🌢
Duncan Hines, fudge, chewy	1 brownie	170	8	1	T	🌢
Duncan Hines, milk chocolate chunk	1 brownie	170	7	0	T	🌢
Pillsbury, Thick'n Fudgy, chocolate chunk deluxe	$1/16$ pkg.	120	4	0	T	🌢
Pillsbury, Thick'n Fudgy, double chocolate deluxe	$1/16$ pkg.	120	3	0	T	🌢
Pillsbury, Thick'n Fudgy, walnut	$1/12$ pkg.	190	5	1	T	🌢
Pillsbury, Thick'n Fudgy, walnut deluxe	$1/12$ pkg.	150	5	1	T	🌢
SnackWell's, fudge, low fat	$1/12$ pkg.	150	3	1	T	🌢

Desserts, Cake

	Portion	Calories	Total Fat	Dietary Fiber	Trans Fat	Guide
Entenmann's, all butter French crumb cake	$1/8$ cake	210	10	0		🌢
Entenmann's, all butter loaf	$1/6$ loaf	210	9	0		🌢
Entenmann's, apple orchard delight	$1/8$ cake	260	10	1	T	🌢
Entenmann's, cheese coffee cake	$1/8$ cake	160	7	1	T	🌢
Entenmann's, cheese filled crumb coffee cake	$1/8$ cake	200	10	0	T	🌢
Entenmann's, chocolate fudge	$1/6$ cake	310	14	2	T	🌢
Entenmann's, crumb coffee cake	$1/10$ cake	250	12	1	T	🌢
Entenmann's, iced devil's food	$1/6$ cake	340	17	1	T	🌢
Entenmann's, light, Louisiana crunch, fat free	$1/6$ cake	210	0	0		✂
Entenmann's, light, banana loaf	$1/8$ loaf	140	0	1		✂
Entenmann's, light, chocolate loaf	$1/8$ loaf	120	0	1		✂
Entenmann's, light, cinnamon apple coffee	$1/9$ cake	120	0	2		✂
Entenmann's, light, crumb delight	$1/9$ cake	210	6	1	T	🌢
Entenmann's, light, fudge iced chocolate cake	$1/6$ cake	190	0	2		✂
Entenmann's, light, golden loaf	$1/8$ loaf	130	0	0		✂
Entenmann's, light, marble loaf	$1/8$ loaf	130	0	0		✂
Entenmann's, light, marshmallow iced devil's food	$1/6$ cake	190	0	1		✂
Entenmann's, marshmallow iced devil's food	$1/6$ cake	340	18	0	T	🌢
Entenmann's, ultimate crumb cake	$1/10$ cake	250	13	0	T	🌢

Desserts, Cake Mix

	Portion	Calories	Total Fat	Dietary Fiber	Trans Fat	Guide
Aunt Jemima, coffee	$1/8$ pkg.	180	5	1	T	🌢
Betty Crocker, Stir'n Bake, carrot cake w/cream cheese frosting	$1/6$ pkg.	250	7	0	T	🌢

🌢 = Avoid • 🌢 = Add for flavor

	Portion	Calories	Total Fat	Dietary Fiber	Trans Fat	Guide
Betty Crocker, Stir'n Bake, coffee cake, w/cinnamon streusel	$1/6$ pkg.	200	6	0	T	🌢
Betty Crocker, Stir'n Bake, devil's food w/chocolate frosting	$1/6$ pkg.	240	4	1	T	🌢
Betty Crocker, Super Moist, French vanilla	$1/12$ pkg.	250	3	0	T	🌢
Betty Crocker, Super Moist, German chocolate	$1/12$ pkg.	250	4	0	T	🌢
Betty Crocker, Super Moist, butter recipe yellow	$1/12$ pkg.	260	2	0	T	🌢
Betty Crocker, Super Moist, carrot	$1/10$ pkg.	320	3	0	T	🌢
Betty Crocker, Super Moist, chocolate fudge	$1/12$ pkg.	270	3	1	T	🌢
Betty Crocker, Super Moist, double chocolate swirl	$1/12$ pkg.	250	4	1	T	🌢
Betty Crocker, Sweet Rewards, lemon	$1/8$ pkg.	170	0	0		✂
Betty Crocker, angel food	$1/12$ pkg.	140	0	0		✂
Betty Crocker, pound	$1/8$ pkg.	270	7	0	T	🌢
Dromedary, pound	$1/8$ cake	260	8	0	T	🌢
Duncan Hines, Moist Deluxe, French vanilla	$1/12$ pkg.	250	11	0	T	🌢
Duncan Hines, Moist Deluxe, butter recipe golden	$1/10$ pkg.	320	16	2	T	🌢
Duncan Hines, Moist Deluxe, dark chocolate fudge	$1/12$ pkg.	290	15	1	T	🌢
Duncan Hines, Moist Deluxe, fudge marble	$1/12$ pkg.	250	11	0	T	🌢
Duncan Hines, Moist Deluxe, pineapple supreme	$1/12$ pkg.	250	11	0	T	🌢
Duncan Hines, Moist Deluxe, white	$1/12$ pkg.	190	6	0	T	🌢
Duncan Hines, Moist Deluxe, yellow	$1/12$ pkg.	250	11	0	T	🌢
Duncan Hines, angel food	$1/12$ pkg.	140	0	0		✂
Jell-O, cheesecake, cherry	$1/8$ pkg.	340	4	0	T	🌢
Jell-O, cheesecake, real	$1/6$ cake	360	5	1	T	🌢
Jell-O, cheesecake, strawberry swirl, reduced fat	$1/8$ pkg.	250	2	0	T	🌢
Jell-O, chocolate silk pie	$1/6$ pkg.	310	5	1	T	🌢
Jell-O, cookies & cream dessert	$1/6$ pkg.	390	8	1	T	🌢
Jell-O, double layer chocolate dessert	$1/8$ pkg.	260	4	1	T	🌢
Jell-O, peanut butter cup dessert	$1/8$ pkg.	380	15	1	T	🌢
Pillsbury, Moist Supreme, devils food	$1/12$ pkg.	270	4	1	T	🌢
Pillsbury, Moist Supreme, funfetti	$1/12$ pkg.	240	5	0	T	🌢
Pillsbury, Moist Supreme, lemon	$1/10$ pkg.	300	4	1	T	🌢
Pillsbury, Moist Supreme, yellow	$1/12$ pkg.	240	4	0	T	🌢
Pillsbury, streusel coffee, choc chip	$1/16$ pkg.	270	6	0	T	🌢

Desserts, Cake, Frozen

	Portion	Calories	Total Fat	Dietary Fiber	Trans Fat	Guide
Oregon Farms, carrot	$1/6$ cake	280	15	3	T	🌢
Pepperidge Farm, 3 Layer	$1/8$ cake	250	12	0	T	🌢
Pepperidge Farm, cream cheese carrot	$1/9$ cake	320	20	1	T	🌢
Sara Lee, cheesecake, French	$1/5$ cake	410	25	1	T	🌢
Sara Lee, cheesecake, strawberry French	$1/6$ cake	320	14	1	T	🌢
Sara Lee, chocolate swirl	$1/4$ cake	330	16	0	T	🌢
Sara Lee, coffee, butter streusel	$1/6$ cake	220	12	0		🌢
Sara Lee, coffee, pecan	$1/6$ cake	230	12	0	T	🌢
Sara Lee, double chocolate layer	$1/8$ cake	260	13	2	T	🌢
Sara Lee, flaky coconut layer	$1/8$ cake	280	14	2	T	🌢

☺ = Eat as much as you want • ✂ = Cut Back

	Portion	Calories	Total Fat	Dietary Fiber	Trans Fat	Guide
Sara Lee, pound, all butter	1/4 cake	320	16	0	T	🌰

Desserts, Cupcake

	Portion	Calories	Total Fat	Dietary Fiber	Trans Fat	Guide
Entenmann's, light, creme filled chocolate	1 cupcake	160	0	1		✂
Hostess Cupcakes, chocolate	1 cake	180	6	1	T	🌰
Hostess, lights, chocolate	1 cake	140	2	0	T	🌰
Hostess, orange flavored	1 cake	160	5	0	T	🌰
Little Debbie, chocolate creme-filled	1 cupcake	180	9	0	T	🌰
Little Debbie, strawberry creme-filled	1 cupcake	200	9	0	T	🌰
Tastykake, chocolate	2 cakes	200	6	1	T	🌰
Tastykake, creme filled chocolate	2 cakes	230	8	1	T	🌰

Desserts, Jell-O

	Portion	Calories	Total Fat	Dietary Fiber	Trans Fat	Guide
Hunt's, Juicygels, raspberry/mixed berry	1 cup	100	0	0		✂
Hunt's, Juicygels, strawberry/orange	1 cup	100	0	0		✂
Jell-O, Americana custard dessert	1/4 pkg.	80	0	0		✂
Jell-O, gelatin Snacks, all flavors	1 snack	70	0	0		👍
Jell-O, gelatin Snacks, sugar free, strawberry	1 snack	10	0	0		👍
Jell-O, naturally fat free, assorted flavors	1/4 pkg.	80	0	0		✂
Jell-O, sugar free, all flavors	1/4 pkg.	10	0	0		👍
Knox, drinking gelatin for nails	1 env.	35	0	0		👍
Knox, original unflavored gelatin	1 env.	25	0	0		👍

Desserts, Other

	Portion	Calories	Total Fat	Dietary Fiber	Trans Fat	Guide
Baklava	2.5 pieces	540	31	2	T	🌰
Dessert shells	2 shells	150	2	0		✂
Entenmann's, apple puffs	1 puff	260	13	1	T	🌰
Entenmann's, guava cheese puffs	1 puff	290	16	1	T	🌰
Entenmann's, homestyle apple pie	1/6 pie	300	13	2	T	🌰
Rich's, eclairs, frozen	1 eclair	190	9	0	T	🌰

Desserts, Pie, Frozen

	Portion	Calories	Total Fat	Dietary Fiber	Trans Fat	Guide
Mrs. Smith's, Boston cream	1/8 pie	180	7	0	T	🌰
Mrs. Smith's, French silk chocolate	1/9 pie	560	40	2	T	🌰
Mrs. Smith's, apple cobbler	1/8 cobbler	240	9	3	T	🌰
Mrs. Smith's, apple, Dutch crumb	1/8 pie	350	14	1	T	🌰
Mrs. Smith's, apple, deep dish	1/10 pie	370	16	2	T	🌰
Mrs. Smith's, banana cream	1/4 pie	290	15	1	T	🌰
Mrs. Smith's, cherry	1/8 pie	310	14	1	T	🌰
Mrs. Smith's, chocolate cream	1/4 pie	330	17	1	T	🌰
Mrs. Smith's, key lime, authentic	1/9 pie	420	19	0	T	🌰
Mrs. Smith's, lemon cream	1/4 pie	300	15	0	T	🌰
Mrs. Smith's, lemon meringue	1/5 pie	300	8	0	T	🌰
Mrs. Smith's, peach cobbler	1/8 cobbler	240	9	3	T	🌰
Mrs. Smith's, peach, deep dish	1/10 pie	330	14	1	T	🌰
Sara Lee, apple, Dutch	1/8 pie	350	15	2	T	🌰
Sara Lee, chocolate silk supreme	1/5 pie	500	32	2	T	🌰
Sara Lee, coconut cream	1/5 pie	480	31	2	T	🌰
Sara Lee, lemon meringue	1/6 pie	350	11	5	T	🌰

🌰 = *Avoid* • 👍 = *Add for flavor*

	Portion	Calories	Total Fat	Dietary Fiber	Trans Fat	Guide

Desserts, Pudding Cup

	Portion	Calories	Total Fat	Dietary Fiber	Trans Fat	Guide
Healthy Choice, low fat, French vanilla	1 cup	110	2	0	T	🌢
Healthy Choice, low fat, double chocolate fudge	1 cup	110	2	0	T	🌢
Hunt's, Snack Pack fat free, chocolate	1 cup	90	0	0		✂
Hunt's, Snack Pack fat free, tapioca	1 cup	90	0	0		✂
Hunt's, Snack Pack fat free, vanilla	1 cup	80	0	0		✂
Hunt's, Snack Pack, chocolate	1 cup	140	5	0	T	🌢
Hunt's, Snack Pack, milk chocolate variety swirl	1 cup	140	5	0	T	🌢
Hunt's, Snack Pack, tapioca	1 cup	130	4	0	T	🌢
Hunt's, Snack Pack, vanilla	1 cup	130	5	0	T	🌢
Jell-O, cheesecake snacks, blueberry	1 snack	140	5	0	T	🌢
Jell-O, cheesecake snacks, strawberry	1 snack	150	5	0	T	🌢
Jell-O, fat free, chocolate	1 snack	100	0	0		✂
Jell-O, fat free, chocolate vanilla swirls	1 snack	100	0	0		✂
Kozy Shack, banana	4 oz.	130	3	0		🌢
Kozy Shack, chocolate	4 oz.	140	4	1		🌢
Kozy Shack, chocolate, lite	1 container	110	1	1		✂
Kozy Shack, flan cream caramel	4 oz.	150	4	0		🌢
Kozy Shack, rice	4 oz.	130	3	1		🌢
Kraft, Handi-Snacks, butterscotch	1 snack	130	5	0	T	🌢
Kraft, Handi-Snacks, chocolate	1 snack	130	5	0	T	🌢
Kraft, Handi-Snacks, chocolate fudge	1 snack	130	5	0	T	🌢
Kraft, Handi-Snacks, tapioca	1 snack	120	4	0	T	🌢
Kraft, Handi-Snacks, vanilla	1 snack	140	5	0	T	🌢
Swiss Miss, Pie Lovers, chocolate cream pie	1 cup	150	6	0	T	🌢
Swiss Miss, Pie Lovers, coconut cream pie	1 cup	150	7	0	T	🌢
Swiss Miss, butterscotch	1 cup	130	5	0	T	🌢
Swiss Miss, chocolate	1 cup	150	5	0	T	🌢
Swiss Miss, fat free, chocolate	1 cup	90	0	0		✂
Swiss Miss, fat free, tapioca	1 cup	90	0	0		✂
Swiss Miss, vanilla	1 cup	140	5	0	T	🌢
Tapioca cup	1 cup	130	4	0	T	🌢

Desserts, Pudding Mix

	Portion	Calories	Total Fat	Dietary Fiber	Trans Fat	Guide
Alsa, mousse mix, milk chocolate	2 1/2 tbsp.	90	4	0	T	🌢
Alsa, mousse mix, white chocolate	2 tbsp.	70	4	0	T	🌢
Jell-O, Cook & Serve, butterscotch	1/4 pkg.	100	0	0		✂
Jell-O, Cook & Serve, chocolate	1/4 pkg.	90	0	1		✂
Jell-O, Cook & Serve, lemon	1/6 pkg.	50	0	0	T	🌢
Jell-O, Cook & Serve, vanilla	1/4 pkg.	80	0	0		✂
Jell-O, instant, banana cream	1/4 pkg.	90	0	0		✂
Jell-O, instant, chocolate	1/4 pkg.	100	0	1		✂
Jell-O, instant, fat free sugar free, banana cream	1/4 pkg.	25	0	0		✂
Jell-O, instant, fat free sugar free, chocolate fudge	1/4 pkg.	35	0	1		✂
Jell-O, instant, fat free sugar free, vanilla	1/4 pkg.	25	0	0		✂
Jell-O, instant, fat free, vanilla	1/4 pkg.	90	0	0		✂
Jell-O, instant, lemon	1/4 pkg.	90	0	0		✂

☺ = Eat as much as you want • ✂ = Cut Back

	Portion	Calories	Total Fat	Dietary Fiber	Trans Fat	Guide
Jell-O, instant, pistachio	1/4 pkg.	100	1	0		✂
Jell-O, instant, stir 'n snack, chocolate	1 scoop	100	0	0		✂
Jell-O, instant, vanilla	1/4 pkg.	90	0	0		✂
Jell-O, instant, white chocolate	1/4 pkg.	90	0	0		✂
Minute, tapioca, quick cooking	1 1/2 tsp.	20	0	0		✂
Nestlé, mousse mix, milk chocolate	1/4 pkg.	90	3	2	T	🌢
Nestlé, mousse mix, milk chocolate Irish creme	1/4 pkg.	90	3	2	T	🌢
Sans Sucre, mousse mix, cheesecake, low fat	1/8 pkg.	60	2	0	T	🌢
Sans Sucre, mousse mix, chocolate, low fat	1/8 pkg.	50	3	1	T	🌢

Desserts, Snack Bar Mix

	Portion	Calories	Total Fat	Dietary Fiber	Trans Fat	Guide
Betty Crocker, Sunkist lemon	1/16 pkg.	140	4	0	T	🌢
Pillsbury, Oreo	1/18 pkg.	180	4	0	T	🌢

Desserts, Snack Cake

	Portion	Calories	Total Fat	Dietary Fiber	Trans Fat	Guide
Hostess Fruit Pie, apple	1 pie	480	22	2	T	🌢
Hostess Fruit Pie, blueberry	1 pie	480	21	2	T	🌢
Hostess Fruit Pie, cherry	1 pie	470	22	1	T	🌢
Hostess Fruit Pie, lemon	1 pie	500	24	0	T	🌢
Hostess HoHos	3 cakes	380	18	2		🌢
Hostess King Dons	2 cakes	340	17	2	T	🌢
Hostess Lights, cinnamon crumb cake	1 cake	90	1	0	T	🌢
Hostess Suzy Q's	1 cake	230	9	1	T	🌢
Hostess Twinkies	1 cake	150	5	0	T	🌢
Hostess Twinkies, lights	1 cake	130	2	0		✂
Little Debbie, Apple Flips	1 cookie	150	5	0	T	🌢
Little Debbie, Apple Streusel Coffee Cake	2 cakes	230	7	0	T	🌢
Little Debbie, Banana Twins	2 cakes	250	10	0	T	🌢
Little Debbie, Breakfast, muffin loaves, banana nut	1 muffin	220	10	0	T	🌢
Little Debbie, Breakfast, muffin loaves, bluberry	1 muffin	230	11	0	T	🌢
Little Debbie, Caramel Cookie Bars	1 cookie	160	8	0	T	🌢
Little Debbie, Chocolate Chip Cakes	2 cakes	290	14	1	T	🌢
Little Debbie, Coconut Creme Cakes	1 cake	210	10	0	T	🌢
Little Debbie, Coconut Rounds w/creme jelly	1 cookie	150	7	0	T	🌢
Little Debbie, Devil Squares	2 cakes	270	13	1	T	🌢
Little Debbie, Donut Sticks	1 donut	220	13	0	T	🌢
Little Debbie, Fig Bars	1 cookie	150	4	1	T	🌢
Little Debbie, Frosted Fudge Fake	1 cake	200	10	0	T	🌢
Little Debbie, Fudge Rounds	1 cookie	140	6	0	T	🌢
Little Debbie, German Chocolate Cookie Ring w/caramel	1 cookie	140	8	1	T	🌢
Little Debbie, Homestyle brownie loaves, chocolate	1 cake	260	15	1		🌢
Little Debbie, Homestyle ginger cookies	1 cookie	90	3	0	T	🌢
Little Debbie, Honey Buns	1 pastry	220	11	1	T	🌢
Little Debbie, Marshmallow Pie, banana	1 pie	180	6	0	T	🌢
Little Debbie, Marshmallow Pie, vanilla	1 pie	190	7	0	T	🌢
Little Debbie, Marshmallow Pies	1 cookie	160	6	1	T	🌢

🌢 = Avoid • 🌢 = Add for flavor

	Portion	Calories	Total Fat	Dietary Fiber	Trans Fat	Guide
Little Debbie, Marshmallow Supremes	1 cookie	130	5	0	T	🌢
Little Debbie, Nutty Bars	2 cookies	310	18	1	T	🌢
Little Debbie, Oatmeal Creme Pies	1 cookie	170	7	0	T	🌢
Little Debbie, Oatmeal Lights	1 cookie	130	3	0	T	🌢
Little Debbie, Peanut Butter Bars	2 cookies	270	15	1	T	🌢
Little Debbie, Peanut Clusters	1 cookie	190	11	0	T	🌢
Little Debbie, Pecan Spinwheels	1 roll	110	4	0	T	🌢
Little Debbie, Raisin Creme Pies	1 cookie	140	5	0	T	🌢
Little Debbie, Snack Cakes	2 cakes	310	15	1	T	🌢
Little Debbie, Snack Smart, iced soft, choc fudge	1 cookie	110	2	0	T	🌢
Little Debbie, Snack Smart, iced soft, oatmeal spce	1 cookie	110	2	0	T	🌢
Little Debbie, Starcrunch	1 cookie	140	6	0	T	🌢
Little Debbie, Strawberry Shortcake Rolls	1 shortcake	230	8	0	T	🌢
Little Debbie, Swiss Cake Rolls	2 cakes	260	12	1	T	🌢
Little Debbie, Zebra Cakes	2 cakes	330	16	0	T	🌢
Pepperidge Farm, fat free, blondie, chocolate chip	1 blondie	120	0	0		✂
Tastykake, Chocolate Creamies	1 cake	180	7	0	T	🌢
Tastykake, Kandy Kakes, chocolate	2 cakes	160	8	1	T	🌢
Tastykake, Kandy Kakes, peanut butter	2 cakes	180	9	0	T	🌢
Tastykake, Koffee Kakes, creme filled	2 cakes	240	9	0	T	🌢
Tastykake, Koffee Kakes, lemon filled	2 cakes	160	2	0	T	🌢
Tastykake, Krimpets, butterscotch	2 cakes	210	5	0	T	🌢
Tastykake, Krimpets, jelly	2 cakes	190	3	1	T	🌢
Tastykake, Krimpets, strawberry	2 cakes	210	5	1	T	🌢
Tastykake, Krimpies, creme	2 cakes	230	9	0	T	🌢
Tastykake, Krimpies, creme chocolate	2 cakes	240	9	1	T	🌢
Tastykake, Sparkle Kakes	1 cake	150	5	0	T	🌢

Toppings, Butterscotch/Caramel

	Portion	Calories	Total Fat	Dietary Fiber	Trans Fat	Guide
Smucker's, fat free, butterscotch	2 tbsp.	130	0	0		✂
Smucker's, fat free, caramel	2 tbsp.	130	0	0		✂
Smucker's, sundae Syrup, caramel	2 tbsp.	110	0	0		✂

Toppings, Chocolate/Fudge

	Portion	Calories	Total Fat	Dietary Fiber	Trans Fat	Guide
Heath Shell, Chocolate w/toffee bits	2 tbsp.	230	17	0	T	🌢
Hershey's, Chocolate Shoppe, double chocolate	2 tbsp.	120	2	0	T	🌢
Hershey's, Chocolate Shoppe, hot fudge	2 tbsp.	130	5	0	T	🌢
Hershey's, Krackel shell topping	2 tbsp.	190	14	0	T	🌢
Hershey's Syrup	2 tbsp.	100	0	0		✂
Hershey's Syrup, Chocolate Shoppe, fudge, fat free	2 tbsp.	100	0	1		✂
Hershey's Syrup, chocolate malt	2 tbsp.	100	0	0		✂
Hershey's Syrup, double chocolate, fat free	2 tbsp.	110	0	0		✂
Hershey's Syrup, genuine chocolate flavor, lite	2 tbsp.	50	0	0		✂
Hershey's Syrup, special dark	2 tbsp.	110	0	0		✂
Nestlé Quik, chocolate syrup	2 tbsp.	100	1	0		✂
Smucker's, Dove, dark chocolate	2 tbsp.	140	5	1	T	🌢

☺ = Eat as much as you want • ✂ = Cut Back

	Portion	Calories	Total Fat	Dietary Fiber	Trans Fat	Guide
Smucker's, Dove, milk chocolate	2 tbsp.	130	4	1	T	🍢
Smucker's, Guilt Free, Hot Fudge Topping	2 tbsp.	100	0	1		✂
Smucker's, Magic Shell, chocolate fudge	2 tbsp.	200	14	1	T	🍢
Smucker's, Magic Shell, cookie dough crunch	2 tbsp.	210	16	0	T	🍢
Smucker's, hot fudge	2 tbsp.	140	4	1	T	🍢
Smucker's, hot fudge, fat free	2 tbsp.	90	0	2		✂

Toppings, Frosting, Canned

	Portion	Calories	Total Fat	Dietary Fiber	Trans Fat	Guide
Betty Crocker, Rich & Creamy, French vanilla	2 tbsp.	140	5	0	T	🍢
Betty Crocker, Rich & Creamy, chocolate	2 tbsp.	130	5	0	T	🍢
Betty Crocker, Rich & Creamy, coconut pecan	2 tbsp.	150	8	0	T	🍢
Betty Crocker, Rich & Creamy, cream cheese	2 tbsp.	140	5	0	T	🍢
Betty Crocker, Rich & Creamy, dark chocolate	2 tbsp.	150	6	0	T	🍢
Betty Crocker, Rich & Creamy, rainbow chip	2 tbsp.	160	6	0	T	🍢
Betty Crocker, Rich & Creamy, vanilla	2 tbsp.	140	5	0	T	🍢
Betty Crocker, Soft Whipped, chocolate	2 tbsp.	100	5	0	T	🍢
Betty Crocker, Soft Whipped, cream cheese	2 tbsp.	100	5	0	T	🍢
Betty Crocker, Soft Whipped, fluffy lemon	2 tbsp.	110	5	0	T	🍢
Betty Crocker, Soft Whipped, strawberry	2 tbsp.	110	5	0	T	🍢
Betty Crocker, Soft Whipped, vanilla	2 tbsp.	100	5	0	T	🍢
Betty Crocker, Sweet Rewards, chocolate, reduced fat	2 tbsp.	120	3	0	T	🍢
Betty Crocker, Sweet Rewards, vanilla, reduced fat	2 tbsp.	120	2	0	T	🍢
Duncan Hines, Homestyle, chocolate	2 tbsp.	130	5	0	T	🍢
Duncan Hines, Homestyle, milk chocolate	2 tbsp.	130	5	0	T	🍢
Duncan Hines, Homestyle, vanilla	2 tbsp.	140	5	0	T	🍢
Duncan Hines, chocolate butter cream	2 tbsp.	130	5	0	T	🍢
Pillsbury, Creamy Supreme, chocolate fudge	2 tbsp.	140	6	0	T	🍢
Pillsbury, Creamy Supreme, coconut pecan	2 tbsp.	160	10	0	T	🍢
Pillsbury, Creamy Supreme, milk chocolate	2 tbsp.	140	6	0	T	🍢
Pillsbury, Creamy Supreme, vanilla	2 tbsp.	150	6	0	T	🍢
SnackWell's, chocolate fudge	2 tbsp.	120	3	0	T	🍢
SnackWell's, vanilla	2 tbsp.	130	3	0	T	🍢

Toppings, Frosting, Mix

	Portion	Calories	Total Fat	Dietary Fiber	Trans Fat	Guide
Washington, fudge frosting	$1/4$ cup	150	2	0	T	🍢
Washington, white frosting	$1/4$ cup	150	2	0	T	🍢

Toppings, Fruit

	Portion	Calories	Total Fat	Dietary Fiber	Trans Fat	Guide
Cherries, maraschino	1 cherry	10	0	0		👍
Hershey's Syrup, strawberry	2 tbsp.	100	0	0		✂
Nestlè Quik, strawberry	2 tbsp.	110	0	0		✂
Smucker's, pineapple	2 tbsp.	110	0	0		✂
Smucker's, strawberry	2 tbsp.	100	0	0		✂

Toppings, Nut

	Portion	Calories	Total Fat	Dietary Fiber	Trans Fat	Guide
Betty Crocker, Parlor Perfect, cookie 'n nut crunch	2 tbsp.	80	3	0	T	🍢

🍢 = *Avoid* • 👍 = *Add for flavor*

	Portion	Calories	Total Fat	Dietary Fiber	Trans Fat	Guide
Betty Crocker, Parlor Perfect, praline nut crunch	2 tbsp.	100	5	1		🌢
Diamond, toasted walnut topping	2 tbsp.	110	10	2		🌢
Smucker's, walnuts in syrup	2 tbsp.	170	9	0		🌢

Toppings, Peanut Butter

Hershey's, Chocolate Shoppe, Reese's sprinkles	2 tbsp.	150	7	0	T	🌢
Reese's Shell	2 tbsp.	220	17	1	T	🌢
Smucker's, Magic Shell, peanut butter	2 tbsp.	220	17	0	T	🌢

Toppings, Sprinkles

Betty Crocker, Parlor Perfect, confetti sprinkles	2 tbsp.	110	2	0	T	🌢
Betty Crocker, Parlor Perfect, ice cream critters	2 tbsp.	90	2	0	T	🌢

Toppings, Whipped

Cool Whip	2 tbsp.	25	2	0	T	🌢
Cool Whip, extra creamy	2 tbsp.	25	2	0	T	🌢
Cool Whip, free	2 tbsp.	15	0	0		✂
Cool Whip, lite	2 tbsp.	20	1	0	T	🌢
Dream Whip, whipped topping mix	$1/16$ pouch	15	1	0	T	🌢
Kraft, dairy whip, whipped light cream	2 tbsp.	10	1	0		✂
Kraft, free, whipped topping, fat free	2 tbsp.	15	0	0		✂
Real Whipped, light cream	2 tbsp.	20	2	0		✂
Reddi Whip, Fat free	2 tbsp.	10	0	0		👍
Reddi Whip, extra creamy	2 tbsp.	30	3	0		🌢
Whipped topping, non fat	2 tbsp.	15	0	0		✂

■ FAST FOODS

Arby's

Chicken, chicken fingers	2 pieces	290	16	1		🌢
Chicken sandwich, breaded fillet	1 serv.	536	28	5	T	🌢
Chicken sandwich, grilled chicken BBQ	1 serv.	388	13	2	T	🌢
Chicken sandwich, grilled chicken deluxe	1 serv.	430	20	3	T	🌢
Chicken sandwich, roast chicken club	1 serv.	546	31	2	T	🌢
Chicken sandwich, roast chicken deluxe w/sesame bun	1 serv.	433	22	2	T	🌢
Condiments, dressing, blue cheese	1 serv.	290	31	0		🌢
Condiments, dressing, buttermilk ranch reduced calorie	1 serv.	50	0	0		✂
Condiments, dressing, honey French	1 serv.	280	23	0		🌢
Condiments, dressing, thousand island	1 serv.	260	26	0		🌢
Condiments, sauce, Arby's	1 serv.	15	0	0		✂
Condiments, sauce, barbeque	1 serv.	30	0	0		✂
Condiments, sauce, horsey	1 serv.	60	5	0		🌢
Condiments, sressing, Italian reduced calorie	1 serv.	20	1	0		✂
Curly fries	1 serv.	300	15	0	T	🌢
French fries	1 serv.	246	13	0	T	🌢
Polar Swirl, Butterfinger	1 serv.	457	18	0	T	🌢

☺ = Eat as much as you want • ✂ = Cut Back

	Portion	Calories	Total Fat	Dietary Fiber	Trans Fat	Guide
Polar Swirl, Heath	1 serv.	543	22	0	T	💣
Polar Swirl, Oreo	1 serv.	482	22	0	T	💣
Polar Swirl, Snickers	1 serv.	511	19	1		💣
Polar Swirl, peanut butter cup	1 serv.	517	24	1		💣
Potato, baked, broccoli 'n chedar	1 serv.	571	20	9	T	💣
Potato, baked, deluxe	1 serv.	736	36	7		💣
Potato, baked, plain	1 serv.	355	0	7		☺
Roast beef sandwich, Arby-Q	1 serv.	431	18	3	T	💣
Roast beef sandwich, beef 'n cheddar	1 serv.	487	28	2	T	💣
Roast beef sandwich, giant roast beef	1 serv.	555	28	5	T	💣
Roast beef sandwich, regular	1 serv.	388	19	3	T	💣
Salad, garden	1 serv.	61	1	5		☺
Salad, side	1 serv.	23	0	2		☺
Shake, chocolate	1 serv.	451	12	0	T	💣
Shake, jamocha	1 serv.	384	10	0	T	💣
Shake, vanilla	1 serv.	360	12	0		💣
Sub roll sandwich, Italian sub	1 serv.	675	36	2	T	💣
Sub roll sandwich, Philly beef 'n swiss	1 serv.	755	47	3	T	💣
Sub roll sandwich, roast beef sub	1 serv.	700	42	4	T	💣
Sub roll sandwich, turkey	1 serv.	550	27	2	T	💣

Boston Market

	Portion	Calories	Total Fat	Dietary Fiber	Trans Fat	Guide
Chicken, $^1/_2$, w/skin	1 serv.	630	37	0	n.a.	💣
Chicken, dark meat, $^1/_4$, no skin	1 serv.	210	10	0	n.a.	💣
Chicken, dark meat, $^1/_4$, w/skin	1 serv.	330	22	0	n.a.	💣
Chicken, white meat, $^1/_4$, no skin or wing	1 serv.	160	4	0	n.a.	💣
Chicken, white meat, $^1/_4$, w/skin	1 serv.	330	17	0	n.a.	💣
Chicken sandwich, chicken salad	1 serv.	680	30	4	n.a.	💣
Chicken sandwich, no sauce or cheese	1 serv.	430	5	5	n.a.	💣
Chicken sandwich, w/cheese & sauce	1 serv.	750	33	5	n.a.	💣
Dessert, brownie	1 piece	450	27	3	n.a.	💣
Dessert, cookie, chocolate chip	1 cookie	320	13	1	n.a.	💣
Dessert, cookie, oatmeal raisin	1 cookie	340	17	1	n.a.	💣
Ham, w/cinnamon apples	8 oz.	350	13	2	n.a.	💣
Ham & turkey club sandwich, no cheese or sauce	1 serv.	430	6	4	n.a.	💣
Ham & turkey club sandwich, w/cheese & sauce	1 serv.	890	44	4	n.a.	💣
Ham sandwich, no cheese or sauce	1 serv.	450	9	4	n.a.	💣
Ham sandwich, w/cheese & sauce	1 serv.	760	35	5	n.a.	💣
Meat loaf, & brown gravy	7 oz.	390	22	1	n.a.	💣
Meat loaf, & chunky tomato sauce	8 oz.	370	18	2	n.a.	💣
Meat loaf sandwich, no cheese	1 serv.	690	21	6	n.a.	💣
Meat loaf sandwich, w/cheese	1 serv.	860	33	6	n.a.	💣
Pot pie, chicken, original	1 serv.	750	34	6	n.a.	💣
Potato, mashed, homestyle w/gravy	$^3/_4$ cup	200	9	2	n.a.	💣
Potato, new	$^3/_4$ cup	130	3	2	n.a.	💣
Salad, caesar, chicken	13 oz.	670	47	3	n.a.	💣
Salad, caesar, entree	10 oz.	520	43	3	n.a.	💣

💣 = Avoid • 💧 = Add for flavor

	Portion	Calories	Total Fat	Dietary Fiber	Trans Fat	Guide
Salad, caesar, side	4 oz.	210	17	1	n.a.	🍔
Salad, chunky chicken	³/₄ cup	370	27	1	n.a.	🍔
Salad, coleslaw	³/₄ cup	280	16	3	n.a.	🍔
Salad, fruit	³/₄ cup	70	1	2	n.a.	☺
Salad, pasta, Mediterranean	³/₄ cup	170	10	2	n.a.	🍔
Salad, tortellini	³/₄ cup	380	24	2	n.a.	🍔
Side, apples, hot cinnamon	³/₄ cup	250	5	3	n.a.	🍔
Side, beans, BBQ baked	³/₄ cup	330	9	9	n.a.	🍔
Side, bread, corn	1 loaf	200	6	1	n.a.	🍔
Side, corn, whole kernel	³/₄ cup	180	4	2	n.a.	🍔
Side, green bean casserole	³/₄ cup	90	5	2	n.a.	🍔
Side, macaroni & cheese	³/₄ cup	280	10	1	n.a.	🍔
Side, spinach, creamed	³/₄ cup	280	21	2	n.a.	🍔
Side, squash, butternut	³/₄ cup	160	6	3	n.a.	🍔
Side, stuffing	³/₄ cup	310	12	3	n.a.	🍔
Side, vegetables, steamed	²/₃ cup	35	1	3	n.a.	☺
Side, zucchini marinara	³/₄ cup	80	4	2	n.a.	🍔
Soup, chicken	³/₄ cup	80	3	1	n.a.	🍔
Soup, chicken tortilla	1 cup	220	11	2	n.a.	🍔
Turkey breast, skinless rotisserie	5 oz.	170	1	0	n.a.	✂
Turkey sandwich, no cheese or sauce	1 serv.	400	4	4	n.a.	🍔
Turkey sandwich, w/cheese & sauce	1 serv.	710	28	4	n.a.	🍔

Burger King

	Portion	Calories	Total Fat	Dietary Fiber	Trans Fat	Guide
Breakfast, French toast sticks	1 serv.	500	27	1	T	🍔
Breakfast, biscuit	1 serv.	330	18	1	T	🍔
Breakfast, biscuit w/bacon, egg & cheese	1 serv.	510	31	1	T	🍔
Breakfast, biscuit w/egg	1 serv.	420	24	1	T	🍔
Breakfast, biscuit w/sausage	1 serv.	530	36	1	T	🍔
Breakfast, biscuit w/sausage & cheese	1 serv.	450	35	1	T	🍔
Breakfast, biscuit w/sausage, egg & cheese	1 serv.	550	42	1	T	🍔
Breakfast, hash browns, small	1 serv.	240	15	2	T	🍔
Burger, Big King	1 serv.	660	43	1	T	🍔
Burger, Double cheeseburger w/bacon	1 serv.	640	39	1	T	🍔
Burger, Whopper	1 serv.	640	39	3	T	🍔
Burger, Whopper w/cheese	1 serv.	730	46	3	T	🍔
Burger, Whopper, Jr.	1 serv.	420	24	2	T	🍔
Burger, Whopper, Jr. w/cheese	1 serv.	460	28	2	T	🍔
Burger, Whopper, double	1 serv.	870	56	3	T	🍔
Burger, Whopper, double w/cheese	1 serv.	960	63	3	T	🍔
Burger, cheeseburger	1 serv.	380	19	1	T	🍔
Burger, double cheeseburger	1 serv.	600	36	1	T	🍔
Burger, hamburger	1 serv.	330	15	1	T	🍔
Chicken, Chicken tenders, 8 piece	1 serv.	350	22	1	T	🍔
Chicken sandwich	1 serv.	710	43	2	T	🍔
Chicken sandwich, BK broiler	1 serv.	530	26	2	T	🍔
Condiments, dressing, French	1 serv.	140	10	0		🍔
Condiments, dressing, Italian, light reduced calorie	1 pkg.	15	1	0		✂

☺ = Eat as much as you want • ✂ = Cut Back

	Portion	Calories	Total Fat	Dietary Fiber	Trans Fat	Guide
Condiments, dressing, bleu cheese	1 serv.	160	16	0		🛢
Condiments, dressing, ranch	1 pkg.	180	19	0		🛢
Condiments, dressing, thousand island	1 pkg.	140	12	0		🛢
Condiments, sauce, barbecue	1 serv.	35	0	0		✂
Condiments, sauce, honey	1 serv.	90	0	0		✂
Condiments, sauce, ranch	1 serv.	170	17	0		🛢
Condiments, sauce, sweet & sour	1 pkg.	45	0	0		✂
Dessert, pie, Dutch apple	1 serv.	300	15	2	T	🛢
Fish sandwich, BK big	1 serv.	720	43	3	T	🛢
French Fries, medium, salted	1 serv.	400	21	4	T	🛢
Onion rings	1 serv.	310	14	6	T	🛢
Salad, broiled chicken	1 serv.	190	8	3	T	🛢
Salad, garden	1 serv.	100	5	3		🛢
Salad, side	1 serv.	60	3	2		🛢
Shake, chocolate, medium	1 serv.	320	7	3		🛢
Shake, strawberry, medium, syrup added	1 serv.	420	6	1		🛢
Shake, vanilla, medium	1 serv.	300	6	1		🛢

Chik-fil-A

	Portion	Calories	Total Fat	Dietary Fiber	Trans Fat	Guide
Chicken, Chick-n-Strips, 4 count	1 serv.	230	8	0		🛢
Chicken, Nuggets, 8 pack	1 serv.	290	14	0		🛢
Chicken sandwich	1 serv.	290	9	1	T	🛢
Chicken sandwich, chargrilled	1 serv.	280	3	1	T	🛢
Chicken sandwich, chargrilled club, no dressing	1 serv.	390	12	2	T	🛢
Chicken sandwich, chargrilled deluxe	1 serv.	290	3	2	T	🛢
Chicken sandwich, chicken salad on whole wheat	1 serv.	320	5	1	T	🛢
Chicken sandwich, deluxe	1 serv.	300	9	2	T	🛢
Dessert, Icedream, small cone	1 serv.	140	4	0	T	🛢
Dessert, brownie, fudge w/nuts	1 serv.	350	16	0	T	🛢
Dessert, cheesecake slice	1 serv.	270	21	0		🛢
Dessert, cheesecake slice, w/blueberry topping	1 serv.	290	23	0		🛢
Dessert, cheesecake slice, w/strawberry topping	1 serv.	290	23	0		🛢
Dessert, pie, lemon, slice	1 serv.	320	16	1	T	🛢
Fries, waffle potato, salted, small	1 serv.	290	10	0	T	🛢
Salad, Chargrilled chicken garden	1 serv.	170	3	5	T	🛢
Salad, Chick-n-Strips	1 serv.	290	9	5		🛢
Salad, carrot & raisin, small	1 serv.	150	2	2		✂
Salad, chicken plate	1 serv.	290	5	6		🛢
Salad, cole slaw, cup, small	1 serv.	130	6	1		🛢
Salad, tossed	1 serv.	70	0	1		☺
Soup, hearty breast of chicken, cup	1 serv.	110	1	1		✂

Dairy Queen

	Portion	Calories	Total Fat	Dietary Fiber	Trans Fat	Guide
Burger, Homestyle, cheeseburger	1 serv.	340	17	n.a.	n.a.	🛢
Burger, Homestyle, cheeseburger, double	1 serv.	540	31	n.a.	n.a.	🛢
Burger, Homestyle, double hamburger, deluxe	1 serv.	440	22	n.a.	n.a.	🛢
Burger, Homestyle, hamburger	1 serv.	290	12	n.a.	n.a.	🛢

🛢 = Avoid • 💧 = Add for flavor

	Portion	Calories	Total Fat	Dietary Fiber	Trans Fat	Guide
Chicken, chicken strip basket, w/BBQ sauce, fries & toast	1 serv.	840	37	n.a.	n.a.	🌢
Chicken, chicken strip basket, w/gravy, fries & toast	1 serv.	860	42	n.a.	n.a.	🌢
Chicken fillet sandwich, breast	1 serv.	430	20	n.a.	n.a.	🌢
Chicken fillet sandwich, grilled breast	1 serv.	310	10	n.a.	n.a.	🌢
Dessert, Blizzard, Butterfinger, regular	1 serv.	750	26	1	n.a.	🌢
Dessert, Blizzard, Heath, regular	1 serv.	820	33	1	n.a.	🌢
Dessert, Blizzard, Reese's peanut butter cup, regular	1 serv.	790	33	2	n.a.	🌢
Dessert, Blizzard, strawberry, regular	1 serv.	570	16	1	n.a.	🌢
Dessert, Breeze, Heath, regular	1 serv.	710	18	1	n.a.	🌢
Dessert, Breeze, strawberry, regular	1 serv.	460	1	1	n.a.	🌢
Dessert, DIlly Bar, chocolate	1 serv.	210	13	0	n.a.	🌢
Dessert, DQ sandwich, ice cream	1 serv.	150	5	1	n.a.	🌢
Dessert, Misty, slush, regular	1 serv.	290	0	0	n.a.	✂
Dessert, Parfait, peanut buster	1 serv.	730	31	2	n.a.	🌢
Dessert, banana split	1 serv.	510	12	3	n.a.	🌢
Dessert, bar, caramel & nut	1 serv.	260	13	0	n.a.	🌢
Dessert, bar, fudge	1 serv.	50	0	0	n.a.	✂
Dessert, bar, vanilla orange	1 serv.	60	0	0	n.a.	✂
Dessert, cone, chocolate, regular	1 serv.	360	11	0	n.a.	🌢
Dessert, cone, vanilla, regular	1 serv.	350	10	0	n.a.	🌢
Dessert, malt, chocolate, regular	1 serv.	880	22	0	n.a.	🌢
Dessert, shake, chocolate, regular	1 serv.	770	20	0	n.a.	🌢
Dessert, soft serve, chocolate	$1/2$ cup	150	5	0	n.a.	🌢
Dessert, soft serve, vanilla	$1/2$ cup	140	5	0	n.a.	🌢
Dessert, sundae, chocolate, regular	1 serv.	410	10	0	n.a.	🌢
Dessert, yogurt cone, regular	1 serv.	280	1	0	n.a.	✂
Dessert, yogurt, frozen, nonfat	$1/2$ cup	100	0	0	n.a.	✂
Fish fillet sandwich	1 serv.	370	16	n.a.	n.a.	🌢
French fries, regular	1 serv.	300	14	n.a.	n.a.	🌢
Hot dog	1 serv.	240	14	n.a.	n.a.	🌢
Hot dog, w/cheese	1 serv.	290	18	n.a.	n.a.	🌢
Hot dog, w/chili	1 serv.	280	16	n.a.	n.a.	🌢
Onion rings	1 serv.	240	12	n.a.	n.a.	🌢

Einstein Bros Bagels

	Portion	Calories	Total Fat	Dietary Fiber	Trans Fat	Guide
Bagel, chocolate chip	1 serv.	370	3	3		🌢
Bagel, cinnamon raisin swirl	1 serv.	350	1	2		✂
Bagel, everything	1 serv.	340	2	2		✂
Bagel, plain	1 serv.	320	1	2		✂
Bagel, poppy dip'd	1 serv.	350	2	2		✂
Bagel, sesame dip'd	1 serv.	380	5	3		🌢
Bagel, wild blueberry	1 serv.	350	1	3		✂
Cinnamon bun, iced	1 serv.	545	16	3	T	🌢
Cookie, chocolate chunk	1 serv.	510	24	2	T	🌢
Cookie, oatmeal raisin	1 serv.	470	18	3	T	🌢
Cream Cheese, plain	2 tbsp.	100	10	0		🌢
Cream Cheese, plain lite	2 tbsp.	60	5	0		🌢

☺ = Eat as much as you want   •   ✂ = Cut Back

	Portion	Calories	Total Fat	Dietary Fiber	Trans Fat	Guide
Cream Cheese, veggie lite	2 tbsp.	60	5	0		🌢
Muffin, banana nut	1 serv.	220	12	0	T	🌢
Muffin, blueberry	1 serv.	200	10	0	T	🌢
Muffin, chocolate chip	1 serv.	240	13	0	T	🌢
Muffin, fat-free, cranberry orange	1 serv.	130	1	1		✂
Muffin, fat-free, wildberry	1 serv.	120	1	1		✂
Muffin, low-fat, apple date raisin bran	1 serv.	160	2	2		✂
Muffin, low-fat, lemon poppyseed	1 serv.	150	3	0		🌢
Salad, Idaho potato, regular	1 serv.	150	7	1		🌢
Salad, caesar, regular	1 serv.	210	18	1		🌢
Salad, fruit	1 serv.	110	1	2		✂
Salad, veggie cup	1 serv.	230	20	3		🌢
Sandwich, chicken salad, low-fat	1 serv.	510	9	4		🌢
Sandwich, ham & cheese	1 serv.	580	15	3		🌢
Sandwich, pepperoni pizza melt	1 serv.	740	30	3		🌢
Sandwich, scrambled egg	1 serv.	540	16	2		🌢
Sandwich, tasty turkey	1 serv.	600	21	3		🌢
Sandwich, tuna melt	1 serv.	840	36	3		🌢
Sandwich, tuna salad, low fat	1 serv.	510	8	4		🌢
Sandwich, veg-out	1 serv.	420	6	3		🌢
Scone, blueberry	1 serv.	295	9	2	T	🌢

Kentucky Fried Chicken

	Portion	Calories	Total Fat	Dietary Fiber	Trans Fat	Guide
Chicken, Chicken Twister	1 serv.	480	20	2	n.a.	🌢
Chicken, Crispy Strips, Colonel's	3 pieces	261	16	3	n.a.	🌢
Chicken, Crispy Strips, spicy buffalo	3 pieces	350	19	2	n.a.	🌢
Chicken, extra tasty crispy, breast	1 serv.	470	28	1	n.a.	🌢
Chicken, extra tasty crispy, drumstick	1 serv.	190	11	0	n.a.	🌢
Chicken, extra tasty crispy, thigh	1 serv.	370	25	2	n.a.	🌢
Chicken, extra tasty crispy, whole wing	1 serv.	200	13	0	n.a.	🌢
Chicken, hot & spicy, breast	1 serv.	530	35	2	n.a.	🌢
Chicken, hot & spicy, drumstick	1 serv.	190	11	0	n.a.	🌢
Chicken, hot & spicy, thigh	1 serv.	370	27	1	n.a.	🌢
Chicken, hot & spicy, whole wing	1 serv.	210	15	0	n.a.	🌢
Chicken, hot wing pieces, 6 pieces	1 serv.	471	33	2	n.a.	🌢
Chicken, original recipe, breast	1 serv.	400	24	1	n.a.	🌢
Chicken, original recipe, drumstick	1 serv.	140	9	0	n.a.	🌢
Chicken, original recipe, thigh	1 serv.	250	18	1	n.a.	🌢
Chicken, original recipe, whole wing	1 serv.	140	10	0	n.a.	🌢
Chicken, tender roast, breast w/out skin	1 serv.	169	4	0	n.a.	🌢
Chicken, tender roast, breast w/skin	1 serv.	251	11	0	n.a.	🌢
Chicken, tender roast, drumstick w/out skin	1 serv.	67	2	0	n.a.	🌢
Chicken, tender roast, drumstick w/skin	1 serv.	97	4	0	n.a.	🌢
Chicken, tender roast, thigh w/out skin	1 serv.	106	6	0	n.a.	🌢
Chicken, tender roast, thigh w/skin	1 serv.	207	12	0	n.a.	🌢
Chicken, tender roast, wing w/skin	1 serv.	121	8	0	n.a.	🌢
Chicken Sandwich, original recipe	1 serv.	497	22	3	n.a.	🌢
Chicken Sandwich, value BBQ flavored	1 serv.	256	8	2	n.a.	🌢
Pot Pie, chunky chicken	1 serv.	770	42	5	n.a.	🌢

🌢 = Avoid • ⚖ = Add for flavor

	Portion	Calories	Total Fat	Dietary Fiber	Trans Fat	Guide
Side, beans, BBQ baked	1 serv.	190	3	6	n.a.	🌢
Side, biscuit	1 serv.	180	10	0	n.a.	🌢
Side, cole slaw	1 serv.	180	9	3	n.a.	🌢
Side, corn on the cob	1 serv.	150	2	2	n.a.	✂
Side, cornbread	1 serv.	228	13	1	n.a.	🌢
Side, green beans	1 serv.	45	2	3	n.a.	☺
Side, macaroni & cheese	1 serv.	180	8	2	n.a.	🌢
Side, mean greens	1 serv.	70	3	5	n.a.	🌢
Side, potato salad	1 serv.	230	14	3	n.a.	🌢
Side, potato wedges	1 serv.	280	13	5	n.a.	🌢
Side, potatoes mashed w/gravy	1 serv.	120	6	2	n.a.	🌢

Little Caesars

	Portion	Calories	Total Fat	Dietary Fiber	Trans Fat	Guide
Big!Big!, Italian sausage, large	1 slice	250	9	2	n.a.	🌢
Big!Big!, Meatsa, small	1 slice	260	12	2	n.a.	🌢
Big!Big!, cheese, large	1 slice	230	8	1	n.a.	🌢
Big!Big!, cheese, medium	1 slice	210	7	1	n.a.	🌢
Big!Big!, cheese, small	1 slice	230	8	1	n.a.	🌢
Big!Big!, pepperoni, large	1 slice	270	11	2	n.a.	🌢
Big!Big!, pepperoni, medium	1 slice	230	9	1	n.a.	🌢
Big!Big!, pepperoni, small	1 slice	210	8	1	n.a.	🌢
Big!Big!, stuffed crust, cheese, small	1 slice	240	10	1	n.a.	🌢
Big!Big!, stuffed crust, pepperoni, small	1 slice	260	12	1	n.a.	🌢
Big!Big!, supreme, small	1 slice	230	10	2	n.a.	🌢
Big!Big!, veggie, small	1 slice	200	7	2	n.a.	🌢
Bread, Crazy	1 piece	110	3	1	n.a.	🌢
Pan!Pan!, cheese	1 slice	250	8	2	n.a.	🌢
Pan!Pan!, pepperoni	1 slice	310	12	2	n.a.	🌢
Pizza!Pizza!, cheese	1 slice	180	6	1	n.a.	🌢
Pizza!Pizza!, pepperoni	1 slice	200	8	1	n.a.	🌢
Sauce, Crazy	1 serv.	40	1	2	n.a.	✂

McDonald's

	Portion	Calories	Total Fat	Dietary Fiber	Trans Fat	Guide
Breakfast, McMuffin, egg	1 serv.	290	12	1	T	🌢
Breakfast, McMuffin, sausage	1 serv.	360	23	1	T	🌢
Breakfast, McMuffin, sausage w/egg	1 serv.	440	28	1	T	🌢
Breakfast, biscuit	1 serv.	290	15	1	T	🌢
Breakfast, biscuit, bacon, egg, & cheese	1 serv.	470	28	1	T	🌢
Breakfast, biscuit, sausage	1 serv.	470	31	1	T	🌢
Breakfast, biscuit, sausage w/egg	1 serv.	550	37	1	T	🌢
Breakfast, breakfast burrito	1 serv.	320	20	2	T	🌢
Breakfast, cinnamon roll	1 serv.	390	18	2	T	🌢
Breakfast, danish, apple	1 serv.	360	16	1	T	🌢
Breakfast, danish, cheese	1 serv.	410	22	0	T	🌢
Breakfast, eggs, scrambled	2 eggs	160	11	0	T	🌢
Breakfast, hash browns	1 serv.	130	8	1	T	🌢
Breakfast, hotcakes w/syrup & margarine (2 pats)	1 serv.	570	16	2	T	🌢
Breakfast, hotcakes, plain	1 serv.	310	7	2		🌢

☺ = Eat as much as you want • ✂ = Cut Back

	Portion	Calories	Total Fat	Dietary Fiber	Trans Fat	Guide
Breakfast, muffin, English	1 serv.	140	2	1	T	🌢
Breakfast, muffin, apple bran, lowfat	1 serv.	300	3	3	T	🌢
Breakfast, sausage	1 serv.	170	16	0	T	🌢
Burger, Arch Deluxe	1 serv.	550	31	4	T	🌢
Burger, Arch Deluxe w/bacon	1 serv.	590	34	4	T	🌢
Burger, Big Mac	1 serv.	560	31	3	T	🌢
Burger, Quarter Pounder	1 serv.	420	21	2	T	🌢
Burger, Quarter Pounder w/cheese	1 serv.	530	30	2	T	🌢
Burger, cheeseburger	1 serv.	320	13	2	T	🌢
Burger, hamburger	1 serv.	260	9	2	T	🌢
Chicken, McNuggets	4 pieces	190	11	0	T	🌢
Chicken sandwich, crispy deluxe	1 serv.	500	25	4	T	🌢
Chicken sandwich, grilled, deluxe	1 serv.	440	20	4	T	🌢
Chicken sandwich, grilled, deluxe (plain w/o mayo)	1 serv.	300	5	4	T	🌢
Condiments, Dressing, red French, reduced calorie	1 pkg.	160	8	0		🌢
Condiments, dressing, caesar	1 pkg.	160	14	0		🌢
Condiments, dressing, herb vinaigrette, fat free	1 pkg.	50	0	0		✂
Condiments, dressing, ranch	1 pkg.	230	21	0		🌢
Condiments, sauce, barbeque	1 pkg.	45	0	0		✂
Condiments, sauce, honey	1 pkg.	45	0	0		✂
Condiments, sauce, honey mustard	1 pkg.	50	5	0		🌢
Condiments, sauce, hot mustard	1 pkg.	60	4	0		🌢
Condiments, sauce, sweet'n sour	1 pkg.	50	0	0		✂
Dessert, apple pie, baked	1 serv.	260	13	0	T	🌢
Dessert, cookies, McDonaldland	1 pkg.	180	5	1	T	🌢
Dessert, cookies, chocolate chip	1 serv.	170	10	1		🌢
Dessert, ice cream cone, vanilla, reduced fat	1 serv.	150	5	0	T	🌢
Dessert, sundae, hot caramel	1 serv.	360	10	0		🌢
Dessert, sundae, hot fudge	1 serv.	340	12	1	T	🌢
Dessert, sundae, strawberry	1 serv.	290	7	0		🌢
Fish Sandwich, Filet-O-Fish	1 serv.	450	25	2	T	🌢
Fish Sandwich, fish filet deluxe	1 serv.	560	28	4	T	🌢
French Fries, large	1 serv.	450	22	5	T	🌢
French Fries, small	1 serv.	210	10	2	T	🌢
French Fries, super size	1 serv.	540	26	6	T	🌢
Salad, garden	1 serv.	35	0	3		☺
Salad, grilled chicken deluxe	1 serv.	120	2	3		☺
Shake, chocolate, small	1 serv.	360	9	1		🌢
Shake, strawberry, small	1 serv.	360	9	0		🌢
Shake, vanilla, small	1 serv.	360	9	0		🌢

Pizza Hut

	Portion	Calories	Total Fat	Dietary Fiber	Trans Fat	Guide
Hand Tossed, Italian sausage	1 med. slice	300	12	3	T	🌢
Hand Tossed, Meat Lover's	1 med. slice	290	11	3	T	🌢
Hand Tossed, Pepperoni Lover's	1 med. slice	320	13	4	T	🌢
Hand Tossed, Super Supreme	1 med. slice	290	10	4	T	🌢
Hand Tossed, Supreme	1 med. slice	270	9	3	T	🌢

🌢 = Avoid • 🌢 = Add for flavor

	Portion	Calories	Total Fat	Dietary Fiber	Trans Fat	Guide
Hand Tossed, Veggie Lover's	1 med. slice	240	7	3	T	🌢
Hand Tossed, beef	1 med. slice	280	10	3	T	🌢
Hand Tossed, chicken supreme	1 med. slice	240	6	3	T	🌢
Hand Tossed, pepperoni	1 med. slice	260	9	3	T	🌢
Hand Tossed, pork	1 med. slice	290	11	3	T	🌢
Pan, Italian sausage	1 med. slice	350	18	3	T	🌢
Pan, Meat Lover's	1 med. slice	360	19	3	T	🌢
Pan, Pepperoni Lover's	1 med. slice	350	17	2	T	🌢
Pan, Super Supreme	1 med. slice	340	16	4	T	🌢
Pan, Supreme	1 med. slice	300	13	3	T	🌢
Pan, Veggie Lover's	1 med. slice	240	9	3	T	🌢
Pan, beef	1 med. slice	310	14	2	T	🌢
Pan, cheese	1 med. slice	300	14	2	T	🌢
Pan, chicken supreme	1 med. slice	280	11	3	T	🌢
Pan, ham	1 med. slice	250	9	2	T	🌢
Pan, pepperoni	1 med. slice	280	12	3	T	🌢
Pan, pork	1 med. slice	300	13	3	T	🌢
Personal Pan, cheese	whole pizza	630	24	4	T	🌢
Personal Pan, pepperoni	whole pizza	670	29	4	T	🌢
Personal Pan, supreme	whole pizza	710	31	5	T	🌢
Stuffed Crust, Italian sausage	1 med. slice	430	19	4	T	🌢
Stuffed Crust, Meat Lover's	1 med. slice	500	23	4	T	🌢
Stuffed Crust, Pepperoni Lover's	1 med. slice	480	22	4	T	🌢
Stuffed Crust, Super Supreme	1 med. slice	470	20	5	T	🌢
Stuffed Crust, Supreme	1 med. slice	440	16	4	T	🌢
Stuffed Crust, Veggie Lover's	1 med. slice	390	14	5	T	🌢
Stuffed Crust, beef	1 med. slice	410	14	4	T	🌢
Stuffed Crust, cheese	1 med. slice	380	11	4	T	🌢
Stuffed Crust, Chicken Supreme	1 med. slice	390	13	4	T	🌢
Stuffed Crust, ham	1 med. slice	380	14	4	T	🌢
Stuffed Crust, pepperoni	1 med. slice	410	17	4	T	🌢
Stuffed Crust, pork	1 med. slice	420	16	4	T	🌢
Thin 'N Crispy, Italian sausage	1 med. slice	300	16	3	T	🌢
Thin 'N Crispy, Meat Lover's	1 med. slice	310	16	3	T	🌢
Thin 'N Crispy, Pepperoni Lover's	1 med. slice	270	12	2	T	🌢
Thin 'N Crispy, Super Supreme	1 med. slice	280	13	4	T	🌢
Thin 'N Crispy, Supreme	1 med. slice	250	11	3	T	🌢
Thin 'N Crispy, Veggie Lover's	1 med. slice	170	6	3	T	🌢
Thin 'N Crispy, beef	1 med. slice	240	11	2	T	🌢
Thin 'N Crispy, cheese	1 med. slice	210	9	2	T	🌢
Thin 'N Crispy, Chicken Supreme	1 med. slice	220	7	2	T	🌢
Thin 'N Crispy, ham	1 med. slice	190	6	1	T	🌢
Thin 'N Crispy, pepperoni	1 med. slice	220	9	2	T	🌢
Thin 'N Crispy, pork	1 med. slice	270	13	2	T	🌢

Roy Rogers

	Portion	Calories	Total Fat	Dietary Fiber	Trans Fat	Guide
Breakfast, 3 pancakes	1 serv.	280	2	n.a.	n.a.	✂
Breakfast, 3 pancakes w/1 sausage	1 serv.	430	16	n.a.	n.a.	🌢
Breakfast, 3 pancakes w/2 bacon	1 serv.	350	9	n.a.	n.a.	🌢

☺ = Eat as much as you want • ✂ = Cut Back

	Portion	Calories	Total Fat	Dietary Fiber	Trans Fat	Guide
Breakfast, biscuit	1 serv.	390	21	n.a.	n.a.	🌢
Breakfast, biscuit, bacon	1 serv.	420	23	n.a.	n.a.	🌢
Breakfast, biscuit, bacon & egg	1 serv.	470	26	n.a.	n.a.	🌢
Breakfast, biscuit, cinnamon 'n' raisin	1 serv.	370	18	n.a.	n.a.	🌢
Breakfast, biscuit, ham & cheese	1 serv.	450	24	n.a.	n.a.	🌢
Breakfast, biscuit, ham, egg, & cheese	1 serv.	500	27	n.a.	n.a.	🌢
Breakfast, biscuit, sausage	1 serv.	510	31	n.a.	n.a.	🌢
Breakfast, biscuit, sausage & egg	1 serv.	560	35	n.a.	n.a.	🌢
Breakfast, biscuits 'n' gravy	1 serv.	510	28	n.a.	n.a.	🌢
Breakfast, breakfast platter, big country w/bacon	1 serv.	740	43	n.a.	n.a.	🌢
Breakfast, breakfast platter, big country w/ham	1 serv.	710	39	n.a.	n.a.	🌢
Breakfast, breakfast platter, big country w/sausage	1 serv.	920	60	n.a.	n.a.	🌢
Breakfast, sourdough, ham, egg, & cheese	1 serv.	480	24	n.a.	n.a.	🌢
Burger, bacon cheeseburger	1 serv.	520	33	n.a.	n.a.	🌢
Burger, cheeseburger	1 serv.	393	22	n.a.	n.a.	🌢
Burger, hamburger	1 serv.	343	18	n.a.	n.a.	🌢
Chicken, fried breast	1 serv.	370	15	n.a.	n.a.	🌢
Chicken, fried leg	1 serv.	170	7	n.a.	n.a.	🌢
Chicken, fried thigh	1 serv.	330	15	n.a.	n.a.	🌢
Chicken, fried wing	1 serv.	200	8	n.a.	n.a.	🌢
Chicken, nuggets, 6 piece	1 serv.	290	18	n.a.	n.a.	🌢
Chicken sandwich, Gold Rush	1 serv.	558	30	n.a.	n.a.	🌢
Chicken sandwich, grilled	1 serv.	294	8	n.a.	n.a.	🌢
Dessert, frozen yogurt, vanilla cone	1 serv.	180	4	n.a.	n.a.	🌢
Dessert, strawberry shortcake	1 serv.	440	19	n.a.	n.a.	🌢
Dessert, sundae, hot fudge	1 serv.	320	10	n.a.	n.a.	🌢
Dessert, sundae, strawberry	1 serv.	260	6	n.a.	n.a.	🌢
Fish sandwich	1 serv.	490	21	n.a.	n.a.	🌢
Fry, large	1 serv.	430	18	n.a.	n.a.	🌢
Fry, regular	1 serv.	350	15	n.a.	n.a.	🌢
Potato, baked	1 serv.	130	1	n.a.	n.a.	☺
Potato, baked w/margarine	1 serv.	240	13	n.a.	n.a.	🌢
Potato, mashed	5 oz.	92	0	n.a.	n.a.	✄
Roast beef sandwich	1 serv.	329	10	n.a.	n.a.	🌢
Salad, cole slaw	5 oz.	295	25	n.a.	n.a.	🌢
Salad, garden	1 serv.	110	5	n.a.	n.a.	🌢
Salad, grilled chicken	1 serv.	221	9	n.a.	n.a.	🌢
Salad, side	1 serv.	20	0	n.a.	n.a.	☺

Subway

	Portion	Calories	Total Fat	Dietary Fiber	Trans Fat	Guide
6-inch cold sub, BLT	1 serv.	327	10	n.a.	n.a.	🌢
6-inch cold sub, Veggie Delite	1 serv.	237	3	n.a.	n.a.	🌢
6-inch cold sub, classic Italian BMT	1 serv.	460	22	n.a.	n.a.	🌢
6-inch cold sub, club	1 serv.	312	5	n.a.	n.a.	🌢
6-inch cold sub, cold cut trio	1 serv.	378	13	n.a.	n.a.	🌢
6-inch cold sub, ham	1 serv.	302	5	n.a.	n.a.	🌢
6-inch cold sub, roast beef	1 serv.	303	5	n.a.	n.a.	🌢

🌢 = Avoid   •   ☖ = Add for flavor

FOOD LISTS

	Portion	Calories	Total Fat	Dietary Fiber	Trans Fat	Guide
6-inch cold sub, seafood & crab w/light mayo	1 serv.	347	10	n.a.	n.a.	🌢
6-inch cold sub, tuna w/light mayo	1 serv.	391	15	n.a.	n.a.	🌢
6-inch cold sub, turkey breast	1 serv.	289	4	n.a.	n.a.	🌢
6-inch hot sub, meatball	1 serv.	419	16	n.a.	n.a.	🌢
6-inch hot sub, roasted chicken breast	1 serv.	348	6	n.a.	n.a.	🌢
6-inch hot sub, steak & cheese w/out cheese	1 serv.	398	10	n.a.	n.a.	🌢
Cookie, chocolate chip	1 cookie	210	10	n.a.	n.a.	🌢
Cookie, chocolate chunk	1 cookie	210	10	n.a.	n.a.	🌢
Cookie, oatmeal raisin	1 cookie	200	8	n.a.	n.a.	🌢
Cookie, peanut butter	1 cookie	220	12	n.a.	n.a.	🌢
Cookie, sugar	1 cookie	230	12	n.a.	n.a.	🌢
Cookie, white chocolate macademia nut	1 cookie	230	12	n.a.	n.a.	🌢
Deli style sandwich, ham	1 serv.	234	4	n.a.	n.a.	🌢
Deli style sandwich, roast beef	1 serv.	245	4	n.a.	n.a.	🌢
Deli style sandwich, tuna w/light mayo	1 serv.	279	9	n.a.	n.a.	🌢
Deli style sandwich, turkey breast	1 serv.	235	4	n.a.	n.a.	🌢
Dressing, French	1 tbsp.	65	5	n.a.	n.a.	🌢
Dressing, French, fat free	1 tbsp.	15	0	n.a.	n.a.	✂
Dressing, Italian, creamy	1 tbsp.	65	6	n.a.	n.a.	🌢
Dressing, Italian, fat free	1 tbsp.	5	0	n.a.	n.a.	👍
Dressing, ranch	1 tbsp.	87	9	n.a.	n.a.	🌢
Dressing, ranch, fat free	1 tbsp.	12	0	n.a.	n.a.	✂
Dressing, thousand island	1 tbsp.	65	6	n.a.	n.a.	🌢
Salad, w/out dressing, BLT	1 serv.	140	8	n.a.	n.a.	🌢
Salad, w/out dressing, Veggie delite	1 serv.	51	1	n.a.	n.a.	✂
Salad, w/out dressing, classic Italian BMT	1 serv.	274	20	n.a.	n.a.	🌢
Salad, w/out dressing, club	1 serv.	126	3	n.a.	n.a.	🌢
Salad, w/out dressing, cold cut trio	1 serv.	191	11	n.a.	n.a.	🌢
Salad, w/out dressing, ham	1 serv.	116	3	n.a.	n.a.	🌢
Salad, w/out dressing, meatball	1 serv.	233	14	n.a.	n.a.	🌢
Salad, w/out dressing, roast beef	1 serv.	117	3	n.a.	n.a.	🌢
Salad, w/out dressing, roasted chicken breast	1 serv.	162	4	n.a.	n.a.	🌢
Salad, w/out dressing, seafood & crab w/light mayo	1 serv.	161	8	n.a.	n.a.	🌢
Salad, w/out dressing, steak & cheese w/out cheese	1 serv.	212	8	n.a.	n.a.	🌢
Salad, w/out dressing, tuna w/light mayo	1 serv.	205	13	n.a.	n.a.	🌢
Salad, w/out dressing, turkey breast	1 serv.	102	2	n.a.	n.a.	✂

Taco Bell

	Portion	Calories	Total Fat	Dietary Fiber	Trans Fat	Guide
Breakfast, burrito, country	1 serv.	270	14	2	n.a.	🌢
Breakfast, burrito, double bacon & egg	1 serv.	480	27	2	n.a.	🌢
Breakfast, burrito, fiesta	1 serv.	280	16	2	n.a.	🌢
Breakfast, burrito, grande	1 serv.	420	22	3	n.a.	🌢
Breakfast, hash brown nuggets	1 serv.	280	18	1	n.a.	🌢
Breakfast, quesadilla w/bacon	1 serv.	450	27	2	n.a.	🌢
Breakfast, quesadilla w/sausage	1 serv.	430	25	1	n.a.	🌢
Breakfast, quesadilla, cheese	1 serv.	380	21	1	n.a.	🌢
Burrito, 7-Layer	1 serv.	530	23	13	n.a.	🌢
Burrito, Big Beef Supreme	1 serv.	520	23	11	n.a.	🌢

☺ = Eat as much as you want • ✂ = Cut Back

	Portion	Calories	Total Fat	Dietary Fiber	Trans Fat	Guide
Burrito, Big Chicken Supreme	1 serv.	510	24	4	n.a.	♦
Burrito, Supreme	1 serv.	440	19	10	n.a.	♦
Burrito, bean	1 serv.	380	12	13	n.a.	♦
Burrito, grilled chicken	1 serv.	410	15	4	n.a.	♦
Condiments, pico de gallo	1 serv.	5	0	0	n.a.	♦
Condiments, sauce: border; fire, hot or mild	1 serv.	0	0	0	n.a.	♦
Condiments, sauce, fajita	1 serv.	70	7	0	n.a.	♦
Condiments, sauce, green	1 serv.	5	0	0	n.a.	♦
Condiments, sauce, nacho cheese	1 serv.	230	10	0	n.a.	♦
Condiments, sauce, picante	1 serv.	0	0	0	n.a.	♦
Condiments, sauce, red	1 serv.	10	0	0	n.a.	♦
Dessert, cinnamon twists	1 serv.	140	6	0	n.a.	♦
Dessert, ice cream, choco taco	1 serv.	310	17	1	n.a.	♦
Fajita Wrap, Chicken Supreme	1 serv.	520	26	4	n.a.	♦
Fajita Wrap, Steak Supreme	1 serv.	540	25	3	n.a.	♦
Fajita Wrap, Veggie Supreme	1 serv.	470	22	3	n.a.	♦
Fajita Wrap, chicken	1 serv.	470	22	4	n.a.	♦
Fajita Wrap, steak	1 serv.	470	21	3	n.a.	♦
Fajita Wrap, veggie	1 serv.	420	19	3	n.a.	♦
MexiMelt, Big Beef	1 serv.	290	15	4	n.a.	♦
Nachos	1 serv.	320	18	3	n.a.	♦
Nachos, BellGrande	1 serv.	770	39	17	n.a.	♦
Nachos, Big Beef Supreme	1 serv.	450	24	9	n.a.	♦
Pizza, Mexican	1 serv.	570	35	8	n.a.	♦
Quesadilla, cheese	1 serv.	350	18	2	n.a.	♦
Quesadilla, chicken	1 serv.	410	21	3	n.a.	♦
Side, pintos 'n cheese	1 serv.	190	9	10	n.a.	♦
Soft Taco	1 serv.	220	10	3	n.a.	♦
Soft Taco, BLT	1 serv.	340	23	2	n.a.	♦
Soft Taco, Grilled Steak Supreme	1 serv.	290	14	3	n.a.	♦
Soft Taco, Supreme	1 serv.	260	14	3	n.a.	♦
Soft Taco, grilled chicken	1 serv.	240	12	3	n.a.	♦
Soft Taco, grilled steak	1 serv.	230	10	2	n.a.	♦
Taco	1 serv.	180	10	3	n.a.	♦
Taco, Double Decker Supreme	1 serv.	390	19	9	n.a.	♦
Taco, Supreme	1 serv.	220	14	3	n.a.	♦
Taco, double decker	1 serv.	340	15	9	n.a.	♦
Taco Salad, w/salsa	1 serv.	850	52	16	n.a.	♦
Taco Salad, w/salsa, w/out shell	1 serv.	420	22	15	n.a.	♦
Tostada	1 serv.	300	15	12	n.a.	♦

Wendy's

	Portion	Calories	Total Fat	Dietary Fiber	Trans Fat	Guide
Burger, Big Bacon Classic	1 serv.	580	30	3		♦
Burger, cheeseburger, Jr.	1 serv.	320	13	2		♦
Burger, cheeseburger, Jr., bacon	1 serv.	380	19	2		♦
Burger, cheeseburger, Jr., deluxe	1 serv.	360	17	3		♦
Burger, hamburger, Jr.	1 serv.	270	10	2		♦
Burger, hamburger, plain single	1 serv.	360	16	2		♦
Burger, hamburger, single w/everythng	1 serv.	420	20	3		♦

♦ = Avoid • ♦ = Add for flavor

	Portion	Calories	Total Fat	Dietary Fiber	Trans Fat	Guide
Chicken, nuggets, 5 piece	1 serv.	230	16	0	T	💧
Chicken sandwich, breaded	1 serv.	440	18	2	T	💧
Chicken sandwich, club	1 serv.	470	20	2	T	💧
Chicken sandwich, grilled	1 serv.	310	8	2	T	💧
Chicken sandwich, spicy	1 serv.	410	15	2	T	💧
Condiments, dressing, French	2 tbsp.	120	10	0		💧
Condiments, dressing, French, fat free	2 tbsp.	35	0	0		✂
Condiments, dressing, Hidden Valley Ranch	2 tbsp.	100	10	0		💧
Condiments, dressing, Hidden Valley Ranch, reduced fat	2 tbsp.	60	5	0		💧
Condiments, dressing, Italian caesar	2 tbsp.	150	16	0	T	💧
Condiments, dressing, Italian, reduced fat	2 tbsp.	40	3	0		💧
Condiments, dressing, blue cheese	2 tbsp.	180	19	0		💧
Condiments, dressing, caesar vinaigrette	1 tbsp.	70	7	0		💧
Condiments, dressing, thousand island	2 tbsp.	90	8	0		💧
Condiments, sauce, barbecue	1 pkt.	45	0	0		✂
Condiments, sauce, garden ranch	1 tbsp.	50	5	0		💧
Condiments, sauce, honey mustard	1 pkt.	130	12	0		💧
Condiments, sauce, spicy buffalo wing	1 pkt.	25	1	0	T	💧
Condiments, sauce, sweet & sour	1 pkt.	50	0	0		✂
Dessert, Frosty, large	1 serv.	540	14	0		💧
Dessert, Frosty, medium	1 serv.	440	11	0		💧
Dessert, Frosty, small	1 serv.	330	8	0		💧
Dessert, cookie, chocolate chip	1 serv.	270	13	1	T	💧
French fries, Biggie	1 serv.	470	23	6	T	💧
French fries, Great Biggie	1 serv.	570	27	7	T	💧
French fries, medium	1 serv.	390	19	5	T	💧
French fries, small	1 serv.	270	13	3	T	💧
Pita, fresh stuffed, garden ranch chicken	1 serv.	480	18	5		💧
Pita, fresh stuffed, garden veggie	1 serv.	400	17	5		💧
Pita, fresh stuffed, chicken caesar	1 serv.	490	18	4		💧
Pita, fresh stuffed, classic Greek	1 serv.	440	20	4		💧
Potato, baked, bacon & cheese	1 serv.	530	1	7	T	💧
Potato, baked, broccoli & cheese	1 serv.	470	14	9	T	💧
Potato, baked, cheese	1 serv.	570	23	7	T	💧
Potato, baked, chili & cheese	1 serv.	630	24	9	T	💧
Potato, baked, plain	1 serv.	220	0	7		☺
Potato, baked, sour cream & chives	1 serv.	380	6	8		💧
Salad, caesar side w/out dressing	1 serv.	100	4	1	T	💧
Salad, deluxe garden w/out dressing	1 serv.	110	6	3		💧
Salad, grilled chicken caesar	1 serv.	260	9	2	T	💧
Salad, grilled chicken w/out dressing	1 serv.	200	8	3	T	💧
Salad, side w/out dressing	1 serv.	60	3	2		💧
Salad, taco w/out dressing	1 serv.	380	19	7	T	💧
Side, breadstick, soft	1 serv.	130	3	1	T	💧
Side, chili, small	1 serv.	210	7	5		💧

☺ = Eat as much as you want • ✂ = Cut Back

FOOD LISTS

	Portion	Calories	Total Fat	Dietary Fiber	Trans Fat	Guide
■ Fats, Oils & Salad Dressings						
Fats						
Lard	1 tbsp.	120	13	0		🌢
Fats, Butter						
Breakstone's	1 tbsp.	100	11	0		🌢
Land O Lakes, honey butter	1 tbsp.	90	8	0	T	🌢
Land O Lakes, roasted garlic w/olive oil	1 tbsp.	100	11	0		🌢
Land O Lakes, salted	1 tbsp.	100	11	0		🌢
Land O Lakes, salted light	1 tbsp.	50	6	0		🌢
Land O Lakes, salted light whipped	1 tbsp.	35	4	0		🌢
Land O Lakes, salted whipped	1 tbsp.	60	7	0		🌢
Land O Lakes, unsalted sweet	1 tbsp.	100	11	0		🌢
Land O Lakes, unsweetened	1 tbsp.	100	11	0		🌢
Move Over Butter	1 tbsp.	60	6	0	T	🌢
Organic Valley	1 tbsp.	100	11	0		🌢
Fats, Margarine						
Fleischmann's, lower fat, no cholesterol	1 tbsp.	50	6	0	T	🌢
Land O Lakes	1 tbsp.	100	11	0	T	🌢
Land O Lakes, Country Morning Blend	1 tbsp.	100	11	0	T	🌢
Promise, Ultra, fat free, non fat	1 tbsp.	5	0	0		👌
Shedd's, soy bean, willow run	1 tbsp.	100	11	0	T	🌢
Smart Beat, super light, trans fat free	1 tbsp.	20	2	0		✂
Fats, No-Stick Spray						
Baker's Joy, vegetable oil & flour	1/2 sec. spray	5	1	0		👌
Canola oil	1/3 sec. spray	0	0	0		👌
Country Crock, cooking & topping spray	1.25 sprays	0	0	0		👌
I Can't Believe It's Not Butter	1.25 sprays	0	0	0		👌
Mazola, butter flavor	1/3 sec. spray	0	0	0		👌
Mazola, corn oil	1/3 sec. spray	0	0	0		👌
Pam, butter flavor	1/3 sec. spray	0	0	0		👌
Pam, olive oil	1/3 sec. spray	0	0	0		👌
Pam, original canola	1/3 sec. spray	0	0	0		👌
Fats, Shortening						
Crisco	1 tbsp.	110	12	0	T	🌢
Crisco, butter flavor	1 tbsp.	110	12	0	T	🌢
Fats, Spread						
Blue Bonnet, vegetable oil	1 tbsp.	70	7	0	T	🌢
Brummel & Brown, made w/yogurt	1 tbsp.	50	5	0	T	🌢
Brummel & Brown, sticks, made w/yogurt	1 tbsp.	90	10	0	T	🌢
Country Crock	1 tbsp.	60	7	0	T	🌢
Country Crock, churn style	1 tbsp.	60	7	0	T	🌢
Country Crock, spreadable sticks	1 tbsp.	80	9	0	T	🌢

🌢 = *Avoid* • 👌 = *Add for flavor*

	Portion	Calories	Total Fat	Dietary Fiber	Trans Fat	Guide
Fleischmann's, original	1 tbsp.	90	10	0	T	🌢
Fleischmann's, soft	1 tbsp.	80	9	0	T	🌢
Fleischmann's, unsalted	1 tbsp.	90	10	0	T	🌢
I Can't Believe It's Not Butter, light	1 tbsp.	50	6	0	T	🌢
I Can't Believe It's Not Butter, sweet cream buttermilk	1 tbsp.	90	10	0	T	🌢
I Can't Believe It's Not Butter, sweet unsalted	1 tbsp.	90	10	0	T	🌢
Land O Lakes, Country Morning Blend, light, sticks	1 tbsp.	50	6	0		🌢
Land O Lakes, w/sweet cream	1 tbsp.	80	8	0	T	🌢
Lawry's, garlic	2 tbsp.	50	6	0	T	🌢
McCormick, garlic & herb	1/2 tbsp.	45	5	0	T	🌢
Parkay, vegetable	1 tbsp.	90	10	0	T	🌢
Promise, Ultra, vegetable oil	1 tbsp.	30	4	0	T	🌢
Promise, buttery light	1 tbsp.	50	6	0	T	🌢
Promise, sticks	1 tbsp.	90	10	0	T	🌢
Smart Balance	1 tbsp.	80	9	0		🌢

Fats, Squeeze

	Portion	Calories	Total Fat	Dietary Fiber	Trans Fat	Guide
Fleischmann's, fat free	1 tbsp.	5	0	0		👍
I Can't Believe It's Not Butter, easy squeeze	1 tbsp.	80	9	0	T	🌢
Parkay	1 tbsp.	80	9	0	T	🌢

Oils

	Portion	Calories	Total Fat	Dietary Fiber	Trans Fat	Guide
Canola & corn oil	1 tbsp.	120	14	0		🌢
Canola oil	1 tbsp.	120	14	0		🌢
Corn oil	1 tbsp.	120	14	0		🌢
Grapeseed oil	1 tbsp.	120	14	0		🌢
Hazelnut oil	1 tbsp.	120	14	0		🌢
Kame, Sesame oil	1 tbsp.	120	14	0		🌢
Olive oil	1 tbsp.	120	14	0		🌢
Orville Redenbacher's, popping & topping buttery flavor	1 tbsp.	120	14	0		🌢
Planters, peanut oil, 100% pure	1 tbsp.	120	14	0		🌢
Safflower oil	1 tbsp.	120	14	0		🌢
Seasoned wok oil	1 tbsp.	130	14	0		🌢
Smucker's, Baking Healthy, oil & shortening replacement	1 tbsp.	30	0	0		✂
Sunflower oil	1 tbsp.	120	14	0		🌢
Sunsweet, Lighter Bake, butter & oil replacement	1 tbsp.	35	0	0		✂
Vegetable oil	1 tbsp.	120	14	0		🌢

Salad Dressings

	Portion	Calories	Total Fat	Dietary Fiber	Trans Fat	Guide
Hellmann's, Italian	2 tbsp.	110	11	0		🌢
Hellmann's, Italian, fat free	2 tbsp.	15	0	0		✂
Hellmann's, caesar	2 tbsp.	100	9	0		🌢
Hellmann's, chunky bleu cheese	2 tbsp.	140	15	0		🌢
Hellmann's, creamy ranch	2 tbsp.	140	15	0		🌢
Hellmann's, creamy thousand island	2 tbsp.	130	13	0		🌢

☺ = Eat as much as you want • ✂ = Cut Back

	Portion	Calories	Total Fat	Dietary Fiber	Trans Fat	Guide
Hidden Valley, caesar	2 tbsp.	110	11	0		●
Hidden Valley, fat free, Italian herb & cheese	2 tbsp.	30	0	0		✂
Hidden Valley, fat free, original ranch	2 tbsp.	30	0	0		✂
Hidden Valley, fat free, red wine & herb vinaigrette	2 tbsp.	45	0	0		✂
Hidden Valley, fat free, roasted garlic Italian	2 tbsp.	40	0	0		✂
Hidden Valley, honey & bacon French	2 tbsp.	150	12	0		●
Hidden Valley, original ranch	2 tbsp.	140	14	0		●
Hidden Valley, original ranch, light	2 tbsp.	80	7	0		●
Ken's Steak House, Italian w/aged romano	2 tbsp.	110	12	0		●
Ken's Steak House, thousand island	2 tbsp.	140	13	0		●
Ken's Steak House, burgundy basil vinaigrette	2 tbsp.	100	11	0		●
Ken's Steak House, caesar	2 tbsp.	170	18	0		●
Ken's Steak House, chunky blue cheese	2 tbsp.	140	15	0		●
Ken's Steak House, fat free, peppercorn ranch	2 tbsp.	25	0	0		✂
Ken's Steak House, fat free, raspberry pecan	2 tbsp.	45	0	0		✂
Ken's Steak House, fat free, sun-dried tomato vinaigrette	2 tbsp.	60	0	0		✂
Ken's Steak House, ranch	2 tbsp.	180	20	0		●
Ken's Steak House Lite, caesar	2 tbsp.	70	6	0		●
Ken's Steak House Lite, country French w/Vermont honey	2 tbsp.	90	5	0		●
Ken's Steak House Lite, creamy parmesan	2 tbsp.	90	9	0		●
Ken's Steak House Lite, honey mustard	2 tbsp.	70	5	0		●
Ken's Steak House Lite, raspberry walnut vinaigrette	2 tbsp.	80	6	0		●
Ken's Steak House Lite, red wine vinegar & olive oil	2 tbsp.	50	5	0		●
Kraft, zesty Italian	2 tbsp.	110	11	0		●
Kraft, catalina	2 tbsp.	130	11	0		●
Kraft, classic caesar	2 tbsp.	110	11	0		●
Kraft, creamy French	2 tbsp.	160	15	0		●
Kraft, fat free, Italian	2 tbsp.	20	0	0		✂
Kraft, fat free, blue cheese	2 tbsp.	45	0	0		✂
Kraft, fat free, classic caesar	2 tbsp.	45	0	0		✂
Kraft, fat free, thousand island	2 tbsp.	40	0	0		✂
Kraft Free, French style	2 tbsp.	45	0	0		✂
Kraft Free, catalina	2 tbsp.	35	0	0		✂
Kraft Free, ranch	2 tbsp.	50	0	1		✂
Kraft Free, zesty Italian	2 tbsp.	15	0	0		✂
Kraft, parmesan Italian	2 tbsp.	120	12	0		●
Kraft, ranch	2 tbsp.	170	18	0		●
Kraft, roka blue cheese	2 tbsp.	130	13	0		●
Kraft, thousand island	2 tbsp.	110	10	0		●
Newman's Own, balsamic vinaigrette	2 tbsp.	90	9	0		●
Newman's Own, caesar	2 tbsp.	150	16	0		●
Newman's Own, olive oil & vinager dressing	2 tbsp.	150	16	0		●
Olympia Dukakis', creamy feta	2 tbsp.	140	15	0		●
Olympia Dukakis', Greek	2 tbsp.	150	16	0		●
Pritikin, fat free, honey dijon	2 tbsp.	45	0	1		✂

● = Avoid • ✂ = Add for flavor

	Portion	Calories	Total Fat	Dietary Fiber	Trans Fat	Guide
Pritikin, fat free, kitchen classic French	2 tbsp.	30	0	0		✄
Pritikin, fat free, zesty Italian	2 tbsp.	30	0	0		✄
Weight Watchers, French style	2 tbsp.	40	0	0		✄
Weight Watchers, caesar, fat free	2 tbsp.	10	0	0		👍
Weight Watchers, honey dijon	2 tbsp.	45	0	0		✄
Weight Watchers, ranch	2 tbsp.	35	0	0		✄
Wishbone, French, deluxe	2 tbsp.	120	11	0		🌢
Wishbone, Italian	2 tbsp.	80	8	0		🌢
Wishbone, Italian, lite	2 tbsp.	15	1	0		✄
Wishbone, Russian	2 tbsp.	110	6	0		🌢
Wishbone, chunky blue cheese	2 tbsp.	170	17	0		🌢
Wishbone, classic caesar	2 tbsp.	110	10	0		🌢
Wishbone, creamy Italian	2 tbsp.	110	10	0		🌢
Wishbone, fat free, Italian	2 tbsp.	10	0	0		👍
Wishbone, fat free, chunky blue cheese	2 tbsp.	35	0	0		✄
Wishbone, fat free, red wine vinaigrette	2 tbsp.	35	0	0		✄
Wishbone, fat free, thousand island	2 tbsp.	35	0	0		✄
Wishbone, oriental	2 tbsp.	70	5	0		🌢
Wishbone, ranch	2 tbsp.	160	17	0		🌢
Wishbone, red wine vinaigrette	2 tbsp.	90	5	0		🌢
Wishbone, robusto Italian	2 tbsp.	90	8	0		🌢

Salad Dressings, Dry Mix

	Portion	Calories	Total Fat	Dietary Fiber	Trans Fat	Guide
Good Seasons, Italian, prepared	2 tbsp.	140	15	0		🌢
Good Seasons, cheese garlic, prepared	2 tbsp.	140	16	0		🌢
Good Seasons, garlic & herb, prepared	2 tbsp.	140	15	0		🌢
Hidden Valley, fiesta ranch, prepared	1/6 pkt.	70	0	0		✄
Hidden Valley, original ranch, prepared	1/6 pkt.	35	0	0		✄

■ FISH & SHELLFISH

Fish, Canned

	Portion	Calories	Total Fat	Dietary Fiber	Trans Fat	Guide
Bonavita, snails, natural	6 snails	80	1	0		✄
Bumble Bee, albacore tuna, fancy in veg. oil	2 oz.	90	3	0		🌢
Bumble Bee, albacore tuna, fancy in water	2 oz.	70	1	0		✄
Bumble Bee, salmon, pink in water	1/4 cup	70	2	0		✄
Bumble Bee, salmon, red	1/4 cup	110	7	0		✄
Empress, anchovies, roll fillets in olive oil	4 pieces	25	2	0		✄
Empress, mackerel, jack	1/4 cup	90	4	0		✄
Gorton's, codfish cakes	4 oz.	100	1	0		✄
Iceland Waters, herring, smoked, kipper snacks	1 can	200	13	0		✄
Iceland Waters, trout, brook	1/4 cup	70	3	0		✄
Marina, smoked salmon pâté	1/2 tub	126	10	0		🌢
Progresso, tuna, solid packed in olive oil	1/4 cup	160	12	0		🌢
Reese, sardines, hot & spicy w/veg.	1/2 can	100	6	0		✄
Season, salmon, pink	1/4 cup	90	5	0		✄
Season, sardines in pure olive oil	1 can	240	14	0		🌢
Season, sardines in tomato sauce	1/2 can	110	6	0		✄

☺ = Eat as much as you want • ✄ = Cut Back

	Portion	Calories	Total Fat	Dietary Fiber	Trans Fat	Guide
Season, sardines, skinless & boneless in water	1 can	160	8	0		✂
Starkist, fancy albacore, in pure vegetable oil	2 oz.	90	3	0		⚫
Starkist, fancy albacore, white tuna in spring water	2 oz.	70	1	0		✂
Underwood, sardines in mustard sauce	1 can	180	12	1		✂
Underwood, sardines, fancy, in soya oil	1 can	220	16	0		⚫

Fish, Fresh or Thawed

	Portion	Calories	Total Fat	Dietary Fiber	Trans Fat	Guide
Amberjack	3.5 oz.	106	8	0		✂
Bass, Chilean sea	3 oz.	97	2	0		✂
Bass, hybrid striped	3 oz.	82	2	0		✂
Bass, sea	3 oz.	82	2	0		✂
Butter fish	3 oz.	124	7	0		✂
Carp	3 oz.	108	5	0		✂
Catfish	4 oz.	140	9	0		✂
Catfish, skinless	3 oz.	140	9	0		✂
Cod	4 oz.	90	1	0		✂
Cod, skinless	3 oz.	90	1	0		✂
Croaker	3 oz.	89	3	0		✂
Drum	3 oz.	101	4	0		✂
Flounder	4 oz.	100	2	0		✂
Flounder, skinless	3 oz.	100	2	0		✂
Grouper	3 oz.	78	1	0		✂
Haddock	4 oz.	100	1	0		✂
Haddock, skinless	3 oz.	100	1	0		✂
Hake	3.5 oz.	90	1	0		✂
Halibut	4 oz.	110	2	0		✂
Halibut, skinless	3 oz.	110	2	0		✂
Hoki	3 oz.	85	2	0		✂
Mackerel	4 oz.	210	13	0		✂
Mackerel, Atlantic/Pacific, skinless	3 oz.	210	13	0		✂
Mahi-mahi	3 oz.	73	1	0		✂
Marlin	3 oz.	109	3	0		✂
Monkfish	3 oz.	64	1	0		✂
Mullet	3 oz.	99	3	0		✂
Ocean perch, skinless, baked	3 oz.	110	2	0		✂
Orange roughy	4 oz.	80	1	0		✂
Orange roughy, skinless	3 oz.	80	1	0		✂
Perch, Lake Victoria	3 oz.	77	1	0		✂
Perch, ocean	4 oz.	110	2	0		✂
Pollock	4 oz.	90	1	0		✂
Pollock, skinless	3 oz.	90	1	0		✂
Pompano	3 oz.	140	8	0		✂
Rockfish	4 oz.	100	2	0		✂
Rockfish, skinless	3 oz.	100	2	0		✂
Salmon, Atlantic	4 oz.	160	7	0		✂
Salmon, Atlantic/Coho, skinless	3 oz.	160	7	0		✂
Salmon, chum	4 oz.	130	4	0		✂
Salmon, Coho	4 oz.	160	7	0		✂

⚫ = *Avoid* • 💧 = *Add for flavor*

	Portion	Calories	Total Fat	Dietary Fiber	Trans Fat	Guide
Salmon, chum/pink, skinless	3 oz.	130	4	0		✂
Salmon, sockeye	4 oz.	180	9	0		✂
Salmon, sockeye, skinless	3 oz.	180	9	0		✂
Shark	3 oz.	111	4	0		✂
Sheepshead	3 oz.	92	2	0		✂
Smelt	3 oz.	83	2	0		✂
Snapper	3 oz.	85	1	0		✂
Sole	4 oz.	100	2	0		✂
Sole, skinless	3 oz.	100	2	0		✂
Squid	3 oz.	78	1	0		✂
Sturgeon	3 oz.	90	3	0		✂
Swordfish	4 oz.	130	5	0		✂
Swordfish, skinless	3 oz.	130	5	0		✂
Tilapia	3 oz.	93	1	0		✂
Trout, lake	3 oz.	126	6	0		✂
Trout, rainbow	4 oz.	140	6	0		✂
Trout, rainbow, skinless	3 oz.	140	6	0		✂
Trout, sea	3 oz.	88	3	0		✂
Tuna	3 oz.	92	1	0		✂
Turbot	3 oz.	100	3	0		✂
Walleye	3 oz.	79	1	0		✂
Whitefish	3 oz.	114	5	0		✂
Whiting	4 oz.	110	3	0		✂
Whiting, skinless	3 oz.	110	3	0		✂

Shellfish, Canned

	Portion	Calories	Total Fat	Dietary Fiber	Trans Fat	Guide
Chicken of the Sea, crabmeat, fancy	2 oz.	40	0	0		✂
Doxsee, clams, minced	1/4 cup	25	0	0		✂
Dynasty, clams, baby	2 oz.	30	0	0		✂
Geisha, oysters, fancy smoked	1/2 cup	120	7	2		✂
Geisha, oysters, whole	1/3 cup	60	3	2		✂
Gold Boat, mussels, marinated	1/3 cup	60	0	0		✂
Gorton's, Chesapeake classics, clams, cocktail, steamer	1/4 cup	30	0	0		✂
Orleans, crabmeat, fancy white	2 oz.	28	0	0		✂
Orleans, shrimp, deviled large	2 oz.	44	0	0		✂
Sun of Italy, clams, minced	1/4 cup	30	0	0		✂

Shellfish, Fresh or Thawed

	Portion	Calories	Total Fat	Dietary Fiber	Trans Fat	Guide
Blue crab, shell-less	3 oz.	100	1	0		✂
Clams, hard shell	4 oz.	100	2	0		✂
Clams, shell-less	12 small	100	2	0		✂
Crab, blue	4 oz.	100	1	0		✂
Crab, Dungeness	3 oz.	73	1	0		✂
Crab, king	3 oz.	71	1	0		✂
Crab, snow	3 oz.	76	1	0		✂
Crab, softshell	3 oz.	63	1	0		✂
Crabmeat, imitation	3 oz.	84	1	0		✂
Crawfish	3 oz.	76	1	0		✂

☺ = Eat as much as you want • ✂ = Cut Back

	Portion	Calories	Total Fat	Dietary Fiber	Trans Fat	Guide
Lobster, American	4 oz.	80	1	0		✂
Lobster, shell-less	3 oz.	80	1	0		✂
Lobster, spiny	3 oz.	95	1	0		✂
Mussels	3 oz.	73	2	0		✂
Oysters	6 med.	100	4	0		✂
Oysters, shell-less	12 med.	100	4	0		✂
Scallop, shell-less	6 large	120	1	0		✂
Scallops, Bay	4 oz.	120	1	0		✂
Scallops, sea	4 oz.	120	1	0		✂
Shrimp, Gulf	4 oz.	80	2	0		✂
Shrimp, black tiger	4 oz.	80	1	0		✂
Shrimp, pink, cold water	3 oz.	90	2	0		✂
Shrimp, rock	3 oz.	90	2	0		✂
Shrimp, skinless	3 oz.	80	1	0		✂

■ FRUITS

Canned

	Portion	Calories	Total Fat	Dietary Fiber	Trans Fat	Guide
Apricot halves, unpeeled in heavy syrup	$^1/_4$ cup	100	0	1		✂
Bing cherries, glazed	1 piece	15	0	0		✂
Blueberries, filling in heavy syrup	$^1/_2$ cup	130	0	1		✂
Cherries, glazed	1 piece	15	0	0		✂
Cherries, red, pitted tart filling	$^2/_3$ cup	60	0	2		✂
Comstock, More Fruit, apple filling	$^1/_3$ cup	80	0	1		✂
Comstock, More Fruit, blueberry filling	$^1/_3$ cup	80	0	1		✂
Comstock, More Fruit, peach filling	$^1/_3$ cup	80	4	1		●
Comstock, Original, cherry, light filling	$^1/_3$ cup	60	0	1		✂
Comstock, Original, cherry, red ruby filling	$^1/_3$ cup	90	0	1		✂
Comstock, strawberry, premium filling	$^1/_3$ cup	100	0	1		✂
Del Monte, peaches, sliced, lite	$^1/_2$ cup	60	0	1		☺
Del Monte, fruit cocktail, lite	$^1/_2$ cup	60	0	1		☺
Del Monte, mixed fruit, very cherry	$^1/_2$ cup	90	0	0		☺
Del Monte, peaches, freestone sliced	$^1/_2$ cup	100	0	1		☺
Del Monte, peaches, harvest spice sliced	$^1/_2$ cup	80	0	0		☺
Del Monte, peaches, sliced, fruit naturals	$^1/_2$ cup	60	0	1		☺
Del Monte, pear halves, Fruit Naturals	$^1/_2$ cup	60	0	1		☺
Del Monte, pear halves, lite	$^1/_2$ cup	60	0	1		☺
Del Monte, pineapple wedges	$^1/_2$ cup	70	0	1		☺
Del Monte, pineapple, fresh cut chunks	$^1/_2$ cup	70	0	1		☺
Dole, fruit salad, tropical	$^1/_2$ cup	80	0	1		☺
Dole, oranges, mandarin	$^1/_2$ cup	80	0	0		☺
Dole, pineapple chunks	$^1/_2$ cup	90	0	1		☺
Dole, pineapple, crushed	$^1/_2$ cup	90	0	1		☺
Grapefruit, sections in light syrup	$^2/_3$ cup	100	0	0		✂
Kame, lychees, whole pitted	15 pieces	130	0	0		☺
Libby's, apricot halves in fruit juice, lite	$^1/_2$ cup	60	0	1		✂
Libby's, mixed fruits, chunky, light	$^1/_2$ cup	60	0	1		☺
Libby's, peaches, sliced, lite	$^1/_2$ cup	60	0	1		☺

● = *Avoid* • ◔ = *Add for flavor*

	Portion	Calories	Total Fat	Dietary Fiber	Trans Fat	Guide
Libby's, pear halves, lite	1/2 cup	60	0	1		☺
Libby's, pumpkin, solid packed filling	1/2 cup	40	1	5		☺
Lucky Leaf, apples, Dutch baked	1/2 cup	170	0	3		☺
Mott's, Fruitsations, cherry	4 oz.	70	0	1		✂
Mott's, Fruitsations, mango peach	4 oz.	70	0	1		✂
Mott's, Fruitsations, mixed berry	4 oz.	90	0	1		✂
Mott's, applesauce	1/2 cup	100	0	1		✂
Musselman's, applesauce	1/2 cup	90	0	2		☺
Ocean Spray, Cranfruit, cranberry orange	1/4 cup	120	0	1		☺
Ocean Spray, Cranfruit, cranberry raspberry	1/4 cup	120	0	2		☺
Ocean Spray, Cranfruit, cranberry strawberry	1/4 cup	120	0	2		☺
Ocean Spray, cranberry sauce, crushed berry	1/4 cup	120	0	1		☺
Ocean Spray, cranberry sauce, jellied	1/4 cup	110	0	0		✂
Oregon Fruit Products, blackberries in light syrup, filling	1/2 cup	120	0	6		☺
Oregon Fruit Products, kadota figs in heavy syrup, filling	1/2 cup	130	1	3		☺
Prunes, in heavy syrup	1/2 cup	123	0	4		☺
Seneca, applesauce, macintosh	1/2 cup	100	0	2		☺
Solo, apricot filling	2 tbsp.	80	0	1		✂
Sunfresh, citrus salad	1/2 cup	70	0	0		☺
Sunfresh, grapefruit, pink	1/2 cup	45	0	2		☺
Sunfresh, grapefruit, red sections	1/2 cup	70	0	1		☺
Sunfresh, mango slices	1/2 cup	100	1	0		☺
Sunfresh, orange sections	1/2 cup	80	0	2		☺
Sunfresh, tropical salad in extra light syrup	1/2 cup	80	0	0		☺
White House, Fruitastics, apple banana	4 oz.	100	0	1		✂
White House, Fruitastics, apple peach	4 oz.	100	0	1		✂
White House, apple rings, spiced	1 ring	30	0	0		✂
White House, apples, escalloped	1/2 cup	160	0	0		✂
Whole dates	5–6 dates	120	0	3		☺

Dried

	Portion	Calories	Total Fat	Dietary Fiber	Trans Fat	Guide
Apple, organic rings	1/3 cup	110	0	3		☺
Banana chips	1/4 cup	150	8	1		◖
Cranberries	1/3 cup	120	0	2		☺
Dates, natural	10 dates	228	0	6		☺
Dole, chopped dates	1/4 cup	120	0	3		☺
Dole, raisins, California seedless	1/4 cup	130	0	2		☺
Goya, plantain chips	38 pieces	170	11	2		◖
Ocean Spray, craisins (cranberries)	1/3 cup	130	0	2		☺
Orchard Choice, Calimyrni figs	1.5 oz.	120	0	5		☺
Prunes, large	1.5 oz.	100	0	3		☺
Raisin, golden, seedless, unpacked	1/4 cup	110	0	2		☺
Raisins, seedless, not packed	1/4 cup	109	0	2		☺
Sun-Maid, raisins, California golden	1/4 cup	130	0	2		☺
Sun-Maid, raisins, California sun-dried	1/4 cup	130	0	2		☺
Sunsweet, apricots	1/4 cup	110	0	2		☺
Sunsweet, mixed fruit	1/4 cup	110	0	3		☺

☺ = *Eat as much as you want* • ✂ = *Cut Back*

	Portion	Calories	Total Fat	Dietary Fiber	Trans Fat	Guide
Sunsweet, prunes, bite size pitted	1.5 oz.	110	0	3		☺
Sunsweet, prunes, large	1.5 oz.	100	0	3		☺
Sunsweet, prunes, pitted	1.5 oz.	110	0	3		☺
Sunsweet, prunes, ready to serve	$2/3$ cup	150	0	3		☺

Fresh

	Portion	Calories	Total Fat	Dietary Fiber	Trans Fat	Guide
Apple	1 med.	80	0	5		☺
Apricot	3 med.	51	0	3		☺
Avocado	1 med.	306	30	5		●
Banana	1 med.	110	0	4		☺
Blackberries	1 cup	84	1	6		☺
Blueberries	$1/2$ cup	41	0	2		☺
Cantaloupe	$1/4$ med.	50	0	1		☺
Cherry, Bing	10 cherries	47	0	1		☺
Cranberries	$1/2$ cup	23	0	2		☺
Currant	$1/4$ cup	100	0	2		☺
Fig	1 med.	37	0	2		☺
Grapefruit	$1/2$ med.	60	0	6		☺
Grapes	$1 1/2$ cups	90	1	1		☺
Honeydew	$1/10$ med.	50	0	1		☺
Kiwi	1 med.	46	0	3		☺
Lemon	1 med.	15	0	1		☺
Lime	1 med.	20	0	2		☺
Mango	1 med.	135	1	4		☺
Nectarine	1 med.	70	1	2		☺
Orange	1 med.	70	0	7		☺
Papaya	1 med.	119	0	3		☺
Peach	1 med.	40	0	2		☺
Pear	1 med.	100	1	4		☺
Pineapple	1 cup	80	0	2		☺
Plantain	1 med.	218	1	4		☺
Plum	1 med.	36	0	1		☺
Raspberry	1 cup	98	2	7		☺
Rhubarb	$1/2$ cup	13	0	1		☺
Strawberry	1 cup	55	1	2		☺
Tangerine	1 med.	50	1	3		☺
Watermelon	2 cups	80	0	2		☺

Frozen

	Portion	Calories	Total Fat	Dietary Fiber	Trans Fat	Guide
Blackberry	$3/4$ cup	90	0	4		☺
Blueberry	$3/4$ cup	70	0	4		☺
Cherry, pitted dark	$3/4$ cup	140	2	7		☺
Peach, sliced	$3/4$ cup	60	1	3		☺
Raspberry, red	$1/2$ cup	130	0	2		☺
Raspberry, red in sugar syrup	$1/2$ cup	200	1	7		☺
Strawberry	$2/3$ cup	50	0	2		☺
Strawberry, sliced in sugar	$1/2$ cup	150	0	2		☺

● = Avoid • ⬟ = Add for flavor

	Portion	Calories	Total Fat	Dietary Fiber	Trans Fat	Guide

■ GRAINS & GRAIN PRODUCTS

Breads

	Portion	Calories	Total Fat	Dietary Fiber	Trans Fat	Guide
Arnold, 100% whole wheat	1 slice	90	1	2	T	✿
Arnold, Bran'nola, 12 grain	1 slice	90	2	3	T	✿
Arnold, Bran'nola, country oat	1 slice	90	3	3	T	✿
Arnold, Bran'nola, nutty grain	1 slice	90	3	3	T	✿
Arnold, Bran'nola, original	1 slice	90	2	3	T	✿
Arnold, Real Jewish rye caraway seed	1 slice	80	1	0	T	✿
Arnold, Real Jewish rye melba thin	2 slices	110	2	1		✂
Arnold, Real Jewish rye w/out seeds	1 slice	80	1	0	T	✿
Arnold, bakery light, Italian	2 slices	80	1	5		✂
Arnold, bakery light, golden wheat	2 slices	80	1	4		✂
Arnold, bakery light, oatmeal	2 slices	80	1	4		✂
Arnold, brick oven, white	2 slices	140	3	1	T	✿
Arnold, buttermilk	1 slice	110	2	0	T	✿
Arnold, country wheat	1 slice	90	2	1	T	✿
Arnold, country white	1 slice	110	2	0	T	✿
Arnold, health nut	1 slice	100	2	2	T	✿
Arnold, honey wheatberry	1 slice	100	1	2	T	✿
Arnold, marble rye & pumpernickel	1 slice	80	1	0	T	✿
Arnold, oatnut	1 slice	110	2	1		✂
Arnold, pumpernickel	1 slice	80	1	0	T	✿
Arnold, raisin cinnamon	1 slice	80	1	0	T	✿
Arnold, stone ground, 100% whole wheat	1 slice	60	1	2	T	✿
B & M, brown bread raisin	2 oz.	130	1	2		✂
Beefsteak, rye, hearty	1 slice	70	1	1		✂
Bread Dujour, French loaves	3 slice	140	1	1		✂
Brownberry, health nut	1 slice	70	2	1	T	✿
Brownberry, wheat, natural	1 slice	90	1	2		✂
Colombo, sourdough	2 oz.	120	0	0		✂
Hawaiian Bread	2 oz.	180	4	2	T	✿
Home Pride, wheat, butter topped	1 slice	80	1	0		✂
Martin's, potato bread	1 slice	100	2	1	T	✿
Monastery Bread, whole wheat	1 slice	70	2	2		✂
New York Flat Breads	1 piece	50	1	1		✂
New York Flat Breads, minis	3 pieces	58	1	1		✂
Pepperidge Farm, Italian	1 slice	90	2	0	T	✿
Pepperidge Farm, Jewish rye, seeded w/caraway	1 slice	80	1	2	T	✿
Pepperidge Farm, Whole natural grain, crunchy grain	1 slice	90	3	2	T	✿
Pepperidge Farm, classic dark pumpernickel	1 slice	80	1	2	T	✿
Pepperidge Farm, crunchy sandwich, oat	1 slice	100	2	2	T	✿
Pepperidge Farm, deli swirl, rye & pumpernickel	1 slice	80	1	1	T	✿
Pepperidge Farm, hearty slices, honey wheatberry	1 slice	100	2	2	T	✿
Pepperidge Farm, hearty slices, sesame wheat	1 slice	100	2	2	T	✿
Pepperidge Farm, hearty slices, seven grain	1 slice	100	2	2	T	✿

☺ = Eat as much as you want • ✂ = Cut Back

	Portion	Calories	Total Fat	Dietary Fiber	Trans Fat	Guide
Pepperidge Farm, hot & crusty, Italian	2 oz.	150	2	1	T	🌢
Pepperidge Farm, light style, 7 grain	3 slices	140	1	5	T	🌢
Pepperidge Farm, light style, oatmeal	3 slices	130	1	5	T	🌢
Pepperidge Farm, light style, wheat	3 slices	130	1	5	T	🌢
Pepperidge Farm, oatmeal	1 slice	60	1	1	T	🌢
Pepperidge Farm, original, white	1 slice	70	2	0	T	🌢
Pepperidge Farm, sandwich swirl, wheat & 7 grain	1 slice	100	2	2	T	🌢
Pepperidge Farm, sandwich, white	2 slices	130	3	1	T	🌢
Pepperidge Farm, swirl, banana nut	1 slice	100	3	3	T	🌢
Pepperidge Farm, swirl, cinnamon	1 slice	90	3	1	T	🌢
Pepperidge Farm, swirl, raisin cinnamon	1 slice	80	2	1	T	🌢
Pepperidge Farm, toasting, white harvest	1 slice	110	1	1	T	🌢
Pepperidge Farm, very thin, wheat	3 slices	120	2	3	T	🌢
Pepperidge Farm, very thin, white	3 slices	120	1	1	T	🌢
Pepperidge Farm, whole natural grain, 9 grain	1 slice	90	1	2	T	🌢
Pepperidge Farm, whole wheat	1 slice	60	1	0	T	🌢
Pepperidge Farm, whole wheat, natural grain	1 slice	90	2	1	T	🌢
Roman Meal, honey wheat berry	1 slice	90	1	2	T	🌢
Roman Meal, sandwich bread, whole grain	2 slices	120	2	2		✂
Roman Meal, sun grain	1 slice	90	2	2	T	🌢
Roman Meal, whole grain	1 slice	90	2	2	T	🌢
Rubschlager, pumpernickel	1 slice	70	1	2		✂
Rubschlager, whole grain	1 slice	70	1	3		✂
Schmidt, butter	1 slice	80	1	0		✂
Schmidt, butter wheat	1 slice	80	1	1		✂
Schmidt's, Italian, seeded	1 slice	80	2	1		✂
Schmidt's, Old Tyme, potato	1 slice	100	2	1		✂
Schmidt's, Old Tyme, wheat, split-top	1 slice	80	1	2		✂
Schmidt's, Sunbeam, pound	1 slice	70	1	0		✂
Schmidt's, Sunbeam, white w/buttermilk	1 slice	70	1	0		✂
Schmidt's, country white potato	1 slice	70	1	1		✂
Steak Light, rye, soft	2 slices	50	1	5		✂
Sunflower crunch loaf	1 slice	140	2	8		✂
Viva de France, baguette, French	6 slice	180	1	2		✂
Viva de France, baguettes, enriched mini	1 baguette	240	2	3		✂
Wonder, Italian seeded	1 slice	70	1	0		✂
Wonder, country potato	1 slice	90	1	0		✂
Wonder, light, Italian, low fat	2 slices	80	1	5		✂
Wonder, light, sourdough, low fat	2 slices	80	1	5		✂
Wonder, light, wheat	2 slices	80	1	5		✂
Wonder, light, white	2 slices	80	1	5		✂
Wonder, thin, white	2 slices	110	2	1		✂
Wonder, white	2 slices	120	2	1		✂
Wonder, white w/buttermilk	1 slice	70	1	0		✂
Wonder, whole wheat, stone ground	1 slice	90	2	3		✂

Breads, Bagel

	Portion	Calories	Total Fat	Dietary Fiber	Trans Fat	Guide
Lender's Bagels, Big'n Crusty, blueberry	1 bagel	220	1	2	T	🌢

🌢 = Avoid • 🌢 = Add for flavor

	Portion	Calories	Total Fat	Dietary Fiber	Trans Fat	Guide
Lender's Bagels, Big'n Crusty, cinnamon raisin	1 bagel	230	2	2		✂
Lender's Bagels, Big'n Crusty, egg	1 bagel	230	2	1		✂
Lender's Bagels, Big'n Crusty, honey wheat	1 bagel	200	1	2		✂
Lender's Bagels, bagelettes, plain	2 bagelettes	140	1	1		✂
Lender's Bagels, blueberry	1 bagel	200	1	2	T	●
Lender's Bagels, blueberry swirl	1 bagel	160	1	1		✂
Lender's Bagels, cinnamon raisin	1 bagel	230	3	2		●
Lender's Bagels, cinnamon swirl	1 bagel	150	1	1		✂
Lender's Bagels, egg	1 bagel	160	2	1		✂
Lender's Bagels, onion	1 bagel	220	2	2		✂
Lender's Bagels, plain	1 bagel	200	2	2		✂
Sara Lee, blueberry, 98% fat free	1 bagel	210	1	3		✂
Sara Lee, cinnamon & raisin, 98% fat free	1 bagel	220	1	3		✂
Sara Lee, oat bran, 98% fat free	1 bagel	210	1	3		✂
Thomas' New York Style, blueberry	1 bagel	290	2	2		✂
Thomas' New York Style, cinnamon raisin	1 bagel	280	2	3		✂
Thomas' New York Style, everything	1 bagel	300	4	3		●
Thomas' New York Style, multi grain	1 bagel	280	2	3		✂
Thomas' New York Style, onion	1 bagel	280	2	2		✂
Thomas' New York Style, plain	1 bagel	280	2	2		✂
Uncle B's, never frozen, cinnamon raisin	1 bagel	210	1	1		✂
Uncle B's, never frozen, honey wheat	1 bagel	210	2	2		✂
Uncle B's, pre-sliced, plain	1 bagel	210	1	1		✂

Breads, Bread Mix

	Portion	Calories	Total Fat	Dietary Fiber	Trans Fat	Guide
Aunt Jemima, easy mix corn bread	1/8 pkg.	140	4	1	T	●
Betty Crocker, gingerbread	1/8 pkg.	230	6	0	T	●
Fleischmann's, bread machine mix, honey oatmeal	1/3 cup dry	160	2	2	T	●
Fleischmann's, bread machine mix, wheat, stone ground	1/3 cup dry	160	2	3	T	●
Fleischmann's, bread machine mix, white, country	1/3 cup dry	160	2	1	T	●
Pillsbury, Quick Bread & Muffin Mix, apple cinnamon	1/12 pkg.	150	2	1	T	●
Pillsbury, Quick Bread Mix, banana	1/12 pkg.	130	2	0	T	●
Pillsbury, Quick Bread Mix, chocolate chip swirl	1/16 pkg.	140	4	0	T	●
Pillsbury, Quick Bread Mix, cinnamon swirl	1/12 pkg.	180	5	0	T	●
Pillsbury, Quick Bread Mix, cranberry	1/12 pkg.	160	2	0	T	●
Pillsbury, Quick Bread Mix, lemon poppyseed	1/12 pkg.	180	5	0	T	●
Pillsbury, Quick Bread Mix, nut	1/12 pkg.	150	4	1	T	●
Pillsbury, Quick Bread Mix, pumpkin	1/12 pkg.	130	2	0	T	●
Pillsbury, specialty mix, hot roll	1 roll	130	1	0	T	●
Quick Loaf, cinnamon raisin	3 tbsp.	120	0	0		✂
Quick Loaf, garlic & herbs	3 tbsp.	110	0	0		✂
Quick Loaf, hearty cracked wheat	3 tbsp.	110	0	0		✂
Quick Loaf, honey oatmeal	3 tbsp.	120	0	1		✂
Quick Loaf, nine grain	3 tbsp.	110	0	1		✂
Washington, biscuit, buttermilk	5 tbsp.	160	5	0	T	●
Washington, buttermilk corn bread	1/9 pkg.	90	2	1	T	●

☺ = Eat as much as you want • ✂ = Cut Back

	Portion	Calories	Total Fat	Dietary Fiber	Trans Fat	Guide
Washington, corn bread	$^1/_9$ pkg.	110	2	1	T	🌢
Washington, spoon bread	$^1/_{17}$ pkg.	70	3	0	T	🌢

Breads, Breadstick

15 Cheese, soft	1 stick	80	2	1	T	🌢
Bread Dujour, original	1 stick	130	1	1		✄

Breads, Bun/Roll

Arnold, Bran'nola, bun	1 bun	150	2	3	T	🌢
Arnold, hamburger bun, original	1 bun	130	2	1	T	🌢
Arnold, hot dog bun, original	1 bun	110	2	1	T	🌢
Arnold, potato roll	1 roll	130	2	0	T	🌢
Arnold, soft roll, sandwich original	1 roll	130	3	1	T	🌢
Bread Dujour, Italian	1 roll	90	1	0		✄
Bread Dujour, cracked wheat	1 roll	100	1	1		✄
Colombo, French, sour	1 roll	120	2	2	T	🌢
King's Hawaiian, honey & wheat	1 roll	90	2	1	T	🌢
Martin's, hoagie rolls	1 roll	250	4	3	T	🌢
Martin's, potato rolls, dinner	1 roll	100	1	0	T	🌢
Martin's, potato rolls, long	1 roll	140	2	0	T	🌢
Martin's, potato rolls, party	3 rolls	150	2	1	T	🌢
Martin's, potato rolls, sandwich	1 roll	150	2	1	T	🌢
Martin's, potato rolls, sliced	1 roll	90	1	0	T	🌢
Martin's, whole wheat sandwich rolls	1 roll	170	2	3	T	🌢
Marty's, large rolls, big	1 roll	190	4	2	T	🌢
Pepperidge Farm, Deli Classic, soft hoagie	1 roll	200	5	2	T	🌢
Pepperidge Farm, dinner, soft	3 rolls	180	5	2	T	🌢
Pepperidge Farm, frankfurter	1 roll	140	3	0	T	🌢
Pepperidge Farm, hot & crusty, French	1 roll	100	1	1	T	🌢
Pepperidge Farm, hot & crusty, club	1 roll	120	2	2	T	🌢
Pepperidge Farm, hot & crusty, sourdough	1 roll	100	1	1	T	🌢
Pepperidge Farm, sandwich bun, onion w/poppyseed	1 roll	150	3	1	T	🌢
Schmidt, Sunbeam, hamburger rolls	1 roll	130	2	1		✄
Schmidt, Sunbeam, hot dog rolls	1 roll	130	2	1		✄
Schmidt, deli steak rolls	1 roll	220	2	2		✄
Schmidt, potato roll, bar-b-que	1 roll	140	2	2		✄
Schmidt, potato roll, dinner	1 roll	90	2	1		✄
Schmidt, potato roll, long	1 roll	140	2	2		✄
Schmidt, potato roll, sandwich	1 roll	140	2	2		✄
Schmidt, potato roll, steak	1 roll	180	3	2		🌢
Schmidt's, Sunbeam, brown 'n serve rolls	1 roll	70	1	1	T	🌢
Schmidt's, soft kaiser rolls	1 roll	170	2	1		✄
Viva de France, French, enriched	1 roll	120	1	1		✄
Wonder, buns, enriched sliced	1 bun	110	2	0		✄
Wonder, light, enriched bun, reduced cal	1 bun	80	1	4		✄
Wonder, light, hot dog buns, rdcd cal	1 roll	80	2	5		✄

🌢 = *Avoid* • 🌢 = *Add for flavor*

	Portion	Calories	Total Fat	Dietary Fiber	Trans Fat	Guide

Breads, Croissant

	Portion	Calories	Total Fat	Dietary Fiber	Trans Fat	Guide
Sara Lee, petite	2 croissants	230	11	1	T	💧
Viva de France, butter	1 croissant	230	12	1	T	💧

Breads, Croutons

	Portion	Calories	Total Fat	Dietary Fiber	Trans Fat	Guide
Hidden Valley, Salad Crispins, Italian parmesan	1 tbsp.	35	1	0	T	💧
Hidden Valley, Salad Crispins, original ranch	1 tbsp.	35	1	0	T	💧
Marie Callender's, cheese & garlic	4 croutons	30	1	0	T	💧
Marie Callender's, herb & onion	4 croutons	30	1	0	T	💧
Marie Callender's, ranch	4 croutons	30	1	0	T	💧
Marie Callender's, seasoned, fat free	2 tbsp.	25	0	0	T	💧
McCormick, Salad Toppins	1 1/3 tbsp.	35	2	0	T	💧
Pepperidge Farm, cracked pepper & parmesan	6 croutons	35	1	0	T	💧
Pepperidge Farm, seasoned crunchy	9 croutons	35	2	0	T	💧
Pepperidge Farm, zesty Italian	6 croutons	35	2	0	T	💧

Breads, Crumbs

	Portion	Calories	Total Fat	Dietary Fiber	Trans Fat	Guide
Arnold, Italian bread crumbs	1/4 cup	50	1	1	T	💧
Devonsheer, bread crumbs, plain	1/4 cup	110	2	1	T	💧
Progresso, bread crumbs, Italian style	1/4 cup	110	2	1	T	💧
Progresso, bread crumbs, garlic & herb	1/4 cup	100	2	1	T	💧

Breads, English Muffin

	Portion	Calories	Total Fat	Dietary Fiber	Trans Fat	Guide
Pepperidge Farm, English muffin	1 muffin	130	1	2	T	💧
Thomas' English Muffins, apple cinnamon	1 muffin	160	1	1	T	💧
Thomas' English Muffins, blueberry	1 muffin	140	2	2		✂
Thomas' English Muffins, cinnamon raisin	1 muffin	140	1	1		✂
Thomas' English Muffins, cranberry	1 muffin	140	1	1	T	💧
Thomas' English Muffins, honey wheat	1 muffin	110	1	3		✂
Thomas' English Muffins, maple French toast	1 muffin	150	2	0	T	💧
Thomas' English Muffins, oat bran	1 muffin	130	1	2		✂
Thomas' English Muffins, original	1 muffin	120	1	1		✂
Thomas' English Muffins, sandwich size, original	1 muffin	190	2	2		✂
Thomas' English Muffins, sandwich size, sourdough	1 muffin	200	2	2		✂
Thomas' English Muffins, sourdough	1 muffin	120	1	1		✂
Thomas' Toast-R-Cakes, blueberry muffin	1 cake	90	3	0		💧
Thomas' Toast-R-Cakes, corn muffin	1 cake	100	3	0		💧
Wonder, original English	1 muffin	130	1	1		✂

Breads, Garlic, Frozen

	Portion	Calories	Total Fat	Dietary Fiber	Trans Fat	Guide
New York, 50% less fat	2, 1" slices	160	4	1	T	💧
New York, Texas toast	1 slice	160	9	1	T	💧
New York, garlic bread	2, 1" slices	190	8	1	T	💧
Pepperidge Farm, crusty Italian	2 1/2"	170	10	1	T	💧
Pepperidge Farm, garlic & olive oil	2 1/2"	180	7	1	T	💧
Pepperidge Farm, garlic, parmesan	2 1/2"	170	7	2	T	💧
Pepperidge Farm, mozzarella cheese	2 1/4"	200	10	1	T	💧

☺ = Eat as much as you want • ✂ = Cut Back

	Portion	Calories	Total Fat	Dietary Fiber	Trans Fat	Guide
Pepperidge Farm, parmesan slices, toast	1 slice	160	9	0	T	🌢

Breads, Muffin

	Portion	Calories	Total Fat	Dietary Fiber	Trans Fat	Guide
Hostess, mini muffins, blueberry	3 pieces	150	8	0		🌢
Hostess, mini muffins, cinnamon apple	3 pieces	160	9	0		🌢
Sara Lee, blueberry, frozen	1 muffin	220	11	0	T	🌢
Sara Lee, corn, frozen	1 muffin	260	14	1	T	🌢
Weight Watchers, Smart Ones, chocolate chocolate chip	1 muffin	190	2	4		✂
Weight Watchers, blueberry, fat free	1 muffin	160	0	2		✂

Breads, Muffin Mix

	Portion	Calories	Total Fat	Dietary Fiber	Trans Fat	Guide
Betty Crocker, Sunkist lemon	1 muffin	190	2	0	T	🌢
Betty Crocker, Sweet Rewards, wild blueberry, fat free	1 muffin	120	0	0	T	🌢
Betty Crocker, banana nut	1 muffin	170	3	0	T	🌢
Betty Crocker, wild blueberry	1 muffin	170	2	0	T	🌢
Duncan Hines, blueberry bakery style	1 muffin	190	6	0	T	🌢
Duncan Hines, chocolate chip	1 muffin	190	7	1	T	🌢
Duncan Hines, cranberry orange	1 muffin	150	5	0	T	🌢
Jiffy, blueberry	1/4 cup	190	5	1	T	🌢
Jiffy, corn	1/4 cup	180	4	1	T	🌢
Mad Batter, blueberry	1/4 cup	130	3	0		🌢
Mrs. Crutchfield's, fat free, blueberry	1/4 cup	150	0	0		✂
Mrs. Crutchfield's, fat free, bran	1/4 cup	140	0	1		✂
Mrs. Crutchfield's, fat free, corn	1/4 cup	140	0	0		✂
Mrs. Crutchfield's, fat free, cranberry	1/4 cup	150	0	0		✂
Pillsbury, banana nut	1/4 cup	170	6	0	T	🌢
Pillsbury, blueberry	1/3 cup	180	5	0	T	🌢
Pillsbury, chocolate chip	1/3 cup	190	6	0	T	🌢
Washington, bran	1/4 cup	140	3	2	T	🌢
Washington, hot	5 tbsp.	170	5	0	T	🌢
Washington, oat bran	1/4 cup	160	4	3	T	🌢
Washington, popover	1/4 cup	140	3	0	T	🌢
Washington, ragamuffin	1/4 cup	170	4	0	T	🌢

Breads, Pita

	Portion	Calories	Total Fat	Dietary Fiber	Trans Fat	Guide
Sesame rings	1/2 ring	210	5	3		🌢
White	1 piece	160	1	3		✂
Whole wheat pocket	1 piece	180	1	3		✂

Breads, Pizza Crust

	Portion	Calories	Total Fat	Dietary Fiber	Trans Fat	Guide
Betty Crocker, pizza crust mix	1/4 crust	160	2	1	T	🌢
Boboli, original pizza crust	1/8 crust	150	3	0	T	🌢
Boboli, thin pizza crust	1/5 crust	160	4	0	T	🌢
Chef Boyardee, quick & easy pizza crust mix	1/3 cup	150	2	1	T	🌢

Breads, Refrigerated Dough

	Portion	Calories	Total Fat	Dietary Fiber	Trans Fat	Guide
Pillsbury, Grands, blueberry biscuits	1 biscuit	210	9	0	T	🌢

🌢 = Avoid • 💧 = Add for flavor

	Portion	Calories	Total Fat	Dietary Fiber	Trans Fat	Guide
Pillsbury, Grands, buttermilk biscuits, reduced fat	1 biscuit	190	7	0	T	💣
Pillsbury, Grands, cinnamon rolls w/icing	1 roll	320	10	1	T	💣
Pillsbury, Grands, cinnamon rolls w/icing, reduced fat	1 roll	300	7	1	T	💣
Pillsbury, Grands, cinnamon rolls w/real cream cheese	1 roll	330	11	1	T	💣
Pillsbury, Grands, golden wheat biscuits	1 biscuit	200	8	2	T	💣
Pillsbury, breadsticks	1 breadstick	110	2	0	T	💣
Pillsbury, cinnamon raisin rolls w/icing	1 roll	170	6	0	T	💣
Pillsbury, cinnamon rolls w/icing, reduced fat	1 roll	140	4	0	T	💣
Pillsbury, corn bread twists	1 twist	130	6	0	T	💣
Pillsbury, crescent, original	1 roll	110	6	0	T	💣
Pillsbury, crusty French loaf	$1/5$ pkg.	150	2	0	T	💣
Pillsbury, fill & bake, apple turnovers, flaky pastry	1 turnover	170	8	0	T	💣
Pillsbury, fill & bake, cherry turnovers, flaky pastry	1 turnover	180	8	0	T	💣
Pillsbury, garlic breadsticks, garlic & herb	1 breadstick	90	4	0	T	💣
Pillsbury, orange sweet rolls w/icing	1 roll	170	7	0	T	💣
Pillsbury, pizza crust	$1/5$ can	150	2	0	T	💣

Breads, Stuffing

	Portion	Calories	Total Fat	Dietary Fiber	Trans Fat	Guide
Arnold, sage & onion, premium	2 cups	240	3	4	T	💣
Brownberry, sage & onion	2 cups	240	4	3	T	💣
Kraft, Stove Top Stuffing Mix, chicken	$1/2$ cup made	180	9	1	T	💣
Kraft, Stove Top Stuffing Mix, cornbread	$1/2$ cup made	170	8	1	T	💣
Kraft, Stove Top Stuffing Mix, pork	$1/2$ cup made	170	9	1	T	💣
Kraft, Stove Top Stuffing Mix, turkey	$1/2$ cup made	170	9	1	T	💣
Pepperidge Farm, cubed country style	$3/4$ cup	140	2	2	T	💣
Pepperidge Farm, top of stove, apple & raisin mix	$1/2$ cup	140	2	2	T	💣
Pepperidge Farm, top of stove, classic chicken mix	$1/2$ cup	130	2	3	T	💣
Pepperidge Farm, top of stove, country garden herb mix	$1/2$ cup	150	5	2	T	💣
Pepperidge Farm, top of stove, honey pecan cornbread mix	$1/2$ cup	140	5	1	T	💣
Pepperidge Farm, wild rice & mushroom mix	$2/3$ cup	170	6	2	T	💣

Breads, Tortilla

	Portion	Calories	Total Fat	Dietary Fiber	Trans Fat	Guide
Chef Garcia, flour, maya	1 tortilla	180	4	2		💣
Chef Garcia, whole wheat	1 tortilla	130	3	2		💣
Mission, flour	1 tortilla	160	4	1	T	💣
Mission, flour, 98% fat free	1 tortilla	80	1	2	T	💣
Pinata, flour	1 tortilla	100	2	1		✂

Flour

	Portion	Calories	Total Fat	Dietary Fiber	Trans Fat	Guide
Arrowhead Mills, brown rice	$1/4$ cup	120	1	2		✂
Arrowhead Mills, buckwheat	$1/4$ cup	100	1	3		✂

☺ = Eat as much as you want • ✂ = Cut Back

	Portion	Calories	Total Fat	Dietary Fiber	Trans Fat	Guide
Arrowhead Mills, rye, whole grain	1/4 cup	100	1	4		✂
Arrowhead Mills, soy flour, whole grain	1/2 cup	200	9	8		🌢
Arrowhead Mills, vital wheat gluten	3 tsp.	35	0	0		✂
Arrowhead Mills, whole grain pastry	1/4 cup	110	1	3		✂
Arrowhead Mills, whole wheat, stone ground	1/4 cup	130	1	4		✂
Gold Medal, whole wheat	1/4 cup	90	1	3		✂
Pillsbury, Best, all purpose	1/4 cup	100	0	0		✂
Pillsbury, Best, bread	1/4 cup	100	0	0		✂
Spelt	28 g.	110	1	0		✂
Swan's Down, cake	1/4 cup	100	0	0		✂
Whole wheat pastry	1/3 cup	100	1	3		✂

Grains

	Portion	Calories	Total Fat	Dietary Fiber	Trans Fat	Guide
Amaranth	1/4 cup dry	170	2	3		☺
Barley	1/4 cup dry	180	1	8		☺
Barley, refined	1/4 cup dry	160	0	2		✂
Bulgur, wheat, coarse	1/3 cup dry	170	1	3		☺
Kamut	1/4 cup dry	212	1	8		☺
Kasha, buckwheat	1/4 cup dry	140	1	3		☺
Millet	1/4 cup dry	150	2	3		☺
Oat Groats, (whole oats)	1/4 cup dry	180	3	4		☺
Oats, rolled	28 g. dry	110	2	3		☺
Oats, steel cut	1/4 cup dry	170	3	5		☺
Quinoa	1/4 cup dry	140	2	4		☺
Rye, flakes	1/3 cup dry	110	1	4		☺
Rye Berries	1/4 cup dry	160	1	6		☺
Spelt	1/4 cup dry	130	1	8		☺
Wheat, bran	1/4 cup dry	30	1	6		☺
Wheat, cracked	1/4 cup dry	140	1	6		☺
Wheat, flakes	1/3 cup dry	110	1	5		☺
Wheat, germ, toasted	3 tbsp. dry	55	2	2		☺
Wheat Berries, (whole wheat)	1/4 cup dry	160	1	7		☺

Grains, Corn, Dry/Meal

	Portion	Calories	Total Fat	Dietary Fiber	Trans Fat	Guide
Arrowhead Mills, yellow, whole grain	1/4 cup	120	1	3		☺
Corn grits, white	1/4 cup	140	0	1		✂
Corn grits, yellow	1/4 cup	130	0	1		✂
Fantastic Foods, polenta fantastica	3/8 cup dry	260	5	4		🌢
Goya, yellow	3 tbsp.	100	0	1		✂
Indian Head, white, stone ground	1/4 cup	100	1	2		✂
Indian Head, yellow, stone ground	1/4 cup	100	2	2		✂
Quaker, masa harina de maiz, corn mix	1/4 cup	110	2	3		✂
Quaker, yellow	3 tbsp.	90	1	2		✂

Grains, Dry Mix

	Portion	Calories	Total Fat	Dietary Fiber	Trans Fat	Guide
Fantastic Foods, Healthy Complements, Jamaican black beans & brown rice	1/3 cup	140	2	5		☺
Fantastic Foods, Healthy Complements, curry basmati rice w/lentils	1/4 cup	140	1	4		☺

🌢 = Avoid • 💧 = Add for flavor

	Portion	Calories	Total Fat	Dietary Fiber	Trans Fat	Guide
Fantastic Foods, Healthy Complements, hacienda spanish rice pilaf	$3/8$ cup	160	1	2		☺
Fantastic Foods, Healthy Complements, roasted garlic & red pepper couscous	$1/3$ cup	200	2	2		☺
Fantastic Foods, Healthy Complements, whole grain pilaf w/wild rice	$1/2$ cup	160	1	2		☺
Fantastic Foods, tabouli	$1/4$ cup	120	1	6		☺
Golden quinoa pilaf	$1/4$ cup	160	2	7		☺
Knorr, Italian rices, vegetable primavera risotto	$1/3$ cup	290	1	1	T	◗
Knorr, pilaf rices, original recipe pilaf	$1/3$ cup	210	1	0	T	◗
Lipton, Rice & Sauce, Spanish	$1/2$ cup	220	2	2		✂
Lipton, Rice & Sauce, cajun style w/beans	$1/2$ cup	260	2	7		☺
Lipton, Rice & Sauce, cheddar broccoli	$1/2$ cup	230	3	1	T	◗
Lipton, Rice & Sauce, chicken	$1/2$ cup	230	3	1		◗
Lipton, Rice & Sauce, chicken & parmesan risotto	$1/2$ cup	220	3	0	T	◗
Lipton, Rice & Sauce, chicken broccoli	$1/2$ cup	230	3	2	T	◗
Lipton, Rice & Sauce, creamy chicken	$1/2$ cup	240	5	1	T	◗
Lipton, Rice & Sauce, herb & butter	$1/2$ cup	230	5	0		◗
Lipton, Rice & Sauce, mushroom	$1/2$ cup	220	2	1	T	◗
Lipton, Seasoned Rice, Southwestern chicken	$1/3$ cup	210	2	1		✂
Lipton, Seasoned Rice, roasted chicken	$1/3$ cup	210	2	1		✂
Lundberg, brown rice & lentils, garlic basil	1 cup	160	1	5		☺
Manischewitz, lentil pilaf mix	$1/4$ cup	160	1	5		☺
Near East, Mediterranean chicken & wild rice	2 oz.	190	1	2		✂
Near East, Spanish rice pilaf mix	2.5 oz.	240	1	2		✂
Near East, barley pilaf mix	2 oz.	180	1	5		☺
Near East, couscous pine nut mix	2 oz.	200	3	2		◗
Near East, toasted almond pilaf mix	2 oz.	200	3	2		◗
Near East, wheat pilaf mix	2 oz.	180	1	5		☺
Old El Paso, Spanish rice	2.5 oz.	250	1	2	T	◗
Old El Paso, cheesy Mexican rice	2.5 oz.	250	2	2	T	◗
Polenta, Italian herb	4 oz.	80	0	2		✂
Polenta, wild mushroom	4 oz.	80	0	2		✂
Uncle Ben's, Brown & Wild Rice, mushroom recipe	2 oz.	190	2	2		✂
Uncle Ben's, Country Inn, Mexican fiesta	2 oz.	190	1	1		✂
Uncle Ben's, Country Inn, Oriental fried rice	2 oz.	190	1	1		✂
Uncle Ben's, Country Inn, broccoli au gratin	2 oz.	200	2	2	T	◗
Uncle Ben's, Country Inn, chicken & vegetables	2 oz.	200	2	1		✂
Uncle Ben's, Country Inn, chicken & wild rice	2 oz.	190	1	1		✂
Uncle Ben's, Country Inn, chicken flavor	2 oz.	200	1	1		✂
Uncle Ben's, Country Inn, rice pilaf	2 oz.	200	1	1		✂
Uncle Ben's, Long Grain & Wild Rice, butter & herb	2 oz.	200	2	1		✂
Uncle Ben's, Long Grain & Wild Rice, original recipe	2 oz.	190	1	1		✂
Uncle Ben's, Long Grain & Wild Rice, roasted garlic	2 oz.	190	1	1		✂
Uncle Ben's, black beans & rice	$1/3$ cup dry	210	1	4	T	◗

☺ = *Eat as much as you want* • ✂ = *Cut Back*

FOOD LISTS

	Portion	Calories	Total Fat	Dietary Fiber	Trans Fat	Guide
Uncle Ben's, pinto beans & rice	1/3 cup dry	210	1	4	T	💧
Uncle Ben's, red beans & rice	1/3 cup dry	210	1	4	T	💧
Uncle Ben's, spicy cajun-style beans & rice	1/3 cup dry	210	2	5	T	💧

Grains, Rice

	Portion	Calories	Total Fat	Dietary Fiber	Trans Fat	Guide
10 Minute Success Rice, brown & wild mix	2 oz. dry	190	1	3	T	💧
10 Minute Success Rice, brown rice	1/2 cup dry	150	1	2		☺
10 Minute Success Rice, enriched pre-cooked natural long grain	1/2 cup dry	190	0	0		✂
Arborio	1/4 cup dry	170	1	2		✂
Arrowhead Mills, brown rice, quick	1/3 cup dry	150	1	2		☺
Black, japonica	1 cup dry	156	0	3		☺
Brown, basmati	1/4 cup dry	160	2	2		☺
Brown, long grain	1/4 cup dry	170	1	3		☺
Brown, medium grain	1/4 cup dry	170	1	3		☺
Brown, short grain, organic	1/4 cup dry	170	2	3		☺
Brown, sweet	1/4 cup dry	180	1	1		✂
Goya, yellow	1/4 cup dry	170	0	1		☺
Kraft, Minute, instant brown rice	1/2 cup dry	170	2	2		✂
Kraft, Minute, instant enriched white rice	1/2 cup dry	160	0	0		☺
Minnesota, wild, patty-ground	1/4 cup dry	160	0	1		✂
Sushi	51 g. dry	180	1	0		✂
Uncle Ben's, enriched long grain boil-in-bag rice	1/3 cup dry	190	1	1		✂
Uncle Ben's, enriched long grain instant rice	1/2 cup dry	190	1	1		☺
Uncle Ben's, instant brown rice	1/2 cup dry	190	2	2		✂
Uncle Ben's, long grain & wild rice, fast cooking recipe	2 oz. dry	200	1	1		☺
Uncle Ben's, original brown rice	1/4 cup dry	170	2	2		✂
Uncle Ben's, original converted rice, enriched long grain	1/4 cup dry	170	0	0		☺
Wild	28 g. dry	100	0	2		☺
Wild & brown, long grain mix	1/4 cup dry	150	2	3		☺

Pasta & Noodles, Asian

	Portion	Calories	Total Fat	Dietary Fiber	Trans Fat	Guide
China Bowl Select	1/2 cup	150	1	6		☺
China Bowl Select, rice sticks	1/2 cup	150	0	1		✂
Chun King, Chow mein noodles	1/2 cup	140	7	0	T	💧
La Choy, Chow mein noodles	1/2 cup	140	7	0	T	💧
Nanka Seimen, Oriental style noodles	2 oz.	190	1	2		✂
Tomoshiraga Somen, Japanese style noodles	2 oz.	200	2	1		✂
Well Pack, Chow mein stir fry noodles	2 oz.	210	1	1		✂

Pasta & Noodles, Dry

	Portion	Calories	Total Fat	Dietary Fiber	Trans Fat	Guide
Ancient Quinoa Harvest, supergrain pasta, elbows	2 oz. dry	180	2	3		☺
Ancient Quinoa Harvest, supergrain pasta, spaghetti style	2 oz. dry	180	2	3		☺
Barilla, canpanelle bell flowers	2 oz. dry	200	1	2		✂
Barilla, farfalle bow tie	2 oz. dry	200	1	2		✂

💧 = Avoid • 💧 = Add for flavor

	Portion	Calories	Total Fat	Dietary Fiber	Trans Fat	Guide
Barilla, orzo	2 oz. dry	200	1	2		✂
Barilla, pennette rigate	2 oz. dry	200	1	2		✂
Barilla, spaghetti	2 oz. dry	200	1	2		✂
Bionaturae, whole wheat semolina, fusilli	2 oz. dry	190	0	3		☺
Bionaturae, whole wheat semolina, rigatoni	2 oz. dry	190	0	3		☺
Couscous, white	1/4 cup dry	190	0	2		✂
Couscous, whole wheat	1/4 cup dry	210	1	7		☺
Davinci, cut ziti	2 oz. dry	210	1	2		✂
Davinci, sea shells	2 oz. dry	210	1	2		✂
Davinci, spaghetti	2 oz. dry	210	1	2		✂
Davinci, tri-color fusilli springs	4/5 cup dry	210	1	2		✂
De Cecco, spaghetti w/spinach	2 oz. dry	200	1	2		✂
Don Peppe, orzo	1/3 cup dry	210	1	2		✂
Don Peppe, wheels	2 oz. dry	210	1	2		✂
Elbows, organic	1/2 cup dry	210	1	2		✂
Hodgson Hill, yolkless whole wheat pasta ribbons	2 oz. dry	190	1	5		☺
Mueller's, elbows	2 oz. dry	210	1	1		✂
Mueller's, lasagna	2 oz. dry	210	1	1		✂
Mueller's, sea shells	2 oz. dry	210	1	1		✂
Mueller's, spaghetti	2 oz. dry	210	1	1		✂
Mueller's, twist trio	2 oz. dry	210	1	1		✂
Mueller's, twists	2 oz. dry	210	1	1		✂
Mueller's, yolk-free, noodle style pasta	2 oz. dry	210	1	1		✂
Mueller's, ziti	2 oz. dry	210	1	1		✂
No Yolks, egg noodle sub, extra broad, chol free	2 oz. dry	210	1	3		✂
Orzo, organic	1/4 cup dry	210	1	2		✂
Orzo, primavera	2 oz. dry	200	1	1		✂
Penne rigate, organic whole wheat	3/4 cup dry	210	1	6		☺
Quinoa elbows	1/2 cup dry	180	2	0		✂
San Giorgio, elbow macaroni	2 oz. dry	210	1	2		✂
San Giorgio, jumbo shells	2 oz. dry	210	1	2		✂
San Giorgio, rippled edge lasagna	2 oz. dry	210	1	2		✂
San Giorgio, rotelle	2 oz. dry	210	1	2		✂
San Giorgio, spaghetti, thin	2 oz. dry	210	1	2		✂
Spirals, whole wheat veggie	1/2 cup dry	210	1	2		✂
Tinkyada, 100% rice pasta, shells w/rice bran	2 oz. dry	193	0	3		☺
Tinkyada, 100% rice pasta, spirals w/rice bran	2 oz. dry	193	0	3		☺
Vita Spelt, spelt elbows	2 oz. dry	190	2	5		☺
Vita Spelt, spelt spaghetti	2 oz. dry	210	1	2		✂
Westbrae Natural, whole wheat lasagna	2 pieces dry	180	2	7		☺

Pasta & Noodles, Dry Mix

	Portion	Calories	Total Fat	Dietary Fiber	Trans Fat	Guide
Betty Crocker, Hamburger Helper, Southwestern beef	1 cup	150	1	2	T	💣
Betty Crocker, Hamburger Helper, cheddar cheese melt	1 cup	150	2	0	T	💣

☺ = *Eat as much as you want* • ✂ = *Cut Back*

	Portion	Calories	Total Fat	Dietary Fiber	Trans Fat	Guide
Betty Crocker, Hamburger Helper, cheeseburger macaroni	1 cup	180	5	0	T	💣
Betty Crocker, Hamburger Helper, cheesy hash browns	1 cup	170	2	2	T	💣
Betty Crocker, Hamburger Helper, lasagna	1 cup	140	1	0		💣
Betty Crocker, Hamburger Helper, ravioli	1 cup	140	1	1	T	💣
Betty Crocker, Hamburger Helper, stroganoff	1 cup	160	3	0		💣
Betty Crocker, Suddenly Salad, garden Italian	3/4 cup	130	1	2		💣
Betty Crocker, Tuna Helper, cheesy pasta	1 cup	170	3	0	T	💣
Betty Crocker, Tuna Helper, creamy broccoli	1 cup	190	5	1	T	💣
Kraft, Macaroni & Cheese, cheesy alfredo	1 cup	260	3	2		💣
Kraft, Macaroni & Cheese, deluxe	1 cup	320	10	2		💣
Kraft, Macaroni & Cheese, deluxe, 4 cheese	1 cup	320	10	1		💣
Kraft, Macaroni & Cheese, deluxe, light	1 cup	290	5	1		💣
Kraft, Macaroni & Cheese, spirals	1 cup	260	3	1		💣
Kraft, Macaroni & Cheese, thick'n creamy	1 cup	260	3	2		💣
Kraft, Macaroni & Cheese, white cheddar	1 cup	260	3	1		💣
Kraft, Pasta Salad, classic ranch w/bacon	2.5 oz.	350	22	2		💣
Kraft, Pasta Salad, classic Italian garden primavera	2.5 oz.	240	8	2		💣
Kraft, Pasta Salad, creamy caesar	3/4 cup	340	21	2	T	💣
Kraft, Pasta Salad, herb & garlic	2.5 oz.	280	14	2		💣
Kraft, Velveeta, radiatore & cheese, creamy herb & garlic	4 oz.	360	13	2		💣
Kraft, Velveeta, shells & cheese	1 cup	360	13	2		💣
Lipton, Noodles & Sauce, parmesan	2/3 cup	250	8	2		💣
Lipton, Noodles & Sauce, alfredo	2/3 cup	250	7	2	T	💣
Lipton, Noodles & Sauce, alfredo broccoli	2/3 cup	260	7	2	T	💣
Lipton, Noodles & Sauce, beef flavor	2/3 cup	230	4	2		💣
Lipton, Noodles & Sauce, butter	2/3 cup	260	8	2	T	💣
Lipton, Noodles & Sauce, butter & herb	2/3 cup	250	7	2	T	💣
Lipton, Noodles & Sauce, chicken broccoli	2/3 cup	230	4	2		💣
Lipton, Noodles & Sauce, stroganoff	2/3 cup	220	4	2		💣
Lipton, Pasta & Sauce, cheddar broccoli	2/3 cup	260	4	1		💣
Lipton, Pasta & Sauce, creamy garlic	2/3 cup	270	6	1	T	💣
Lipton, Pasta & Sauce, creamy mushroom	3/4 cup	240	4	0		💣
Lipton, Pasta & Sauce, mild cheddar cheese	3/4 cup	210	3	0		💣
Lipton, Pasta & Sauce, roasted garlic chicken	3/4 cup	210	3	0		💣
Lipton, Pasta & Sauce, roasted garlic & olive oil w/tomato	3/4 cup	220	3	2		💣
Rice-A-Roni, Pasta Roni, 4 cheese w/cork screw pasta	1 cup	270	6	2	T	💣
Rice-A-Roni, Pasta Roni, angel hair w/lemon & butter	1 cup	250	4	2	T	💣
Rice-A-Roni, Pasta Roni, chicken & garlic flavor	1 cup	200	3	2	T	💣
Rice-A-Roni, Pasta Roni, fettuccine alfredo	1 cup	260	5	2	T	💣
Rice-A-Roni, Pasta Roni, garlic & olive oil	1 cup	250	4	2	T	💣
Rice-A-Roni, Pasta Roni, herb & butter	1 cup	200	3	2	T	💣
Rice-A-Roni, Pasta Roni, parmesano	2.5 oz.	260	4	2	T	💣
Rice-A-Roni, Pasta Roni, shells & white cheddar	1 cup	270	6	2	T	💣

💣 = *Avoid* • 💧 = *Add for flavor*

	Portion	Calories	Total Fat	Dietary Fiber	Trans Fat	Guide
Rice-A-Roni, Pasta Roni, white cheddar & broccoli	1 cup	270	6	3	T	🌢

Pasta & Noodles, Refrigerated

	Portion	Calories	Total Fat	Dietary Fiber	Trans Fat	Guide
Contadina, angel hair	1 1/4 cups	230	3	2		🌢
Contadina, fettuccine	1 1/4 cups	240	3	2		🌢
Contadina, fettuccine, spinach	1 1/4 cups	260	4	3		🌢
Contadina, light, ravioli, 4 cheese	1 cup	230	4	2		🌢
Contadina, light, ravioli, garden vegetable	1 cup	250	5	2		🌢
Contadina, light, tortellini, 3 cheese	3/4 cup	250	6	2		🌢
Contadina, light, tortellini, garlic & cheese	1 cup	280	5	3		🌢
Contadina, linguine	1 1/4 cups	240	3	2		🌢
Contadina, tortellini, sweet Italian sausage	1 cup	320	8	3		🌢
DiGiorno, angel's hair	2 oz.	160	2	2		✂
DiGiorno, fettuccine	2.5 oz.	200	2	2		✂
DiGiorno, linguine	2.5 oz.	200	2	2		✂
DiGiorno, tortellini, 3 cheese	3/4 cup	250	7	2		🌢

■ MEAT & POULTRY

Meat, Bacon

	Portion	Calories	Total Fat	Dietary Fiber	Trans Fat	Guide
Butterball, turkey, thin & crispy	3 slices	60	5	0		🌢
Esskay, sliced, lower fat	2 slices	50	3	0		🌢
Esskay, sliced, lower sodium	2 slices	60	5	0		🌢
Gwaltney, brown sugar Virginia cured	2 slices	60	5	0		🌢
Gwaltney, center cut, 40% less fat	2 slices	50	3	0		🌢
Gwaltney, hardwood smoked Virgina cured	2 slices	60	5	0		🌢
Hormel, black label original	2 slices	70	6	0		🌢
Louis Rich, turkey	1 slice	35	3	0		🌢
Mr. Turkey, turkey	1 slice	30	2	0		✂
Oscar Mayer	2 slices	70	6	0		🌢
Oscar Mayer, hearty thick cut	1 slice	60	5	0		🌢
Oscar Mayer, lower sodium	2 slices	70	5	0		🌢
Smithfield, regular sliced	2 slices	70	6	0		🌢
Swift Premium, beef & turkey sizzling	1 slice	70	6	0		🌢

Meat, Beef

	Portion	Calories	Total Fat	Dietary Fiber	Trans Fat	Guide
Brisket, whole, braised	3 oz.	210	11	0		🌢
Chuck, arm pot roast, braised	3 oz.	180	7	0		🌢
Chuck, blade roast, braised	3 oz.	210	11	0		🌢
Ground, broiled, well done, 10% fat	3 oz.	210	11	0		🌢
Ground, broiled, well done, 17% fat	3 oz.	230	13	0		🌢
Ground, broiled, well done, 27% fat	3 oz.	250	17	0		🌢
Loin, sirloin steak, broiled	3 oz.	170	6	0		🌢
Loin, tenderloin steak, broiled	3 oz.	180	9	0		🌢
Loin, top, broiled	3 oz.	180	8	0		🌢
Rib, large end roast, roasted	3 oz.	200	11	0		🌢
Rib, small end steak, broiled	3 oz.	190	10	0		🌢

☺ = Eat as much as you want • ✂ = Cut Back

	Portion	Calories	Total Fat	Dietary Fiber	Trans Fat	Guide
Round, bottom, braised	3 oz.	180	7	0		🌢
Round, eye, roasted	3 oz.	140	4	0		🌢
Round, tip roast, roasted	3 oz.	160	6	0		🌢
Round top steak, broiled	3 oz.	150	4	0		🌢

Meat, Beef, Processed

	Portion	Calories	Total Fat	Dietary Fiber	Trans Fat	Guide
Beardsley, beef, dried	1 oz.	50	2	0		✂
Corned beef brisket	4 oz.	180	13	0		🌢
Slim Jim, hickory smoked, classic	3 pieces	150	14	1		🌢
Slim Jim, hickory smoked, mild	3 pieces	150	14	1		🌢
Underwood, roast beef spread	1/4 cup	130	11	0	T	🌢

Meat, Game

	Portion	Calories	Total Fat	Dietary Fiber	Trans Fat	Guide
Buffalo, roasted	3 oz.	111	2	0		✂
Elk	3.5 oz.	146	2	0		✂
Venison (deer), roasted	3 oz.	134	3	0		🌢
Wild boar	3.5 oz.	160	4	0		🌢

Meat, Hot Dog

	Portion	Calories	Total Fat	Dietary Fiber	Trans Fat	Guide
Ball Park, Smart Creations, lite franks	1 frank	100	7	0		🌢
Ball Park, beef franks	1 frank	180	16	0		🌢
Ball Park, beef franks, bun size	1 frank	180	16	0		🌢
Ball Park, beef knockwurst	1 link	340	32	0		🌢
Ball Park, fat free franks	1 frank	45	0	0		✂
Ball Park, fun franks, microwaveable	2 pkg.	340	20	3		🌢
Ball Park, turkey, smoked white, fat free	1 frank	40	0	0		✂
Gwaltney, chicken frankfurter, great dogs	1 frank	140	10	0		🌢
Healthy Choice, beef frankfurters, low fat	1 frank	60	2	0		✂
Healthy Choice, bun size franks, low fat	1 frank	60	2	0		✂
Hebrew National, beef franks	1 frank	140	13	0		🌢
Hebrew National, beef franks, 97% fat free	1 frank	45	2	0		✂
Hillshire Farm, Lit'l Beef Franks	6 links	170	15	0		🌢
Kahn's, beef corn dogs, crazy dogs	1 corn dog	220	12	1		🌢
Kahn's, beef franks, bun style	1 link	180	16	0		🌢
Mr. Turkey, bun size franks	1 frank	130	11	0		🌢
Oscar Mayer, beef franks	1 link	150	13	0		🌢
Oscar Mayer, beef franks, bun length	1 link	180	17	0		🌢
Oscar Mayer, beef franks, light	1 link	110	8	0		🌢
Oscar Mayer, beef, jumbo franks	1 link	180	17	0		🌢
Oscar Mayer, cheese dogs	1 link	140	13	0		🌢
Oscar Mayer, weiners, big & juicy, hot & spicy	1 link	220	20	0		🌢
Wampler Foods, turkey franks	1 frank	90	8	2		🌢

Meat, Hot Dog, Vegetarian

	Portion	Calories	Total Fat	Dietary Fiber	Trans Fat	Guide
Lightlife, Smart Dogs, vegetarian	1 link	45	0	0		✂
Lightlife, Tofu Pups	1 link	60	3	0		🌢
Morningstar Farms, Veggie Dogs	1 link	80	1	1		✂
Soy Boy, Not Hot Dogs	1 link	95	3	0		🌢
Yves Veggie Cuisine, veggie wieners fat free	1 wiener	55	0	1		✂

🌢 = Avoid • 🌢 = Add for flavor

	Portion	Calories	Total Fat	Dietary Fiber	Trans Fat	Guide
Meat, Lamb						
Leg, whole, roasted	3 oz.	160	7	0		🌢
Loin, chop, broiled	3 oz.	180	8	0		🌢
Rib, roast, roasted	3 oz.	200	11	0		🌢
Shank, braised	3 oz.	160	5	0		🌢
Shoulder, arm chop, broiled	3 oz.	170	8	0		🌢
Shoulder, blade chop, broiled	3 oz.	180	10	0		🌢
Meat, Other, Processed						
Libby's, potted meat food products	1/4 cup	120	8	0		🌢
Sells, liver pâté	1/4 cup	170	14	1		🌢
Spam	2 oz.	170	16	0		🌢
Spam, spread	4 tbsp.	140	12	0		🌢
Meat, Pork						
Ground, broiled	3 oz.	250	18	0		🌢
Hormel, pig's feet	2 oz.	80	6	0		🌢
Loin, center, chop, broiled	3 oz.	170	7	0		🌢
Loin, country style ribs, roasted	3 oz.	210	13	0		🌢
Loin, rib chop, broiled	3 oz.	190	8	0		🌢
Loin, sirloin roast, roasted	3 oz.	180	9	0		🌢
Loin, tenderloin roast, roasted	3 oz.	140	4	0		🌢
Loin, top chop, boneless, broil	3 oz.	170	7	0		🌢
Loin, top roast, boneless, roasted	3 oz.	170	6	0		🌢
Shoulder, blade steak, broiled	3 oz.	190	11	0		🌢
Spareribs, braised	3 oz.	340	26	0		🌢
Meat, Pork, Processed						
Dietz & Watson, boneless, smoked chops	3 oz.	110	3	0		🌢
Gwaltney, country ham	3 oz.	220	10	0		🌢
Gwaltney, fat back	1/2 oz.	90	10	0		🌢
Gwaltney, ham, boneless	3 oz.	120	3	0		🌢
Gwaltney, souse loaf	1 slice	60	5	0		🌢
Hickory Mountain, side meat	2 oz.	370	15	0		🌢
Hormel, chunk lean ham water added	2 oz.	90	6	0		🌢
Hormel, ham, cure/81, boneless	3 oz.	100	5	0		🌢
Hormel, ham, curemaster	3 oz.	80	3	0		🌢
Hormel, salt	2 oz.	320	33	0		🌢
Hormel, smoked chops	3 oz.	100	4	0		🌢
Jones, ham steak	3 oz.	100	4	0		🌢
Underwood, deviled ham spread	1/4 cup	160	14	0		🌢
Underwood, honey ham spread	1/4 cup	140	11	0		🌢
Meat, Sandwich Meat						
Carando, salami, hard, classic Italian	4 slices	70	5	0		🌢
Carl Buddig, beef	10 slices	75	4	0		🌢
Carl Buddig, corned beef	10 slices	75	4	0		🌢
Carl Buddig, ham	10 slices	85	5	0		🌢

☺ = Eat as much as you want • ✂ = Cut Back

	Portion	Calories	Total Fat	Dietary Fiber	Trans Fat	Guide
Carl Buddig, lean slices, ham, oven roasted, honey	1 pkg.	90	2	0		✂
Esskay, chipped beef	1 oz.	50	1	0		✂
Healthy Choice, deli thin, ham, baked	6 slices	60	2	0		✂
Healthy Choice, deli thin, ham, honey	6 slices	60	2	0		✂
Healthy Choice, ham, cooked	1 slice	30	1	0		✂
Healthy Choice, ham, honey	1 slice	30	1	0		✂
Hebrew National, bologna, beef	2 oz.	180	16	0		🌢
Hebrew National, corned beef	4 slices	90	5	0		🌢
Hebrew National, salami, beef	2 oz.	170	14	0		🌢
Hillshire Farm, Deli Select, ham, brown sugar baked	6 slices	60	2	0		✂
Hillshire Farm, Deli Select, ham, honey	6 slices	60	2	0		✂
Hillshire Farm, Deli Select, ham, smoked	6 slices	60	2	0		✂
Jones Dairy Farm, Braunchweiger liverwurst	2 oz.	150	12	0		🌢
Louis Rich, Carving Board Meat, ham, baked	2 slices	50	2	0		✂
Louis Rich, Carving Board Meat, ham, smoked	4 slices	50	2	0		✂
Oscar Mayer, Free, bologna	1 slice	25	0	0		✂
Oscar Mayer, Free, ham, baked cooked	3 slices	35	0	0		✂
Oscar Mayer, bologna	1 slice	90	8	0		🌢
Oscar Mayer, bologna, beef	1 slice	90	8	0		🌢
Oscar Mayer, bologna, beef, light	1 slice	60	4	0		🌢
Oscar Mayer, bologna, light	1 slice	60	4	0		🌢
Oscar Mayer, cotto salami	1 slice	60	5	0		🌢
Oscar Mayer, ham, honey-baked taste	3 slices	70	3	0		🌢
Oscar Mayer, salami, hard	3 slices	100	8	0		🌢
Parson's, air dried beef	1 oz.	50	2	0		✂

Meat, Sausage

	Portion	Calories	Total Fat	Dietary Fiber	Trans Fat	Guide
Bob Evans, links, Italian	1 link	140	11	0		🌢
Bob Evans, links, original	3 links	190	16	0		🌢
Bob Evans, original recipe	2 oz.	210	19	0		🌢
Bob Evans, pork patties	2 patties	240	21	0		🌢
Bob Evans, savory sage	2 oz.	240	20	0		🌢
Eckrich, 3 pepper smoked	2 oz.	180	16	0		🌢
Eckrich, beef smoked	2 oz.	180	16	0		🌢
Eckrich, polska kielbasa	2 oz.	180	16	0		🌢
Eckrich, smoked	2 oz.	180	16	0		🌢
Eckrich, turkey smoked	2 oz.	120	9	0		🌢
Goya, Vienna sausage	3 links	130	12	0		🌢
Gwaltney, pork, fresh	1.5 oz.	150	14	0		🌢
Healthy Choice, beef smoked	2 oz.	70	2	0		✂
Healthy Choice, polska kielbasa	2 oz.	70	2	0		✂
Hebrew National, salami, beef	2 oz.	170	14	0		🌢
Hillshire Farm, beef smoked	2 oz.	190	17	0		🌢
Hillshire Farm, hot links, beef	1 link	260	24	0		🌢
Hillshire Farm, hot links, naturally smoked	1 link	250	23	0		🌢
Hillshire Farm, polska kielbasa	2 oz.	190	17	0		🌢
Hormel, Vienna sausage	2 oz.	150	14	0		🌢

🌢 = *Avoid* • 🌢 = *Add for flavor*

	Portion	Calories	Total Fat	Dietary Fiber	Trans Fat	Guide
Jimmy Dean, pork	4 links	200	17	0		💧
Jimmy Dean, pork, maple	2 oz.	240	21	0		💧
Jimmy Dean, pork, sage	2 oz.	240	21	0		💧
Jimmy Dean, turkey & pork	2.5 oz.	180	14	0		💧
Johnsonville, bratwurst	1 link	290	25	0		💧
Johnsonville, breakfast, Vermont maple syrup	3 links	200	18	0		💧
Johnsonville, breakfast, original	3 links	190	16	0		💧
Johnsonville, mild Italian	1 link	290	25	0		💧
Libby's, Vienna sausage	3 links	150	14	0		💧
Lightlife, lean Italian link	1 link	60	2	0		✂
Mr. Turkey, turkey Polish kielbasa	2 oz.	90	5	0		💧
Mr. Turkey, turkey smoked	2 oz.	90	5	0		💧
Mr. Turkey, turkey smoked, Italian style	2 oz.	90	5	0		💧
Oscar Mayer, Braunschweiger liver sausage	2 oz.	190	17	0		💧
Smithfield, ham	1.5 oz.	180	16	0		💧
Smithfield, pork	1.5 oz.	170	15	0		💧

Meat, Veal

	Portion	Calories	Total Fat	Dietary Fiber	Trans Fat	Guide
Cutlets, roasted	3 oz.	130	3	0		💧
Loin chop, roasted	3 oz.	150	6	0		💧
Rib roast, roasted	3 oz.	150	6	0		💧
Shoulder, arm steak, braised	3 oz.	170	5	0		💧
Shoulder, blade steak, braised	3 oz.	170	6	0		💧

Poultry, Chicken

	Portion	Calories	Total Fat	Dietary Fiber	Trans Fat	Guide
Breast, baked	3 oz.	120	2	0		✂
Drumstick, baked	3 oz.	130	4	0		💧
Thigh, baked	3 oz.	150	7	0		💧
Whole, roasted	3 oz.	130	4	0		💧
Wing, baked	3 oz.	150	6	0		💧

Poultry, Chicken, Processed

	Portion	Calories	Total Fat	Dietary Fiber	Trans Fat	Guide
Hormel, premium chunk breast of chicken in water	2 oz.	60	2	0		✂
Swanson, chicken breast in water	1 can	80	1	0		✂
Swanson, chunk chicken premium white & dark	2 oz.	70	2	0		✂
Swanson, premium chunk chicken in water	2 oz.	70	2	0		✂
Sweet Sue, white chicken premium chunk	2 oz.	90	1	0		✂
Underwood, chicken spread, white meat	1/4 cup	20	8	0	T	💧

Poultry, Sandwich Meat

	Portion	Calories	Total Fat	Dietary Fiber	Trans Fat	Guide
Butterball, turkey bologna	3 slices	150	12	0		💧
Butterball, turkey ham	3 slices	70	3	0		💧
Butterball, turkey salami, cooked	3 slices	120	8	0		💧
Butterball, turkey, smoked, white	3 slices	70	3	0		💧
Carl Buddig, Lean Slices, chicken breast, oven roasted	1 pkg.	60	1	0		✂
Carl Buddig, Lean Slices, turkey breast, smoked	1 pkg.	70	1	0		✂

☺ = Eat as much as you want • ✂ = Cut Back

	Portion	Calories	Total Fat	Dietary Fiber	Trans Fat	Guide
Carl Buddig, chicken	9 slices	80	5	0		🌢
Carl Buddig, turkey	9 slices	80	5	0		🌢
Healthy Choice, deli thin, turkey breast, low fat	6 slices	60	2	0		✂
Healthy Choice, turkey breast	1 slice	30	1	0		✂
Healthy Choice, turkey breast, oven roasted	1 slice	30	1	0		✂
Hebrew National, turkey breast, hickory smoked	5 slices	60	1	0		✂
Hillshire Farm, Deli Select, chicken breast, smoked	6 slices	50	0	0		✂
Hillshire Farm, Deli Select, turkey breast, oven roasted	6 slices	60	1	0		✂
Hillshire Farm, Deli Select, turkey breast, smoked	6 slices	50	1	0		✂
Louis Rich, Carving Board Meat, chicken breast, grilled	2 slices	45	1	0		✂
Louis Rich, Carving Board Meat, turkey breast, oven roast	2 slices	40	1	0		✂
Louis Rich, Carving Board Meat, turkey breast, rotisserie	2 slices	40	1	0		✂
Louis Rich, Carving Board Meat, turkey breast, smoked	4 slices	50	1	0		✂
Louis Rich, Free, turkey breast, oven roasted	1 slice	20	0	0		✂
Louis Rich, chicken breast, oven roasted	4 slices	50	1	0		✂
Louis Rich, turkey bologna	1 slice	50	4	0		🌢
Louis Rich, turkey breast, hickory smoked	1 slice	25	0	0		✂
Louis Rich, turkey breast, oven roasted	1 slice	30	1	0		✂
Louis Rich, turkey ham	1 slice	35	2	0		✂
Louis Rich, turkey, smoked breast	1 slice	50	0	0		✂
Mr. Turkey, turkey bologna	1 slice	70	5	0		🌢
Mr. Turkey, turkey cotto salami	1 slice	50	3	0		🌢
Mr. Turkey, turkey ham, hardwood smoked	1 slice	35	2	0		✂
Mr. Turkey, turkey, white	1 slice	30	1	0		✂
Oscar Mayer, Free, chicken breast, oven roasted	4 slices	45	0	0		✂
Oscar Mayer, Free, turkey breast, oven roasted	4 slices	45	0	0		✂
Oscar Mayer, turkey, oven roasted, white	1 slice	30	1	0		✂

Poultry, Turkey

	Portion	Calories	Total Fat	Dietary Fiber	Trans Fat	Guide
Breast, baked	3 oz.	120	1	0		✂
Drumstick, baked	3 oz.	140	4	0		🌢
Thigh, baked	3 oz.	140	5	0		🌢
Whole, roasted	3 oz.	130	3	0		🌢
Wing, baked	3 oz.	140	3	0		🌢

Poultry, Turkey, Processed

	Portion	Calories	Total Fat	Dietary Fiber	Trans Fat	Guide
Butterball, turkey, breast of	2 oz.	50	0	0		✂
Hormel, chunk turkey in 33% broth	2 oz.	70	3	0		🌢
Jennieo, turkey ham, extra lean	2 oz.	60	3	0		🌢
Louis Rich, turkey, honey roasted breast	2 oz.	60	0	0		✂
Mr. Turkey, turkey breast	2 oz.	50	0	0		✂
Plantation, turkey, hickory smoked	3 oz.	120	5	0		🌢

🌢 = Avoid • 💧 = Add for flavor

FOOD LISTS • CHAPTER 10 237

FOOD LISTS

	Portion	Calories	Total Fat	Dietary Fiber	Trans Fat	Guide
Swanson, premium chunk white turkey in water	1/4 cup	90	2	1		✂

■ PREPARED ENTREES

Canned, Asian

La Choy, chicken chow mein	1 cup	100	3	3		💧
La Choy, Chinese style fried rice	1 cup	290	2	3		✂
Tyling, won ton soup	1 cup	100	3	1	T	💧

Canned, Beef

Hormel, corned beef	2 oz.	120	7	0		💧
Libby's, corned beef	2 oz.	120	7	0		💧
Mary Kitchen, corned beef hash	1 can	370	24	1		💧
Mary Kitchen, roast beef hash	1 cup	390	24	2		💧

Canned, Chicken

Luck's, chicken & dumplings	1 cup	340	17	2		💧
Swanson, chicken a la king	1 cup	320	22	0		💧
Sweet Sue, chicken & dumplings	1 cup	240	7	5		💧

Canned, Chili

Bush's, Chili Magic, chili starter, Texas recipe	1/2 cup	120	2	5	n.a.	☺
Bush's, Chili Magic, chili starter, traditional recipe	1/2 cup	110	1	5	n.a.	☺
Health Valley, fat free, chili w/3 beans	1/2 cup	80	0	7		☺
Health Valley, fat free, chili w/black beans	1/2 cup	80	0	7		☺
Health Valley, mild black beans	1 cup	150	1	12		☺
Health Valley, spicy vegetarian w/black beans	1/2 cup	80	0	7		☺
Hormel Chili, chunky w/beans	1 cup	270	7	7		💧
Hormel Chili, hot no beans	1 cup	210	9	3		💧
Hormel Chili, hot w/beans	1 cup	270	7	7		💧
Hormel Chili, less sodium w/beans	1 cup	270	7	7		💧
Hormel Chili, no beans	1 cup	210	9	3		💧
Hormel Chili, turkey w/beans	1 cup	210	3	5		💧
Hormel Chili, vegetarian w/beans	1 cup	200	1	7		☺
Hormel Chili, w/beans	1 cup	270	7	7		💧

Canned, Pasta

Chef Boyardee, 99% fat free, beef ravioli	1 cup	210	1	3		✂
Chef Boyardee, 99% fat free, cheese ravioli in tomato sauce	1 cup	240	3	2		💧
Chef Boyardee, beef ravioli & tomato & meat sauce	1 cup	230	5	4		💧
Chef Boyardee, cheese tortellini in tomato sauce	1 cup	230	1	4		✂
Chef Boyardee, lasagna, w/chunky tomato & meat sauce	1 cup	270	8	3		💧
Chef Boyardee, mini ravioli, beef in tomato & meat sauce	1 cup	240	7	3		💧
Chef Boyardee, spaghetti & meatballs tomato sauce	1 cup	270	10	2		💧

☺ = Eat as much as you want • ✂ = Cut Back

	Portion	Calories	Total Fat	Dietary Fiber	Trans Fat	Guide
Chef Jr. Boyardee, ABC's & 123's, pasta w/meatballs in tomato sauce	1 cup	290	11	2		💣
Chef Jr. Boyardee, Dinosaurs, tomato pasta & cheese sauce	1 cup	200	1	2		✂
Franco-American, Life w/Louie, shaped pasta w/meatballs	1 cup	250	11	5	T	💣
Franco-American, Raviolios, beef ravioli	1 cup	230	4	2	T	💣
Franco-American, Sonic Hedgehog, pasta w/meatballs	1 cup	280	11	5	T	💣
Franco-American, Spaghetti & tomato sauce w/cheese	1 cup	210	2	3		✂
Franco-American, Spaghettios, pasta w/sliced franks in tomato sauce	1 cup	250	11	4		💣
Franco-American, Superiore, beef ravioli in meat sauce	1 cup	280	9	2	T	💣
Franco-American, Superiore, hearty twists in meat sauce	1 cup	250	5	2		💣
Franco-American, Superiore, mini ravioli, beef in meat sauce	1 cup	280	8	5	T	💣
Franco-American, Superiore, spaghetti & meatballs in tomato sauce	1 cup	270	10	4	T	💣
Franco-American, Where's Waldo, pasta w/meatballs & tomato sauce	1 cup	260	11	5	T	💣

Canned, Stew

	Portion	Calories	Total Fat	Dietary Fiber	Trans Fat	Guide
Dinty Moore, 99% fat free, beef stew, potatoes & carrots	1 cup	230	14	2		💣
Dinty Moore, 99% fat free, turkey stew	1 cup	140	3	2	T	💣

Canned, Tuna

	Portion	Calories	Total Fat	Dietary Fiber	Trans Fat	Guide
Bumble Bee, Ready to Eat Tuna original recipe, tuna only	1 can	190	15	1		💣
Bumble Bee, Ready to Eat Tuna, crackers only	6 crackers	90	2	0		✂
Bumble Bee, Ready to Eat Tuna, fat free tuna only	1 can	70	0	0		✂
Starkist, Charlie's lunch kit, chunk white tuna	1 kit	230	9	1	T	💣
Starkist, Ready-Mixed Tuna Salad & Crackers	1 kit	190	6	2	T	💣

Canned, Vegetarian

	Portion	Calories	Total Fat	Dietary Fiber	Trans Fat	Guide
Bonavita, herb vegetarian pâté	1 tbsp.	30	2	0		✂

Dry Mix, Vegetarian

	Portion	Calories	Total Fat	Dietary Fiber	Trans Fat	Guide
Fantastic Foods, Nature's Burger, natural mix	1/4 cup	170	3	5		☺
Fantastic Foods, Nature's Sausage	2 tbsp.	65	2	2		☺
Fantastic Foods, falafil	1/2 cup	250	4	11		☺
Fantastic Foods, instant black beans	1/3 cup	160	2	7		☺
Fantastic Foods, instant refried beans	1/3 cup dry	160	1	11		☺
Fantastic Foods, tofu burger	1/8 cup	70	2	2		☺
Fantastic Foods, tofu scrambler	2 1/2 tbsp.	60	1	3		☺
Fantastic Foods, vegetarian chili	1/8 cup	50	0	3		☺

💣 = Avoid • 💧 = Add for flavor

	Portion	Calories	Total Fat	Dietary Fiber	Trans Fat	Guide
Dry, Mexican						
Deloro, tostada crowns	1 bowl	226	10	5	T	🖤
Old El Paso, burrito dinner kit	1 tortilla	160	4	1	T	🖤
Old El Paso, fajita dinner kit	2 tortillas	180	5	1	T	🖤
Old El Paso, soft taco dinner kit	2 tortillas	180	5	1	T	🖤
Old El Paso, taco shells	3 shells	150	7	2	T	🖤
Old El Paso, taco shells, white corn	3 shells	150	7	2	T	🖤
Old El Paso, tortillas, flour	2 tortillas	160	5	0	T	🖤
Old El Paso, tostada shells	3 shells	150	7	2	T	🖤
Ortega, taco shells	2 shells	130	6	2	T	🖤
Taco Bell, taco shells	3 shells	150	6	2		🖤
Frozen, Burgers						
Hormel, Quick Meal, bacon cheeseburger	1 sandwich	440	23	2	T	🖤
Hormel, Quick Meal, cheeseburger	1 sandwich	400	20	2	T	🖤
Wampler Foods, turkey burgers	1 burger	210	15	0		🖤
White Castle, hamburgers	2 sandwiches	270	14	5	T	🖤
Frozen, Burgers, Veggie						
Amy's, veggie burger, organic CA	1 burger	100	3	3		☺
Boca Burger	1 burger	110	2	4		☺
Gardenburger, original	2.5 oz.	130	3	5		☺
Gardenburger, savory mushroom	2.5 oz.	120	3	4		☺
Gardenburger, veggie medley	2.5 oz.	100	0	2		☺
Gardenburger, w/cheese	2.5 oz.	110	3	3		✂
Green Giant, Harvest Burger Crumbles	1/2 cup	70	0	3		☺
Green Giant, Harvest Burgers	1 pattie	140	4	5		☺
Ken & Robert's, veggie burger	2.5 oz.	130	1	3		☺
Morningstar Farms, Better'n Burgers	1 pattie	70	0	3		☺
Morningstar Farms, Grillers	1 pattie	140	6	3		☺
Morningstar Farms, garden veggie patties	1 pattie	100	3	4		☺
Morningstar Farms, spicy black bean burger	1 pattie	110	1	5		☺
Natural Touch, garden veggie pattie	1 pattie	100	3	3		☺
Frozen, Chicken						
Banquet, skinless fried chicken	3 oz.	210	13	2		🖤
Banquet, southern fried chicken	3 oz.	280	18	1		🖤
Butterball, Chicken Request, baked breast	1 piece	180	6	2		🖤
Tyson, barbecue style chicken wings	3 pieces	200	13	0	T	🖤
Tyson, breast fillets, breaded chickn	2 fillets	180	8	1	T	🖤
Tyson, crispy baked breast patties	1 pattie	80	0	1		✂
Tyson, crispy baked breast tenders	3 tenders	100	0	1		✂
Tyson, hot & spicy chicken wings	4 pieces	220	15	0	T	🖤
Frozen, Entree, Beef						
Banquet, Hearty Ones, salisbury steak	1 meal	780	54	7	T	🖤
Banquet, Value Meal, salisbury steak meal	1 meal	380	24	4	T	🖤
Banquet, brown gravy salisbury steak	1 pattie	200	14	2	T	🖤
Budget Gourmet, Swedish meatballs w/noodles	1 entree	550	34	3	T	🖤

☺ = Eat as much as you want • ✂ = Cut Back

	Portion	Calories	Total Fat	Dietary Fiber	Trans Fat	Guide
Budget Gourmet, roast beef supreme	1 entree	310	13	3	T	🌢
Healthy Choice, beef macaroni	1 meal	220	4	5		🌢
Healthy Choice, beef peppersteak Oriental	1 meal	250	4	3		🌢
Healthy Choice, beef stroganoff	1 meal	310	7	3	T	🌢
Healthy Choice, traditional beef tips	1 meal	260	6	6		🌢
Marie Callender's, meatloaf & gravy w/mashed potato	1 meal	540	30	6	T	🌢
Marie Callender's, sirloin salisbury steak & gravy	1 meal	550	25	6	T	🌢
Michelina's, salisbury steak & gravy	1 pkg.	300	17	2	T	🌢
Stouffer's, Hearty Portions, beef pot roast	1 pkg.	430	18	8	T	🌢
Stouffer's, Hearty Portions, country fried beef steak	1 meal	750	43	5	T	🌢
Stouffer's, Hearty Portions, meatloaf	1 pkg.	580	30	6	T	🌢
Stouffer's, Hearty Portions, roast beef w/red potatoes	1 pkg.	430	18	5	T	🌢
Stouffer's, Hearty Portions, salisbury steak	1 pkg.	630	30	0	T	🌢
Stouffer's, Homestyle, meatloaf meal	1 pkg.	390	21	3	T	🌢
Stouffer's, Homestyle, sliced beef brisket	1 pkg.	370	18	7		🌢
Stouffer's, Lean Cuisine, Southern beef tips	1 pkg.	290	6	7		🌢
Stouffer's, Lean Cuisine, beef peppercorn	1 pkg.	220	7	2		🌢
Stouffer's, Lean Cuisine, beef pot roast	1 pkg.	210	6	6	T	🌢
Stouffer's, Lean Cuisine, meatloaf	1 pkg.	250	6	4	T	🌢
Stouffer's, Lean Cuisine, oven roasted beef	1 pkg.	260	8	4		🌢
Stouffer's, Welsh rarebit	$1/4$ cup	120	9	0	T	🌢
Stouffer's, cheddar pasta & beef	1 pkg.	500	24	2	T	🌢
Stouffer's, creamed chipped beef	$1/2$ cup	160	11	1	T	🌢
Stouffer's, green pepper steak	1 pkg.	320	9	3	T	🌢
Stouffer's, macaroni & beef w/tomato	1 pkg.	420	20	5		🌢
Stouffer's, swedish meatballs w/pasta	1 pkg.	480	24	3	T	🌢
Swanson, Hungry-Man, salisbury steak meal	1 pkg.	610	33	10	T	🌢
Swanson, Hungry-Man, traditional pot roast meal	1 pkg.	360	6	6	T	🌢
Swanson, Yankee pot roast meal	1 pkg.	250	5	5	T	🌢
Swanson, meatloaf dinner	1 pkg.	380	14	5	T	🌢
Swanson, salisbury steak meal	1 pkg.	360	16	6	T	🌢
Swanson, veal parmigiana meal	1 pkg.	390	18	5	T	🌢

Frozen, Entree, Chicken

	Portion	Calories	Total Fat	Dietary Fiber	Trans Fat	Guide
Banquet, Select Menu, chicken nugget meal	1 meal	430	23	4	T	🌢
Banquet, Select Menu, fried chicken meal, original	1 meal	470	27	2	T	🌢
Budget Gourmet, Italian style vegetables w/chicken	1 entree	250	7	2	T	🌢
Budget Gourmet, chicken Oriental & vegetables	1 entree	290	8	3		🌢
Budget Gourmet, orange glazed chicken breast	1 entree	280	3	2		🌢
Budget Gourmet, rigatoni cream sauce w/broccoli & chicken	1 entree	250	7	1		🌢
Healthy Choice, Southwestern grilled chicken	1 meal	230	6	4	T	🌢
Healthy Choice, cacciatore chicken	1 meal	270	4	5		🌢

🌢 = Avoid • 🌢 = Add for flavor

	Portion	Calories	Total Fat	Dietary Fiber	Trans Fat	Guide
Healthy Choice, chicken & vegetables marsala	1 meal	240	4	3	T	🫗
Healthy Choice, chicken fettucini alfredo	1 meal	280	7	3		🫗
Healthy Choice, chicken parmigiana	1 meal	330	8	3	T	🫗
Healthy Choice, chicken teriyaki	1 meal	270	6	3	T	🫗
Healthy Choice, country breaded chicken	1 meal	350	9	5		🫗
Healthy Choice, country glazed chicken	1 meal	230	4	3		🫗
Healthy Choice, country herb chicken	1 meal	320	6	4	T	🫗
Healthy Choice, ginger chicken hunan	1 meal	380	5	5		🫗
Healthy Choice, grilled chicken sonoma	1 meal	230	4	3	T	🫗
Healthy Choice, honey mustard chicken	1 meal	270	4	2		🫗
Healthy Choice, mesquite chicken BBQ	1 meal	310	5	6		🫗
Healthy Choice, sesame chicken	1 meal	240	3	3		🫗
Healthy Choice, sesame chicken shanghai	1 meal	300	5	6		🫗
Marie Callender's, breaded chicken parmigiana	1 dinner	620	27	9	T	🫗
Marie Callender's, country fried chicken & gravy	1 meal	620	30	6	T	🫗
Stouffer's, Homestyle, baked chicken breast meal	1 pkg.	260	11	3	T	🫗
Stouffer's, Homestyle, chicken parmigiana meal	1 pkg.	460	16	5	T	🫗
Stouffer's, Homestyle, fried chicken breast	1 pkg.	400	17	2	T	🫗
Stouffer's, Lean Cuisine, chicken & vegetables	1 pkg.	250	6	4		🫗
Stouffer's, Lean Cuisine, chicken a l'orange	1 pkg.	250	2	3		✂
Stouffer's, Lean Cuisine, chicken carbonara	1 pkg.	280	8	2		🫗
Stouffer's, Lean Cuisine, chicken chow mein	1 pkg.	220	5	3		🫗
Stouffer's, Lean Cuisine, chicken enchilada suiza	1 pkg.	280	5	3		🫗
Stouffer's, Lean Cuisine, chicken fettucini	1 pkg.	280	6	4		🫗
Stouffer's, Lean Cuisine, chicken in peanut sauce	1 pkg.	290	6	4	T	🫗
Stouffer's, Lean Cuisine, chicken in wine sauce	1 pkg.	210	6	2		🫗
Stouffer's, Lean Cuisine, chicken lasagna	1 pkg.	270	8	5		🫗
Stouffer's, Lean Cuisine, chicken piccata	1 pkg.	270	6	2		🫗
Stouffer's, Lean Cuisine, chicken w/basil cream sauce	1 pkg.	270	7	3	T	🫗
Stouffer's, Lean Cuisine, fiesta chicken	1 pkg.	250	5	3		🫗
Stouffer's, Lean Cuisine, glazed chicken	1 pkg.	240	6	0		🫗
Stouffer's, Lean Cuisine, grilled chicken salsa	1 pkg.	270	7	4		🫗
Stouffer's, Lean Cuisine, herb roasted chicken	1 pkg.	210	5	3		🫗
Stouffer's, Lean Cuisine, honey roasted chicken	1 pkg.	270	6	4	T	🫗
Stouffer's, chicken chow mein w/rice	1 pkg.	260	5	3	T	🫗
Stouffer's, escalloped chicken & noodles	1 pkg.	430	27	3	T	🫗
Swanson, Hungry-Man, boneless chicken meal	1 pkg.	630	22	9	T	🫗
Swanson, Hungry-Man, fried chicken meal	1 pkg.	800	39	6	T	🫗
Swanson, chicken nuggets meal	1 pkg.	590	25	5	T	🫗
Swanson, fried chicken dinner	1 pkg.	630	31	5	T	🫗
Swanson, fried chicken meal	1 pkg.	580	30	5	T	🫗
Tyson, mandarin sesame wraps	1 1/2 wraps	630	15	5	T	🫗
Weight Watchers, Smart Ones, chicken fettucini	1 entree	300	7	4	T	🫗

☺ = Eat as much as you want • ✂ = Cut Back

	Portion	Calories	Total Fat	Dietary Fiber	Trans Fat	Guide
Weight Watchers, Smart Ones, creamy rigatoni w/broccoli & chicken	1 entree	230	2	4	T	🌢
Weight Watchers, Smart Ones, fiesta chicken	1 entree	210	2	5		✂
Weight Watchers, Smart Ones, lemon chicken piccata	1 entree	190	2	3	T	🌢

Frozen, Entree, Pasta

	Portion	Calories	Total Fat	Dietary Fiber	Trans Fat	Guide
Amy's, macaroni & cheese	1 entree	390	14	4		🌢
Amy's, vegetable lasagna	1 lasagna	300	10	5		🌢
Banquet, Meals Made Easy, lasagna w/meat sauce	1 cup	350	11	6	T	🌢
Budget Gourmet, angel hair pasta w/tomatoes	1 entree	230	5	3	T	🌢
Budget Gourmet, cheese manicotti w/meat sauce	1 entree	350	19	3	T	🌢
Budget Gourmet, fettuccine alfredo w/4 cheeses	1 entree	320	12	5	T	🌢
Budget Gourmet, pasta wine & mushroom sauce w/chicken	1 entree	280	7	3	T	🌢
Budget Gourmet, spaghetti marinara	1 entree	260	6	3		🌢
Budget Gourmet, ziti parmesano	1 container	260	7	4		🌢
Healthy Choice, macaroni & cheese	1 meal	320	7	4	T	🌢
Healthy Choice, manicotti w/3 cheeses	1 meal	300	9	5		🌢
Healthy Choice, pasta shells marinara	1 meal	390	8	5		🌢
Healthy Choice, penne pasta in roasted tomato sauce	1 meal	230	5	5	T	🌢
Healthy Choice, spaghetti & sauce w/seasoned beef	1 meal	280	6	5	T	🌢
Marie Callender's, fettucini w/broccoli & chicken	1 cup	410	24	4	T	🌢
Marie Callender's, lasagna w/meat sauce	1 cup	370	18	4	T	🌢
Marie Callender's, spaghetti & meat sauce	1 cup	380	13	5	T	🌢
Michelina's, 4 cheese lasagna	1 pkg.	290	7	3	T	🌢
Michelina's, fettuccine alfredo	1 pkg.	410	16	2	T	🌢
Michelina's, lasagna w/meat sauce	1 pkg.	300	8	3	T	🌢
Michelina's, linguini w/clams	1 pkg.	310	4	3	T	🌢
Michelina's, macaroni & cheese	1 container	340	13	2	T	🌢
Michelina's, wheels & cheese	1 container	300	8	2	T	🌢
Stouffer's, 5 cheese lasagna	1 pkg.	360	13	6	T	🌢
Stouffer's, Lean Cuisine, alfredo pasta primavera	1 pkg.	290	7	3		🌢
Stouffer's, Lean Cuisine, cheese ravioli	1 pkg.	270	7	5		🌢
Stouffer's, Lean Cuisine, lasagna	1 pkg.	290	6	4	T	🌢
Stouffer's, Lean Cuisine, macaroni & cheese	1 pkg.	290	7	4		🌢
Stouffer's, Lean Cuisine, penne pasta w/tomato basil sauce	1 pkg.	270	4	5		🌢
Stouffer's, Lean Cuisine, spaghetti	1 pkg.	290	5	7		🌢
Stouffer's, cheese ravioli	1 pkg.	380	13	6		🌢
Stouffer's, fettucini alfredo	1 pkg.	520	28	4		🌢
Stouffer's, lasagna	1 pkg.	340	12	3		🌢
Stouffer's, lasagna bake w/meat sauce	1 pkg.	370	12	6		🌢

🌢 = Avoid • 🌢 = Add for flavor

	Portion	Calories	Total Fat	Dietary Fiber	Trans Fat	Guide
Stouffer's, macaroni & cheese	1 cup	320	16	3	T	🌢
Stouffer's, spaghetti w/meat sauce	1 pkg.	350	12	5		🌢
Stouffer's, vegetable lasagna	1 pkg.	440	20	5	T	🌢
Swanson, Mac & More, macaroni & cheese	1 pkg.	240	9	2	T	🌢
Weight Watchers, Smart Ones, Santa Fe style rice & beans	1 entree	290	8	6		🌢
Weight Watchers, Smart Ones, angel hair pasta	1 entree	180	2	4		✀
Weight Watchers, Smart Ones, lasagna florentine	1 entree	200	2	5	T	🌢
Weight Watchers, Smart Ones, lasagna w/meat sauce	1 entree	240	2	4	T	🌢
Weight Watchers, Smart Ones, macaroni & cheese	1 entree	220	2	4	T	🌢
Weight Watchers, Smart Ones, penne pasta	1 entree	280	8	3	T	🌢
Weight Watchers, Smart Ones, ravioli floretine	1 entree	220	2	4		✀
Weight Watchers, Smart Ones, tuna noodle casserole	1 entree	270	7	4	T	🌢

Frozen, Entree, Pork

	Portion	Calories	Total Fat	Dietary Fiber	Trans Fat	Guide
Stouffer's, Homestyle, breaded pork cutlet	1 pkg.	420	23	4	T	🌢
Stouffer's, Lean Cuisine, honey roasted pork	1 pkg.	250	6	3		🌢
Swanson, Hungry-Man, boneless pork rib meal	1 pkg.	770	38	9	T	🌢
Swanson, boneless pork rib meal	1 pkg.	470	19	5	T	🌢

Frozen, Entree, Seafood

	Portion	Calories	Total Fat	Dietary Fiber	Trans Fat	Guide
Budget Gourmet, linguini w/clams & shrimp	1 entree	280	8	3		🌢
Healthy Choice, herb baked fish	1 meal	340	7	5	T	🌢
Healthy Choice, lemon pepper fish	1 meal	320	7	5		🌢
Healthy Choice, shrimp & vegetables maria	1 meal	290	5	5		🌢
Stouffer's, Lean Cuisine, baked fish	1 pkg.	270	6	3	T	🌢
Stouffer's, Lean Cuisine, shrimp & angel hair pasta	1 pkg.	290	6	1	T	🌢
Stouffer's, tuna noodle casserole	1 pkg.	340	15	4	T	🌢
Swanson, Hungry-Man, fisherman's platter	1 pkg.	650	26	5	T	🌢
Swanson, fish 'n' chips meal	1 pkg.	490	20	5	T	🌢

Frozen, Entree, Side

	Portion	Calories	Total Fat	Dietary Fiber	Trans Fat	Guide
Marie Callender's, chili & corn bread	1 cup	350	13	5	T	🌢
Matlaw's, egg roll bites	2 bites	45	1	1		✀
Nancy's, mushroom turnovers	12 turnovers	450	30	3		🌢
Nancy's, petite quiche	6 quiches	370	22	1		🌢
Stouffer's, chili w/beans	1 pkg.	290	11	6		🌢

Frozen, Entree, Turkey

	Portion	Calories	Total Fat	Dietary Fiber	Trans Fat	Guide
Banquet, homestyle gravy & sliced turkey	2 slices	150	11	1	T	🌢
Banquet, turkey meal	1 meal	280	10	3	T	🌢
Budget Gourmet, glazed turkey	1 entree	250	5	2	T	🌢
Healthy Choice, country inn roast turkey	1 meal	250	6	4	T	🌢

☺ = Eat as much as you want • ✀ = Cut Back

	Portion	Calories	Total Fat	Dietary Fiber	Trans Fat	Guide
Healthy Choice, country roast turkey w/mushrooms	1 meal	220	4	3		🌢
Healthy Choice, traditional breast of turkey	1 meal	290	5	5		🌢
Marie Callender's, turkey w/gravy & dressing	1 meal	500	19	4	T	🌢
Stouffer's, Hearty Portions, sliced turkey breast	1 pkg.	570	26	7	T	🌢
Stouffer's, Homestyle, roast turkey breast meal	1 pkg.	310	13	3	T	🌢
Stouffer's, Lean Cuisine, homestyle turkey	1 pkg.	230	5	3		🌢
Stouffer's, turkey tetrazzini	1 pkg.	350	18	4	T	🌢
Swanson, Hungry-Man, turkey dinner	1 pkg.	510	15	9	T	🌢
Swanson, Lunch & More, turkey	1 pkg.	240	9	2	T	🌢
Swanson, turkey dinner	1 pkg.	320	8	5	T	🌢

Frozen, Entree, Vegetable

	Portion	Calories	Total Fat	Dietary Fiber	Trans Fat	Guide
Banquet, creamy broccoli chicken & cheese	1 cup	280	14	2		🌢
Birds Eye, New England style in herb butter	1 pkg.	260	14	3		🌢
Birds Eye, side orders, Bavarian style	1 cup	150	8	3		🌢
Birds Eye, side orders, fresh green beans w/toasted almonds	3/4 cup	80	4	3		🌢
Birds Eye, side orders, pearl onions in cream sauce	1/2 cup	60	2	1		✂
Budget Gourmet, cheddar potatoes w/broccoli	5 oz.	160	8	2		🌢
Budget Gourmet, Oriental rice w/vegetables	5.25 oz.	200	11	2	T	🌢
Budget Gourmet, rice pilaf w/green beans	5 oz.	220	10	2	T	🌢
Budget Gourmet, spinach au gratin	5 oz.	160	12	2		🌢
Green Giant, Shoepeg white corn in butter sauce	3/4 cup	120	3	3		🌢
Green Giant, Southwestern style corn	3/4 cup	90	1	1		☺
Green Giant, alfredo	3/4 cup	80	3	3		🌢
Green Giant, baby brussels sprouts & butter	2/3 cup	60	2	4		✂
Green Giant, baby lima beans in butter sauce	2/3 cup	120	3	6		🌢
Green Giant, broccoli & cheese	2/3 cup	70	3	2	T	🌢
Green Giant, creamed spinach	1/2 cup	80	3	2	T	🌢
Green Giant, early June peas & butter sauce	3/4 cup	100	2	4		✂
Green Giant, green beans & almonds	2/3 cup	60	3	2		🌢
Green Giant, honey glazed carrots	1 cup	90	4	2	T	🌢
Green Giant, rice medley, rice, peas & mushrooms	1 pkg.	260	3	3	T	🌢
Green Giant, teriyaki	1 1/4 cups	100	7	2	T	🌢
Mrs. Paul's, eggplant parmesan	1/2 cup	220	14	3	T	🌢
Stouffer's, Lean Cuisine, 3 bean chili	1 pkg.	250	6	9		🌢
Stouffer's, Lean Cuisine, roasted potatoes w/broccoli	1 pkg.	260	6	7		🌢
Stouffer's, Lean Cuisine, teriyaki stir fry	1 pkg.	290	4	4		🌢
Stouffer's, spinach souffle	1/2 cup	140	9	1	T	🌢
Stouffer's, stuffed pepper	1 pkg.	200	5	3	T	🌢
Weight Watchers, Smart Ones, broccoli & cheese baked potato	1 entree	250	6	6		🌢

Frozen, Fish/Seafood

	Portion	Calories	Total Fat	Dietary Fiber	Trans Fat	Guide
Chef's Choice, shrimp stir fry	5 oz.	118	1	1		✂

🌢 = Avoid   •   💧 = Add for flavor

	Portion	Calories	Total Fat	Dietary Fiber	Trans Fat	Guide
Contessa, cooked shrimp	3 oz.	60	0	0		✂
Gorton's, country breaded fillets, lemon herb	2 fillets	220	11	0	T	💧
Gorton's, country golden fillets	2 fillets	250	14	0	T	💧
Gorton's, crispy battered fillets	2 fillets	240	13	0	T	💧
Gorton's, grilled fillets, cajun blackened	1 fillet	120	6	0	T	💧
Gorton's, grilled fillets, garlic butter	1 fillet	120	6	0	T	💧
Gorton's, grilled fillets, lemon butter	1 fillet	120	6	0	T	💧
Gorton's, grilled fillets, lemon pepper	1 fillet	120	6	0	T	💧
Gorton's, homestyle baked fillets, au gratin	1 fillet	130	5	0	T	💧
Gorton's, homestyle baked fillets, garlic butter crumb	1 fillet	230	12	0	T	💧
Gorton's, homestyle baked fillets, primavera	1 fillet	120	5	0	T	💧
Gorton's, popcorn shrimp, original	3.2 oz.	240	13	0	T	💧
Gorton's, southern fried country style fillets	2 fillets	230	14	0	T	💧
Handy, crab cakes	2 pieces	380	27	2	T	💧
Healthy Choice, halibut steaks	4 oz.	120	3	0		✂
Kaptain's Ketch, deviled crab cakes	3 oz.	140	6	1	T	💧
Nancy's, seafood crab cakes	1 pkg.	350	20	2		💧
New Zealand, green shell mussels	3 oz.	100	3	0		✂
Oven Poppers, crabbed stuffed sole	1 piece	250	13	1	T	💧
Oven Poppers, flounder, w/broccoli & cheese	1 piece	150	6	1		💧
Phillips, crab cakes	1 cake	160	9	0		💧
Salmon burger	1 burger	100	1	1		✂
Sea Watch, breaded clam strips	2 oz.	160	8	1		💧
SeaPak, clam strips	1 pkg.	410	23	2		💧
SeaPak, popcorn scallops	13 scallops	190	6	0		💧
SeaPak, popcorn shrimp	3 oz.	210	12	0	T	💧
SeaPak, shrimp poppers	20 pieces	210	12	2	T	💧
Singleton, shrimp poppers	3 oz.	200	7	1	T	💧
Van de Kamp's, breaded flounder fillets	1 fillet	230	11	0		💧
Van de Kamp's, haddock fillets	1 fillet	220	10	0		💧

Frozen, Mexican

	Portion	Calories	Total Fat	Dietary Fiber	Trans Fat	Guide
Amy's, enchilada, black bean and vegetables	1 enchilada	130	4	2		💧
Amy's Organic, beans & rice burrito, cheddar cheese	1 burrito	280	8	6		💧
Healthy Choice, chicken con queso burrito	1 meal	350	6	6		💧
Healthy Choice, fiesta chicken fajitas	1 meal	260	4	4	T	💧
Old El Paso, beef & bean burrito	1 burrito	320	9	4	T	💧
Patio, Mexican style dinner	1 meal	470	19	10	T	💧
Patio, bean & cheese burrito	1 burrito	300	9	4	T	💧
Patio, beef & bean burrito, hot	1 burrito	320	12	4	T	💧
Patio, beef & bean burrito, mild	1 burrito	330	12	4	T	💧
Patio, beef & bean burrito, red hot	1 burrito	320	12	4	T	💧
Patio, chicken burrito	1 burrito	290	8	2	T	💧
Tyson, beef fajitas	3 1/2 fajitas	480	13	5	T	💧
Tyson, chicken fajitas	3 1/2 fajitas	460	11	6	T	💧

☺ = Eat as much as you want • ✂ = Cut Back

	Portion	Calories	Total Fat	Dietary Fiber	Trans Fat	Guide
Frozen, Onion Rings						
Mrs. Paul's, crispy onion rings	7 rings	200	10	1	T	🔴
Ore-Ida, onion ringers	6 pieces	210	11	3	T	🔴
Ore-Ida, onion rings	4 pieces	220	11	2	T	🔴
Frozen, Pizza						
Amy's Organic, cheese	123 g.	310	11	2		🔴
Amy's Organic, roasted vegetable, no cheese	113 g.	270	8	3		🔴
Amy's Organic, spinach	132 g.	320	11	2		🔴
Celeste, Pizza For One, cheese	1 pizza	420	20	3	T	🔴
Celeste, Pizza For One, vegetable	1 pizza	420	21	5	T	🔴
Celeste, cheese	$^1/_4$ pizza	350	18	2		🔴
DiGiorno, Rising Crust, pepperoni	$^1/_3$ pizza	320	14	2		🔴
DiGiorno, Rising Crust, spinach, mushroom & garlic	$^1/_3$ pizza	270	8	2	T	🔴
DiGiorno, Rising Crust, supreme	$^1/_6$ pizza	400	17	3		🔴
DiGiorno, four cheese	$^1/_3$ pizza	280	9	2		🔴
DiGiorno, pepperoni	$^1/_3$ pizza	320	14	2		🔴
Healthy Choice, pepperoni French bread	1 pizza	340	5	6	T	🔴
Hot Pockets, Pizza Minis, double cheese	6 pieces	240	9	3	T	🔴
Hot Pockets, Pizza Minis, pepperoni	6 pieces	250	11	3	T	🔴
Jeno's, Crispy & Tasty, combination	1 pizza	520	28	3	T	🔴
Mama Celeste, fresh baked crust, pepperoni	$^1/_6$ pizza	380	16	6		🔴
Orida, single bites, cheese, sausage & pepperoni	4 pieces	190	7	1		🔴
Pizza Dippers	3 sticks	210	9	0	T	🔴
Red Baron Premium, Baked to Rise, pepperoni	$^1/_6$ pizza	340	15	2	T	🔴
Red Baron Premium, Baked to Rise, special deluxe	$^1/_6$ pizza	350	15	2	T	🔴
Red Baron Premium, Deep Dish Singles, microwave cheese	1 pizza	500	26	2	T	🔴
Red Baron Premium, Deep Dish Singles, microwave meat-trio	1 pizza	490	27	2	T	🔴
Red Baron Premium, Deep Dish Singles, microwave pepperoni	1 pizza	540	31	2	T	🔴
Red Baron Premium, Deep Dish Singles, microwave supreme	1 pizza	490	27	2	T	🔴
Stouffer's, Lean Cuisine, cheese French bread	1 pkg.	320	7	4	T	🔴
Stouffer's, Lean Cuisine, deluxe French bread	1 pkg.	300	6	4	T	🔴
Stouffer's, French Bread, pepperoni	1 pizza	440	20	5	T	🔴
Stouffer's, French Bread, two cheese	1 pizza	370	16	3	T	🔴
Stromboli	5-Jan	410	20	2		🔴
Tombstone, Oven Rising Crust, pepperoni	$^1/_6$ pizza	340	15	2		🔴
Tombstone, extra cheese	$^1/_4$ pizza	350	15	3	T	🔴
Tombstone, pepperoni	$^1/_4$ pizza	400	21	3		🔴
Totino's, pizza rolls	6 rolls	220	11	1	T	🔴
Frozen, Pot Pie						
Amy's, broccoli	1 pie	430	22	4		🔴
Amy's, shephard's pie, organic	1 pie	160	4	5		🔴
Amy's, vegetable	1 pie	360	18	4		🔴

🔴 = *Avoid* • 💧 = *Add for flavor*

	Portion	Calories	Total Fat	Dietary Fiber	Trans Fat	Guide
Banquet, beef	1 pie	400	23	1		🌢
Banquet, chicken	1 pie	380	22	1	T	🌢
Banquet, turkey	1 pie	370	20	3	T	🌢
Marie Callender's, chicken	1 cup	520	32	3	T	🌢
Marie Callender's, chicken & broccoli	1 cup	710	49	4	T	🌢
Marie Callender's, turkey	1 cup	600	36	3	T	🌢
Stouffer's, chicken	1 pkg.	540	33	4		🌢
Swanson, Hungry-Man, beef	1 pkg.	710	38	6	T	🌢
Swanson, Hungry-Man, chicken	1 pkg.	650	35	3	T	🌢
Swanson, Hungry-Man, turkey	1 pkg.	650	34	5	T	🌢
Swanson, beef	1 pkg.	415	23	2	T	🌢
Swanson, chicken	1 pkg.	410	22	2	T	🌢
Swanson, turkey	1 pkg.	400	21	3	T	🌢

Frozen, Potato

	Portion	Calories	Total Fat	Dietary Fiber	Trans Fat	Guide
Cascadian Farm, oven french fries	3 oz.	130	4	2		🌢
Hidden Valley, Fries-to-Go, microwave	1 box	260	14	5	T	🌢
Larry's, Stuffed Potatoes, bacon & cheese	1 potato	200	10	1	T	🌢
Larry's, Stuffed Potatoes, broccoli & cheese	1 potato	190	9	1	T	🌢
McCain, crinkle cut	3 oz.	120	3	3		🌢
Mrs. Paul's, candied sweet potatoes	5 oz.	300	1	3		☺
Ohboy, Stuffed Potatoes, onion, sour cream & chives	1 potato	110	2	2	T	🌢
Ohboy, Stuffed Potatoes, w/cheddar cheese	1 potato	130	4	2	T	🌢
Ore-Ida, Twice Baked Potatoes, butter flavored	1 piece	200	8	5	T	🌢
Ore-Ida, Twice Baked Potatoes, cheddar cheese	1 piece	190	8	3	T	🌢
Ore-Ida, Twice Baked Potatoes, garlic parmesan	1 piece	180	7	2	T	🌢
Ore-Ida, Twice Baked Potatoes, sour cream & chives	1 piece	190	7	3	T	🌢
Ore-Ida, Zesties	3 oz.	160	7	1	T	🌢
Ore-Ida, country fries w/skins	3 oz.	120	4	2	T	🌢
Ore-Ida, country style hash browns	1 1/4 cups	80	0	2	T	🌢
Ore-Ida, country style steak fries	3 oz.	110	4	2	T	🌢
Ore-Ida, crispers	3 oz.	220	13	2	T	🌢
Ore-Ida, fast fries	3 oz.	160	7	2	T	🌢
Ore-Ida, golden crinkles	3 oz.	120	4	2		🌢
Ore-Ida, golden fries	3 oz.	120	4	1	T	🌢
Ore-Ida, golden patties	1 pattie	140	7	1	T	🌢
Ore-Ida, golden twirls	3 oz.	150	6	2		🌢
Ore-Ida, microwave tater tots	1 pkg.	210	9	3	T	🌢
Ore-Ida, mini tater tots	19 pieces	180	10	2	T	🌢
Ore-Ida, onion tater tots	9 pieces	150	7	2	T	🌢
Ore-Ida, oven chips	3 oz.	180	8	1	T	🌢
Ore-Ida, potato wedges w/skin	3 oz.	110	3	2	T	🌢
Ore-Ida, potatoes o'brien	3/4 cup	60	0	2		✂
Ore-Ida, shoestrings	3 oz.	150	6	2	T	🌢
Ore-Ida, tater tots	9 pieces	150	8	2	T	🌢
Ore-Ida, toaster hash browns	2 patties	190	11	1	T	🌢

☺ = Eat as much as you want • ✂ = Cut Back

	Portion	Calories	Total Fat	Dietary Fiber	Trans Fat	Guide
Ore-Ida, topped baked potatoes, broccoli & cheese	$1/2$ baker	160	4	2	T	🔥
Penobscot, baked potato skins	3 oz.	180	11	10	T	🔥

Frozen, Sandwich

	Portion	Calories	Total Fat	Dietary Fiber	Trans Fat	Guide
Amy's, spinach feta pocket sandwich	1 container	200	7	2		🔥
Amy's, vegetable pie pocket sandwich	1 container	230	6	2		🔥
Banquet, Hot Sandwich Toppers, cream chipped beef	1 bag	120	6	0	T	🔥
Banquet, Hot Sandwich Toppers, gravy & salisbury steak	1 bag	220	16	2		🔥
Croissant Pockets, Philly steak & cheese	1 piece	350	16	2	T	🔥
Croissant Pockets, chicken broccoli & cheddar	1 piece	290	9	2	T	🔥
Croissant Pockets, egg sausage & cheese	1 piece	340	15	2	T	🔥
Croissant Pockets, ham & cheese	1 piece	320	12	2	T	🔥
Croissant Pockets, pepperoni pizza	1 piece	360	16	3	T	🔥
Croissant Pockets, supreme pizza	1 piece	390	20	3	T	🔥
Hormel, Quick Meal, grilled chicken sandwich	1 sandwich	300	9	2	T	🔥
Hot Pockets, barbeque	1 piece	330	11	1	T	🔥
Hot Pockets, beef & cheddar	1 piece	350	16	3	T	🔥
Hot Pockets, chicken & cheddar w/broccoli	1 piece	300	10	2	T	🔥
Hot Pockets, ham'n cheese	1 piece	320	12	3	T	🔥
Hot Pockets, meatballs w/mozzarella	1 piece	320	11	4	T	🔥
Hot Pockets, pepperoni & sausage pizza	1 piece	330	14	4	T	🔥
Hot Pockets, pepperoni pizza	1 piece	360	15	4	T	🔥
Ken & Robert's, Veggie Pockets, Indian style	1 pocket	260	8	5		🔥
Ken & Robert's, Veggie Pockets, Tex-Mex style	1 pocket	280	8	6		🔥
Ken & Robert's, Veggie Pockets, barbeque style	1 pocket	290	8	5		🔥
Ken & Robert's, Veggie Pockets, broccoli & cheddar	1 pocket	250	8	4		🔥
Ken & Robert's, Veggie Pockets, pizza style	1 pocket	270	8	4		🔥
Ken & Robert's, Veggie Pockets, potato & cheddar	1 pocket	260	8	2		🔥
Lean Pockets, Philly steak & cheese	1 piece	260	7	1	T	🔥
Lean Pockets, chicken broccoli supreme	1 piece	260	7	3	T	🔥
Lean Pockets, chicken fajita	1 piece	270	7	5	T	🔥
Lean Pockets, chicken parmesan	1 piece	280	7	3	T	🔥
Lean Pockets, ham & cheddar	1 piece	280	8	1	T	🔥
Lean Pockets, pepperoni pizza deluxe	1 piece	270	7	3	T	🔥
Steak-umm	1 steak	190	17	0		🔥
Steak-umm, Sandwich to Go, cheesesteak	1 sandwich	290	13	4		🔥
Steak-umm, reduced fat	1 steak	110	7	0		🔥

Frozen, Vegetarian

	Portion	Calories	Total Fat	Dietary Fiber	Trans Fat	Guide
Cascadian Farm Organic, Aztec vegetarian meal	$1/2$ bag	230	3	10		☺
Cascadian Farm Organic, Indian vegetarian meal	$1/2$ bag	250	4	7		☺
Morningstar Farms, chicken nuggets	4 nuggets	160	4	5		🔥
Morningstar Farms, chicken patties	1 pattie	150	6	2		🔥

🔥 = Avoid • 🝁 = Add for flavor

	Portion	Calories	Total Fat	Dietary Fiber	Trans Fat	Guide
Instant/Microwave						
Chef Boyardee, beefaroni	1 bowl	190	3	4		💧
Chef Boyardee, lasagna	1 bowl	220	6	2		💧
Chef Boyardee, macaroni & cheese	1 bowl	170	2	2		✂
Chef Boyardee, ravioli, beef	1 bowl	290	7	3		💧
Chef Boyardee, rice w/beef & vegetables	1 bowl	250	7	4		💧
Chef Jr. Boyardee, pasta w/meatballs	1 bowl	230	8	2		💧
Dinty Moore, beef stew	1 cup	190	10	2		💧
Dinty Moore, chicken & dumplings, 97% fat free	1 cup	200	6	1	T	💧
Dinty Moore, turkey stew, 99% fat free	1 cup	130	3	2	T	💧
Fantastic Foods, Bombay curry rice & beans	1 pkg.	250	2	5		☺
Fantastic Foods, Ready Set, Pasta!, creamy garlic	1 pkg.	240	4	0		💧
Fantastic Foods, Ready Set, Pasta!, macaroni & cheese	1 pkg.	240	5	0		💧
Fantastic Foods, Ready Set, Pasta!, spicy Thai	1 pkg.	200	2	2		✂
Fantastic Foods, Stuffed-Mashed, broccoli & cheddar	1 pkg.	190	3	3		💧
Fantastic Foods, Stuffed-Mashed, cheddar cheese	1 pkg.	180	3	3		💧
Fantastic Foods, Stuffed-Mashed, garlic & herb	1 pkg.	180	2	3		✂
Fantastic Foods, Stuffed-Mashed, sour cream & chives	1 pkg.	180	3	3		💧
Fantastic Foods, Tex Mex rice & beans	1 pkg.	240	3	6		✂
Fantastic Foods, black bean salsa couscous	1 container	240	2	8		☺
Fantastic Foods, cajun rice & beans	1 pkg.	230	3	8		✂
Fantastic Foods, cha-cha chili	1 pkg.	220	1	13		☺
Fantastic Foods, creole vegetable couscous	1 container	220	2	6		☺
Fantastic Foods, jumpin' black bean	1 pkg.	210	1	8		☺
Fantastic Foods, nacho cheddar couscous	1 container	200	3	6		✂
Fantastic Foods, spicy Jamaican rice & beans	1 pkg.	250	2	6		☺
Fantastic Foods, sweet corn couscous	1 container	180	1	6		☺
Hormel, Kid's Kitchen, beans & weiners	1 cup	310	13	8		💧
Hormel, Kid's Kitchen, beefy macaroni	1 cup	190	6	2		💧
Hormel, Kid's Kitchen, cheesy mac 'n beef	1 cup	260	7	1		💧
Hormel, Kid's Kitchen, noodle rings & chicken	1 cup	150	4	1		💧
Hormel, Kid's Kitchen, ravioli, mini beef	1 cup	240	7	1		💧
Hormel, Kid's Kitchen, spaghetti rings & franks	1 cup	240	9	1		💧
Hormel, chili hot no beans	1 cup	210	9	3		💧
Hormel, chili w/beans	1 cup	270	7	7		💧
Hormel, chili, turkey no beans	1 cup	190	3	3		💧
Nile Spice, couscous parmesan	1 pkg.	200	3	2		💧
Taste Adventure, black bean, South American style	¾ cup dry	210	1	9		☺
Refrigerated, Lunch						
Oscar Mayer, Lunchables, 96% fat free ham, cheddar, Capri, pudding	1 pkg.	390	11	0	T	💧

☺ = *Eat as much as you want* • ✂ = *Cut Back*

	Portion	Calories	Total Fat	Dietary Fiber	Trans Fat	Guide
Oscar Mayer, Lunchables, Taco Bell beef tacos	1 pkg.	310	11	4	T	🌢
Oscar Mayer, Lunchables, Taco Bell beef tacos, Capri, Butterfinger	1 pkg.	470	13	4	T	🌢
Oscar Mayer, Lunchables, Taco Bell cheese & salsa nachos	1 pkg.	380	21	3	T	🌢
Oscar Mayer, Lunchables, Taco Bell nachos, Capri, Crunch bar	1 pkg.	530	24	3	T	🌢
Oscar Mayer, Lunchables, bologna, American, Capri, M&M's	1 pkg.	530	27	1	T	🌢
Oscar Mayer, Lunchables, bologna, American, chocolate chip cakes	1 pkg.	480	33	0	T	🌢
Oscar Mayer, Lunchables, lean ham, American, Capri, Snickers	1 pkg.	440	18	1	T	🌢
Oscar Mayer, Lunchables, lean ham, cheddar, vanilla cream sandwich cake	1 pkg.	420	22	1	T	🌢
Oscar Mayer, Lunchables, lean turkey breast & cheddar	1 pkg.	350	20	1	T	🌢
Oscar Mayer, Lunchables, pizza dunks, soft breadsticks, Capri, Crunch	1 pkg.	510	14	3	T	🌢
Oscar Mayer, Lunchables, pizza swirls, pepperoni, and dessert, Capri, M&M	1 pkg.	480	18	2	T	🌢
Oscar Mayer, Lunchables, pizza, extra cheesy	1 pkg.	300	12	2	T	🌢
Oscar Mayer, Lunchables, pizza, extra cheesy, Capri, Crunch	1 pkg.	460	15	2	T	🌢
Oscar Mayer, Lunchables, pizza, pepperoni sausage	1 pkg.	310	14	2	T	🌢
Oscar Mayer, Lunchables, pizza, pepperoni w/Capri, Butterfinger	1 pkg.	460	16	2	T	🌢
Oscar Mayer, Lunchables, turkey breast, cheddar, Capri, Jell-O	1 pkg.	350	8	0	T	🌢

■ SEASONINGS

Asian

Kikkoman, marin sweet cooking seasoning	1 tbsp.	40	0	0		✂

Batter

McCormick, Golden Dipt, batter all purpose fry mix	1/4 cup mix	120	0	0		✂
McCormick, Golden Dipt, fry easy cajun style	1 1/3 tbsp. mix	35	0	0		✂
McCormick, Golden Dipt, fry easy onion rings	1/4 cup mix	100	0	0		✂
McCormick, Golden Dipt, fry easy tempura	1/4 cup mix	100	0	0		✂
Mrs. Dash, crispy coating mix, original recipe	2 tbsp.	70	1	0	T	🌢

Batter, Seafood

McCormick, Golden Dipt, fry easy fish 'n chips	1/4 cup mix	100	0	0		✂
McCormick, Golden Dipt, fry easy fish fry	1 1/3 tbsp.	35	0	0		✂
McCormick, Golden Dipt, fry easy seafood	1 2/3 tbsp. mix	50	0	0		✂

🌢 = *Avoid* • 🌢 = *Add for flavor*

	Portion	Calories	Total Fat	Dietary Fiber	Trans Fat	Guide
McCormick, Golden Dipt, oven easy cajun style	1/4 cup	90	3	0	T	🌢
McCormick, Golden Dipt, oven easy lemon & pepper	1/4 cup	90	3	0	T	🌢
McCormick, Golden Dipt, oven easy shrimp & seafood	2 tbsp.	70	2	0	T	🌢

Beef

	Portion	Calories	Total Fat	Dietary Fiber	Trans Fat	Guide
McCormick, Bag'n Season, pot roast	1 tsp. dry	10	0	0		👍
McCormick, Swedish meatballs	2 tsp. + 1 tsp.	45	1	0	T	🌢
McCormick, beef stew	2 tsp. dry	15	0	0		✂
McCormick, meat loaf	1 tsp. dry	15	0	0		✂
McCormick, sloppy joe	1 tsp. dry	15	0	0		✂

Chili

	Portion	Calories	Total Fat	Dietary Fiber	Trans Fat	Guide
McCormick, chili seasoning	1 1/3 tbsp.	35	1	2		✂
Old El Paso, chili seasoning mix	2 tsp. dry	15	1	0	T	🌢

Mexican

	Portion	Calories	Total Fat	Dietary Fiber	Trans Fat	Guide
McCormick, fajitas marinade mix	2 tsp. dry	15	0	0		✂
McCormick, taco seasoning	2 tsp. dry	20	0	0		✂
Old El Paso, burrito seasoning mix	2 tsp. dry	20	0	0		✂
Old El Paso, taco seasoning mix	2 tsp. dry	20	0	0		✂
Ortega, taco seasoning mix	1 tsp.	20	0	0		✂
Taco Bell, taco seasoning mix	2 tsp.	20	0	0	T	🌢

Pork

	Portion	Calories	Total Fat	Dietary Fiber	Trans Fat	Guide
Kraft, Shake'n Bake, pork, original	1/8 pkt.	45	1	0	T	🌢
McCormick, Bag'n Season, pork chops	2 tsp. dry	15	0	0		✂
McCormick, Bag'n Season, spare ribs	1 tsp. dry	30	0	0		✂

Poultry

	Portion	Calories	Total Fat	Dietary Fiber	Trans Fat	Guide
Kraft, Shake'n Bake Glazes, barbecue	1/8 pkg.	45	1	0	T	🌢
Kraft, Shake'n Bake Glazes, honey mustard	1/8 pkg.	45	1	0	T	🌢
Kraft, Shake'n Bake Glazes, tangy honey chicken	1/8 pkt.	45	1	0	T	🌢
Kraft, Shake'n Bake, buffalo wings	1/10 pkg.	40	1	0	T	🌢
Kraft, Shake'n Bake, chicken, original	1/8 pkt.	40	1	0	T	🌢
Kraft, Shake'n Bake, classic Italian	1/8 pkt.	40	1	0	T	🌢
Kraft, Shake'n Bake, hot & spicy	1/8 pkg.	40	1	0	T	🌢
McCormick, Bag'n Season, buffalo wings	1 tsp. dry	30	0	0		✂
McCormick, Bag'n Season, roast turkey breast w/gravy	1 tsp. dry	15	0	0		✂
McCormick, Season'n Fry, for chicken	1 tsp. dry	35	0	0		✂
McCormick, chicken fried rice	1 tbsp. dry mix	35	0	0		✂
McCormick, stir fry chicken	2 tsp. dry mix	20	0	0		✂

☺ = Eat as much as you want • ✂ = Cut Back

FOOD LISTS

	Portion	Calories	Total Fat	Dietary Fiber	Trans Fat	Guide
■ SNACK FOODS						
Candy & Gum, Candy Bar						
3 Musketeers	1 bar	260	8	1	T	●
Almond Joy	1 pkg.	240	13	2	T	●
Baby Ruth	1 bar	270	13	2	T	●
Butterfinger	1 bar	270	11	1	T	●
Cadbury's, Caramello	1 bar	220	10	0		●
Cadbury's, Dairy Milk, king size	9 blocks	220	12	0		●
Cadbury's, Fruit & Nut, king size	9 blocks	210	11	1		●
Cadbury's, Krisp, king size	9 blocks	200	10	0		●
Cadbury's, Roast Almond, king size	9 blocks	220	13	1		●
Charleston Chew, vanilla	1 bar	230	7	1	T	●
Heath	1 pkg.	210	13	0	T	●
Hershey's, 5th Avenue	1 bar	280	12	1	T	●
Hershey's, Cookies 'n' Creme	1 bar	220	12	0	T	●
Hershey's, Cookies 'n' Mint, king size	3 blocks	190	10	1	T	●
Hershey's, Mr. Goodbar	1 bar	270	17	2		●
Hershey's, Skor	1 bar	210	12	0		●
Hershey's, Special Dark, king size	3 blocks	200	12	2		●
Hershey's, Sweet Escape	1 bar	150	5	0		●
Hershey's, Whatchamacallit	1 bar	220	10	0	T	●
Hershey's, milk chocolate	1 bar	230	13	1	T	●
Hershey's, milk chocolate w/almonds	1 bar	230	14	1		●
Milky Way	1 bar	270	10	1	T	●
Milky Way, Dark	1 bar	220	8	1	T	●
Milky Way, Lite	1 bar	170	5	0	T	●
Mounds	1 pkg.	250	13	3		●
Nestlé, 100 Grand	1 pkg.	20	8	0		●
Nestlé, Chunky	1 bar	210	11	1		●
Nestlé, Crunch	1 bar	230	12	0		●
Pay Day	1 bar	250	13	2	T	●
Reese's, Nutrageous	1 bar	290	17	2		●
Snickers, Regular	1 bar	280	14	1		●
Twix, 2X chocolate caramel	2 cookies	280	14	1	T	●
Candy & Gum, Gum						
Bazooka, Blasts, soft	1 piece	30	0	0		✂
Bazooka, Sugarless	1 piece	15	0	0		✂
Breath Savers, Ice Breakers	1 stick	10	0	0	T	●
Bubble Yum, Sugarless, assorted	1 piece	15	0	0	T	●
Carefree Sugarless, alpine mint	1 stick	5	0	0	T	●
Carefree Sugarless, spearmint & peppermint	1 stick	5	0	0	T	●
Carefree Sugarless, wintergreen & spicy cinnamon	1 stick	5	0	0		☝
Chiclets, tiny size	1/5 pkg.	10	0	0		☝
Clorets	2 pieces	10	0	0	T	●
Dentyne Ice, Sugarless, all flavors	2 pieces	5	0	0		☝
Stick Free, non-stick sugarless, peppermnt	1 stick	10	0	0	T	●

● = *Avoid* • ☝ = *Add for flavor*

	Portion	Calories	Total Fat	Dietary Fiber	Trans Fat	Guide
Trident, all flavors	1 stick	5	0	0		👍
Wrigley's, Extra, all flavors	1 piece	5	0	0		👍

Candy & Gum, Hard Candy

	Portion	Calories	Total Fat	Dietary Fiber	Trans Fat	Guide
Brach's, Hi-C, fruity hard candy	3 pieces	70	0	0		💧
Breath Savers Sugar Free, all flavors	1 mint	10	0	0		👍
Butterscotch	3 pieces	60	0	0		💧
Certs, Cool Mint Drops	2 pieces	10	0	0	T	💧
Certs Sugar Free, all flavors	1 mint	5	0	0	T	💧
Lemon drops	3 pieces	60	0	0		✂
LifeSavers, Crystomint	2 candies	20	0	0		✂
LifeSavers, assorted	2 candies	20	0	0		✂
Lifesavers, Wintogreen, Spearo- & Pepomint	3 mints	20	0	0		✂
Necco, assorted wafers	3 pieces	15	0	0		✂
Nerds, grape & strawberry	1 tbsp.	60	0	0		✂
Now and Later, classic bar	1 pkg.	270	3	0	T	💧
Peppermint starlites	3 pieces	60	0	0		✂
Spree	8 pieces	60	0	0		✂
Sweetarts	8 pieces	60	0	0		✂
Tastations, caramel	3 pieces	60	2	0		✂
Tastations, chocolate	3 pieces	60	2	0		✂
Tic Tac, all flavors	1 piece	2	0	0		👍
Werther's	3 pieces	60	1	0		✂

Candy & Gum, Marshmallow

	Portion	Calories	Total Fat	Dietary Fiber	Trans Fat	Guide
Jet-Puffed, funmallows	4 pieces	110	0	0	T	💧
Jet-Puffed, original	4 pieces	90	0	0		✂
Jet-Puffed, original miniature	1/2 cup	80	0	0		✂
Marshmallow	4 pieces	100	0	0		✂
Miniature	2/3 cup	110	0	0		✂

Candy & Gum, Other

	Portion	Calories	Total Fat	Dietary Fiber	Trans Fat	Guide
Andes, creme de menthe thins	8 pieces	210	13	1	T	💧
Brach's, HI-C, fruit slices	3 pieces	150	0	0		✂
Candy corn	24 pieces	150	0	0		✂
Caramels	5 pieces	160	3	0	T	💧
Charms, Blow Pop, assorted	1 pop	50	0	0		✂
Dove, Promises, dark chocolate	7 pieces	220	13	2		💧
Dove, Promises, rich milk chocolate miniatures	7 pieces	230	13	1		💧
Ferrero Rocher, fine hazelnut chocolates	3 pieces	220	15	1		💧
Goldenberg's, peanut chews, all natural	3 pieces	180	9	1	T	💧
Goobers	1 box	260	22	5		💧
Good & Plenty	1/5 bag	130	0	0		✂
Gum drops	10 pieces	140	0	0		✂
Gummy bears	22 pieces	150	0	0		✂
Hershey's, Hugs	8 pieces	210	12	0		💧
Hershey's, Hugs w/almonds	9 pieces	230	13	0		💧
Hershey's, Nuggets, Cookies 'n' Creme	4 pieces	220	11	0	T	💧
Hershey's, Nuggets, Cookies 'n' Mint	4 nuggets	200	10	1	T	💧

☺ = Eat as much as you want • ✂ = Cut Back

	Portion	Calories	Total Fat	Dietary Fiber	Trans Fat	Guide
Hershey's, Nuggets, Milk Chocolate	4 pieces	210	12	1		🍶
Hershey's, Nuggets, Milk Chocolate w/Almonds	4 pieces	210	13	1		🍶
Hershey's, Sweet Escapes, chocolate toffee crisp bar	1 bar	80	4	0		🍶
Hershey's, Sweet Escapes, crispy caramel fudge bars	1 bar	80	2	0	T	🍶
Hershey's, Sweet Escapes, triple chocolate wafer bars	1 bar	80	3	0	T	🍶
Hershey's, assorted miniatures	5 pieces	230	13	1		🍶
Hershey's, classic caramels, chocolate cream filled	6 pieces	160	6	0		🍶
Hershey's, classic caramels, soft & chewy	6 pieces	160	5	0		🍶
Hot Tamales	19 pieces	150	0	0		✂
Jelly beans	16 pieces	150	0	0		✂
Juicy Fruits	1 box	240	0	0		✂
Jujubes	58 pieces	150	0	0		✂
Junior Mints	1 box	180	3	0		🍶
Kit Kat	1 pkg.	220	11	0		🍶
Lifesavers, Gummisavers, all flavors	1 pkg.	140	0	0		✂
M & M's, minis	1 tube	180	8	1		🍶
M & M's, peanut butter	1.5 oz.	220	12	2	T	🍶
M & M's, plain	1 pack	240	10	1		🍶
M & M's, w/peanuts	1 pack	250	13	2		🍶
Mentos, mint	1 mint	10	0	0	T	🍶
Mike and Ike	1 pkg.	220	0	0		✂
Milk Duds	13 pieces	180	6	0	T	🍶
Nestlé, Buncha Crunch	1/3 cup	190	10	0		🍶
Nestlé, Butterfinger BB's	1/4 cup	200	9	1	T	🍶
Nestlé, Pretzel Flipz	9 pieces	130	6	0	T	🍶
Nestlé, Raisinets	1 bag	200	8	1		🍶
Nestlé, Sno-Caps	1 box	300	13	3		🍶
Reese's, Crunchy Cookie Cups	1 pkg.	210	12	1	T	🍶
Reese's, Peanut Butter Cup	1 pkg.	250	14	1		🍶
Reese's, Pieces	1 pkg.	230	10	1	T	🍶
Reese's Sticks	1 pkg.	220	13	1	T	🍶
Riesen, Chocolate Chew	1 bar	180	7	3	T	🍶
Rolo	1 pkg.	260	11	0	T	🍶
Skittles	1 pack	240	3	0	T	🍶
SnackWell's candy, caramel nut clusters	3 candies	140	5	0		🍶
SnackWell's candy, chocolate chews	7 pieces	160	3	0		🍶
SnackWell's candy, raisin dips	1/4 cup	160	5	2	T	🍶
Sophie Mae, peanut brittle	1.4 oz.	180	5	1		🍶
Starburst, Fruit Twists	1 pack	190	1	0	T	🍶
Starburst, original	1 pack	240	5	0	T	🍶
Sugar Babies, king size	30 pieces	180	2	0	T	🍶
Thin mints	6 pieces	170	5	3		🍶
Tootsie Roll, Midgees	6 pieces	160	3	0	T	🍶
Tootsie Roll, Pop	1 pop	60	0	0	T	🍶
Twizzlers, Pull-n-Peel, cherry	1 pkg.	190	2	2	T	🍶

🍶 = Avoid • 🥄 = Add for flavor

	Portion	Calories	Total Fat	Dietary Fiber	Trans Fat	Guide
Twizzlers, Twists, strawberry	1 pkg.	230	1	0	T	🩸
Werther's, chocolates	10 pieces	220	14	2	T	🩸
Whoppers, malt milk balls	$1/2$ box	180	7	0	T	🩸
York, peppermint patties	1 pattie	170	3	0		🩸

Chips, Cheese Curl

	Portion	Calories	Total Fat	Dietary Fiber	Trans Fat	Guide
Chee-tos	1 oz.	160	10	1	T	🩸
Chee-tos, Cheesy Checkers	1 oz.	160	10	0	T	🩸
Chee-tos, Crunchy	1 oz.	160	10	0	T	🩸
Chee-tos, Curl	1 oz.	150	10	0	T	🩸
Utz	1 oz.	160	9	0	T	🩸
Weight Watchers, Smart Snackers, cheese curls	1 pkg.	70	3	0	T	🩸

Chips, Corn

	Portion	Calories	Total Fat	Dietary Fiber	Trans Fat	Guide
Bugles, light	1 1/2 cups	130	4	0	T	🩸
Bugles, original	1 1/3 cups	160	9	0		🩸
Doritos, 3Ds, cool rancher	1 oz.	140	6	1	T	🩸
Doritos, 3Ds, nacho cheesier	1 oz.	140	7	1	T	🩸
Doritos, Wow!, nacho cheesier w/olestra	1 oz.	90	1	1	T	🩸
Doritos, cool rancher	1 oz.	140	7	1	T	🩸
Doritos, nacho cheesier	1 oz.	140	7	1	T	🩸
Doritos, spicy nacho	1 oz.	140	7	1	T	🩸
Doritos, taco supreme	1 oz.	150	7	1	T	🩸
Fritos, Bar-B-Q	1 oz.	150	9	1	T	🩸
Fritos, Texas grill	1 oz.	150	9	1	T	🩸
Fritos, original	1 oz.	160	10	1	T	🩸
Guiltless Gourmet, baked, blue corn tortilla	1 oz.	110	2	2		✄
Guiltless Gourmet, baked, mucho nacho tortilla	1 oz.	110	2	2		✄
Guiltless Gourmet, baked, red corn tortilla	1 oz.	110	2	2		✄
Guiltless Gourmet, baked, yellow corn tortilla	1 oz.	110	2	2		✄
Sun Chips	1 oz.	140	6	2	T	🩸
Sun Chips, French onion	1 oz.	140	6	2	T	🩸
Tostitos	1 oz.	110	1	2	T	🩸
Tostitos, Restaurant Style	1 oz.	130	6	1	T	🩸
Tostitos, baked, low fat	1 oz.	110	1	2	T	🩸
Tostitos, baked, salsa & cream cheese bite size	1 oz.	120	3	1	T	🩸
Tostitos, bite size	1 oz.	140	8	1	T	🩸
Tostitos, crispy round	1 oz.	150	8	1	T	🩸
Tostitos, for nachos	1 oz.	140	6	1	T	🩸
Utz, tortillas, baked	1 oz.	120	2	1	T	🩸
Utz, tortillas, cheesier nacho	1 oz.	140	6	1	T	🩸
Utz, tortillas, Restaurant Style	1 oz.	140	7	1	T	🩸
Utz, tortillas, white corn	1 oz.	140	7	1	T	🩸

Chips, Other

	Portion	Calories	Total Fat	Dietary Fiber	Trans Fat	Guide
Funyuns, onion flavor rings	1 oz.	140	7	0	T	🩸
Utz, pork rinds	$1/2$ oz.	80	5	0		🩸

☺ = Eat as much as you want • ✄ = Cut Back

	Portion	Calories	Total Fat	Dietary Fiber	Trans Fat	Guide
Chips, Potato						
Baked Lay's, KC Masterpiece	1 oz.	120	3	2	T	💧
Baked Lay's, original	1 oz.	110	2	2	T	💧
Baked Lay's, sour cream & onion	1 oz.	120	3	2	T	💧
French's, shoestring potato sticks	3/4 cup	180	12	1	T	💧
Lay's, KC Masterpiece barbecue	1 oz.	150	10	1	T	💧
Lay's, Wow!, mesquite b-b-q w/olestra	1 oz.	75	0	1	T	💧
Lay's, classic	1 oz.	150	10	1	T	💧
Lay's, deli style, cheddar	1 oz.	150	10	1	T	💧
Lay's, deli style, hearty chili	1 oz.	150	10	1	T	💧
Lay's, deli style, original	1 oz.	150	10	1	T	💧
Lay's, deli style, salt & vinegar	1 oz.	150	10	1	T	💧
Lay's, salt & vinegar	1 oz.	150	10	1	T	💧
Lay's, sour cream & onion	1 oz.	160	11	1	T	💧
Lay's, wavy, original	1 oz.	150	10	1	T	💧
Pringles, BBQ	1 oz.	150	10	1		💧
Pringles, BBQ w/olestra	1 oz.	70	0	1		✂
Pringles, Right Crisps, original	1 oz.	140	7	1		💧
Pringles, original	1 oz.	160	11	1		💧
Pringles, original w/olestra	1 oz.	70	0	1		✂
Pringles, ridges, original	1 oz.	150	10	1		💧
Pringles, sour cream 'n onion	1 oz.	160	10	1	T	💧
Pringles, sour cream 'n onion w/olestra	1 oz.	70	0	1		✂
Ruffles	1 oz.	160	10	1	T	💧
Ruffles, KC Masterpiece mesquite BBQ	1 oz.	150	10	1	T	💧
Ruffles, Lipton French onion	1 oz.	150	10	1	T	💧
Ruffles, Wow!, original w/olestra	1 oz.	75	0	1		✂
Ruffles, cheddar & sour cream	1 oz.	160	10	1	T	💧
Ruffles, the works	1 oz.	160	11	1	T	💧
Utz	1 oz.	150	9	1		💧
Utz, Carolina style bar-b-que	1 oz.	150	9	1		💧
Utz, Kettle Classics, mesquite bar-b-que	1 oz.	150	9	1		💧
Utz, Kettle Classics, original	1 oz.	150	9	1		💧
Utz, baked crisps, bar-b-que	1 oz.	110	2	2	T	💧
Utz, bar-b-q	1 oz.	150	9	1		💧
Utz, cheddar & sour cream, ripple cut	1 oz.	160	10	1	T	💧
Utz, crab	1 oz.	150	9	1		💧
Utz, grandma's handcooked	1 oz.	140	8	1		💧
Utz, reduced fat, bar-b-que, ripple cut	1 oz.	140	7	1	T	💧
Utz, reduced fat, ripple cut	1 oz.	140	7	1		💧
Utz, ripples	1 oz.	150	10	1		💧
Utz, salt'n vinegar	1 oz.	150	9	1		💧
Utz, sour cream & onion, ripple cut	1 oz.	160	10	1	T	💧
Utz, wavy	1 oz.	150	9	1		💧
Chips, Pretzel						
Combos, oven baked, cheddar cheese pretzel	1 oz.	130	5	1	T	💧
Combos, oven baked, pizzeria pretzel	1 oz.	130	5	1	T	💧
Hanover, baked soft pretzels	1 pretzel	160	0	1		✂

💧 = Avoid   •   ◊ = Add for flavor

	Portion	Calories	Total Fat	Dietary Fiber	Trans Fat	Guide
Newman's Own, salted round	10 pretzels	110	1	0		✂
Snyder's of Hanover, golden cheese	14 nibblers	130	2	0		✂
Snyder's of Hanover, nibblers, fat free	16 nibblers	120	0	0		✂
Snyder's of Hanover, sourdough hard	1 pretzel	100	0	1		✂
Snyder's of Hanover, ultra thin	11 pretzels	110	0	0	T	🌢
Utz, extra thin	1 oz.	100	0	1		✂
Utz, old fashioned sourdough hard	1 pretzel	90	0	0		✂
Yogurt pretzels	8 pieces	190	8	0	T	🌢

Chips, Snack Mix

	Portion	Calories	Total Fat	Dietary Fiber	Trans Fat	Guide
Gardetto's, Snak-ens, Chicago style pizza	1/2 cup	140	5	1	T	🌢
Gardetto's, chips & twists, sour cream & onion, reduced fat	1/2 cup	140	6	1	T	🌢
General Mills, Chex Mix, bold party blend	1/2 cup	140	6	1	T	🌢
General Mills, Chex Mix, cheddar flavor	1/2 cup	130	5	1	T	🌢
General Mills, Chex Mix, traditional	2/3 cup	130	4	1	T	🌢

Cookies, Biscotti

	Portion	Calories	Total Fat	Dietary Fiber	Trans Fat	Guide
Stella D'Oro, French vanilla	1 cookie	90	3	0	T	🌢
Stella D'Oro, chocolate chunk	1 cookie	90	3	0	T	🌢

Cookies, Butter

	Portion	Calories	Total Fat	Dietary Fiber	Trans Fat	Guide
Keebler, Cookie Stix, butter	4 cookies	130	5	0	T	🌢
Pepperidge Farm, Chessman	3 cookies	120	8	0	T	🌢
Rippin' Good, butter thins	10 cookies	110	5	1	T	🌢

Cookies, Chocolate Chip

	Portion	Calories	Total Fat	Dietary Fiber	Trans Fat	Guide
Entenmann's, soft baked, chocolate chip	1 cookie	100	5	0	T	🌢
Entenmann's, soft baked, chocolatey chip, light	2 cookies	120	4	0	T	🌢
Entenmann's, soft baked, double chocolate chip	1 cookie	100	5	0	T	🌢
Entenmann's, soft baked, original recipe chocolate chip	3 cookies	150	7	0	T	🌢
Entenmann's, soft baked, white chocolate macadamia nut	1 cookie	100	6	0	T	🌢
Famous Amos	4 cookies	130	7	1	T	🌢
Famous Amos, & pecans	4 cookies	140	8	0	T	🌢
Famous Amos, chocolate chunk	1 cookie	80	4	0	T	🌢
Health Valley, fat free	3 cookies	100	0	3		✂
Keebler, Chips Deluxe	1 cookie	80	5	0	T	🌢
Keebler, Chips Deluxe, chocolate chewy	2 cookies	130	7	0	T	🌢
Keebler, Chips Deluxe, chocolate lovers	1 cookie	90	5	0	T	🌢
Keebler, Chips Deluxe, coconut	1 cookie	80	5	0	T	🌢
Keebler, Chips Deluxe, rainbow USA	1 cookie	80	4	0	T	🌢
Keebler, Chips Deluxe, soft'n chewy	1 cookie	80	4	0	T	🌢
Keebler, Chips Deluxe, w/peanut butter	1 cookie	80	5	0	T	🌢
Keebler, Cookie Stix, chocolate chip	4 cookies	130	5	0	T	🌢
Keebler, Soft Batch, original	1 cookie	80	4	0	T	🌢
Nabisco, Chips Ahoy!	3 cookies	160	8	1	T	🌢

☺ = Eat as much as you want • ✂ = Cut Back

	Portion	Calories	Total Fat	Dietary Fiber	Trans Fat	Guide
Nabisco, Chips Ahoy!, chewy	3 cookies	170	8	0	T	🌢
Nabisco, Chips Ahoy!, chunky	1 cookie	80	4	0	T	🌢
Nabisco, Chips Ahoy!, munch size	6 cookies	160	8	1	T	🌢
Nabisco, Chips Ahoy!, reduced fat	3 cookies	140	5	0	T	🌢
Nabisco, Chips Ahoy!, star spangled	3 cookies	150	7	0	T	🌢
Pepperidge Farm, chocolate chunk, Chesapeake, pecan	1 cookie	140	8	0	T	🌢
Pepperidge Farm, chocolate chunk, Montauk, milk chocolate chunk	1 cookie	130	7	0	T	🌢
Pepperidge Farm, chocolate chunk, Nantucket	1 cookie	140	7	0	T	🌢
Pepperidge Farm, chocolate chunk, Sausalito, milk chocolate macadamia	1 cookie	140	8	0	T	🌢
Pepperidge Farm, chocolate chunk, Tahoe, white chocolate macadamia	1 cookie	140	8	0	T	🌢
Pepperidge Farm, chocolate chunk, soft baked, reduced fat	1 cookie	110	5	0	T	🌢
Pepperidge Farm, old fashioned	3 cookies	140	7	0	T	🌢
Pepperidge Farm, soft baked, chocolate chunk	1 cookie	130	6	0	T	🌢
Pepperidge Farm, soft baked, chocolate chunk, classic	1 cookie	110	5	0	T	🌢
Rippin' Good	3 cookies	150	7	0	T	🌢
Rippin' Good, chocolate chip thins	10 cookies	110	5	1	T	🌢
SnackWell's	13 cookies	130	4	1	T	🌢
SnackWell's, double chocolate chip	13 cookies	130	4	1	T	🌢

Cookies, Cookie Mix

	Portion	Calories	Total Fat	Dietary Fiber	Trans Fat	Guide
Betty Crocker, chocolate chip	2 cookies	120	3	0	T	🌢
Betty Crocker, double chocolate chunk	2 cookies	150	6	0	T	🌢
Betty Crocker, oatmeal chocolate chip	2 cookies	120	3	0	T	🌢
Betty Crocker, peanut butter	2 cookies	160	8	0	T	🌢
Betty Crocker, sugar	2 cookies	170	8	0	T	🌢
Duncan Hines, chocolate chip	1 cookie	170	8	0	T	🌢
Duncan Hines, golden sugar	$1/_{24}$ pouch	110	3	0	T	🌢

Cookies, Fruit

	Portion	Calories	Total Fat	Dietary Fiber	Trans Fat	Guide
Archway, frosty lemon	1 cookie	110	5	0	T	🌢
Archway, lemon nuggets, fat free	4 cookies	110	0	0		✂
Health Valley, fat free, apple spice	3 cookies	100	0	3		✂
Health Valley, fat free, apricot delight	3 cookies	100	0	3		✂
Health Valley, fat free, date delight	3 cookies	100	0	3		✂
Health Valley, fat free, raisin oatmeal	3 cookies	100	0	3		✂
Nabisco, Fig Newtons	2 cookies	110	3	1	T	🌢
Nabisco, Newtons fat free cobbler, apple cinnamon	1 cookie	70	0	0		✂
Nabisco, Newtons fat free cobbler, peach apricot	1 cookie	70	0	0		✂
Nabisco, Newtons fat free, apple	2 cookies	100	0	0		✂
Nabisco, Newtons fat free, cranberry	2 cookies	100	0	0		✂
Nabisco, Newtons fat free, fig	2 cookies	100	0	2		✂

🌢 = Avoid • ♨ = Add for flavor

	Portion	Calories	Total Fat	Dietary Fiber	Trans Fat	Guide
Nabisco, Newtons fat free, raspberry	2 cookies	100	0	0		✂
Nabisco, Newtons fat free, strawberry	2 cookies	100	0	0		✂
Pepperidge Farm, Fruitful, apricot raspberry cup	3 cookies	140	6	0		💧
Pepperidge Farm, Fruitful, raspberry tart	2 cookies	120	3	0	T	💧
Pepperidge Farm, Fruitful, strawberry cup	3 cookies	140	5	0	T	💧
Pepperidge Farm, lemon nut crunch	3 cookies	170	9	2	T	💧
Rippin' Good, coconut bars	3 cookies	130	6	0	T	💧
Rippin' Good, lemon crisp	3 cookies	160	8	0	T	💧
Sunshine, golden fruit biscuits, cranberry	1 cookie	80	2	0	T	💧
Sunshine, golden fruit biscuits, raisin	1 cookie	80	2	0	T	💧
Sunshine, lemon coolers	5 cookies	140	6	0	T	💧

Cookies, Fudge

	Portion	Calories	Total Fat	Dietary Fiber	Trans Fat	Guide
Keebler, Fudge Shoppe, deluxe grahams	3 pieces	140	7	0	T	💧
Keebler, Fudge Shoppe, fudge sticks	3 pieces	150	8	0	T	💧
Keebler, Fudge Shoppe, fudge stripes	3 cookies	160	8	0	T	💧
Keebler, Fudge Shoppe, fudge stripes, reduced fat	3 cookies	130	5	0	T	
Keebler, Fudge Shoppe, grasshopper mint	4 cookies	150	7	0	T	💧
Nabisco, marshmallow twirls fudge	1 cookie	130	6	0	T	💧

Cookies, Ginger Snap

	Portion	Calories	Total Fat	Dietary Fiber	Trans Fat	Guide
Archway	5 cookies	150	5	0	T	💧
Nabisco, old fashioned	4 cookies	120	3	0	T	💧
Rippin' Good	5 cookies	130	4	0	T	💧
Sunshine	7 cookies	130	5	0	T	💧

Cookies, Oatmeal

	Portion	Calories	Total Fat	Dietary Fiber	Trans Fat	Guide
Archway	1 cookie	110	4	0	T	💧
Archway, apple filled	1 cookie	100	3	0	T	💧
Archway, date filled	1 cookie	100	3	0	T	💧
Archway, gourmet, Ruth's golden oatmeal	1 cookie	120	5	0	T	💧
Archway, iced	1 cookie	120	5	0	T	💧
Archway, raisin	1 cookie	110	4	0	T	💧
Archway, raisin, fat free	1 cookie	110	0	0		✂
Entenmann's, light, oatmeal raisin soft baked	2 cookies	100	0	1		✂
Famous Amos, oatmeal raisin	4 cookies	130	5	1	T	💧
Health Valley, raisin, fat free	3 cookies	100	0	3		✂
Nabisco	1 cookie	80	3	0	T	💧
Pepperidge Farm, soft baked, classic, raisin	1 cookie	100	3	0	T	💧
Rippin' Good	3 cookies	150	6	0	T	💧
Sunshine, w/raisins	2 cookies	120	5	0	T	💧

Cookies, Other

	Portion	Calories	Total Fat	Dietary Fiber	Trans Fat	Guide
Archway, Dutch cocoa	1 cookie	100	3	0	T	💧
Archway, cinnamon honey hearts, fat free	3 cookies	110	0	0		✂
Archway, gourmet, rocky road	1 cookie	130	6	0	T	💧
Archway, old fashioned molasses	1 cookie	100	3	0	T	💧
Fortune cookies	4 cookies	110	0	1		✂

☺ = Eat as much as you want • ✂ = Cut Back

	Portion	Calories	Total Fat	Dietary Fiber	Trans Fat	Guide
Pepperidge Farm, Bordeaux	4 cookies	130	5	0	T	🌢
Pepperidge Farm, Brussels	3 cookies	150	7	1	T	🌢
Pepperidge Farm, Geneva	3 cookies	160	9	1	T	🌢
Pepperidge Farm, Lido	1 cookie	90	5	0	T	🌢
Pepperidge Farm, Milano	3 cookies	180	10	0	T	🌢
Pepperidge Farm, Milano, double chocolate	2 cookies	140	8	0	T	🌢
Pepperidge Farm, Milano, endless chocolate	3 cookies	180	10	1	T	🌢
Pepperidge Farm, Milano, milk chocolate	3 cookies	170	9	0	T	🌢
Pepperidge Farm, Milano, mint	2 cookies	130	7	0	T	🌢
Pepperidge Farm, Milano, orange	2 cookies	130	7	0	T	🌢
Pepperidge Farm, old fashioned, ginger man	4 cookies	130	4	0	T	🌢
Rippin' Good, Rippie cremes chocolate	3 cookies	160	6	1	T	🌢
Rippin' Good, striped dainties	3 cookies	150	7	0	T	🌢
Rippin' Good, toffee 'n creme	2 cookies	150	7	0	T	🌢
SnackWell's, caramel delights	1 cookie	70	2	0	T	🌢
SnackWell's, devil's, fat free	1 cookie	50	0	0		✂
SnackWell's, golden devil's food	1 cookie	50	1	0	T	🌢
SnackWell's, mint creme	2 cookies	110	4	0	T	🌢

Cookies, Peanut Butter

	Portion	Calories	Total Fat	Dietary Fiber	Trans Fat	Guide
Nabisco, Nutter Butter	2 cookies	130	6	0	T	🌢
Nabisco, Nutter Butter bite	10 cookies	150	6	1	T	🌢
Nabisco, Nutter Butter, chocolate	2 cookies	130	5	0	T	🌢
Nabisco, Nutter Butter, peanut creme patties	5 patties	160	9	0	T	🌢
SnackWell's, peanut butter chip	13 cookies	120	4	0	T	🌢

Cookies, Refrigerated Dough

	Portion	Calories	Total Fat	Dietary Fiber	Trans Fat	Guide
Nestlé, Toll House, chocolate chip	2 tbsp.	140	6	0	T	🌢
Pillsbury, chocolate chip	1 oz.	130	6	0	T	🌢
Pillsbury, chocolate chip w/walnuts	1 oz.	140	7	0	T	🌢
Pillsbury, chocolate chip, reduced fat	1 oz.	110	3	0	T	🌢
Pillsbury, double chocolate chip & chunk	1 oz.	130	6	0	T	🌢
Pillsbury, one step cookie, chocolate chip	1/8 pkg.	130	6	0	T	🌢
Pillsbury, sugar	2 cookies	130	5	0	T	🌢
Pillsbury, w/M & M's	1 oz.	130	6	0	T	🌢

Cookies, Sandwich

	Portion	Calories	Total Fat	Dietary Fiber	Trans Fat	Guide
Famous Amos, chocolate	3 cookies	150	7	1	T	🌢
Famous Amos, oatmeal macaroon	3 cookies	160	7	1	T	🌢
Famous Amos, vanilla	3 cookies	160	7	1	T	🌢
Keebler, Classic Collection, French vanilla creme	1 cookie	80	4	0	T	🌢
Keebler, Classic Collection, chocolate fudge creme	1 cookie	80	4	0	T	🌢
Keebler, E.L. Fudge, butter flavor	2 cookies	120	6	0	T	🌢
Keebler, E.L. Fudge, fudge	2 cookies	120	6	0	T	🌢
Nabisco, Oreo	3 cookies	160	7	1	T	🌢
Nabisco, Oreo, Double Stuf	2 cookies	140	7	0	T	🌢
Nabisco, Oreo, reduced fat	3 cookies	130	4	1	T	🌢
Nabisco, cameo creme	2 cookies	130	5	0	T	🌢

🌢 = Avoid • 🌢 = Add for flavor

	Portion	Calories	Total Fat	Dietary Fiber	Trans Fat	Guide
Nabisco, vanilla	3 cookies	160	5	0	T	🌢
Rippin' Good, chocolate chip	2 cookies	150	7	0	T	🌢
Rippin' Good, macaroon	2 cookies	150	7	0	T	🌢
Rippin' Good, peanut butter	2 cookies	150	6	1	T	🌢
Rippin' Good, vanilla	3 cookies	160	6	0	T	🌢
SnackWell's, chocolate	2 cookies	100	3	0	T	🌢
SnackWell's, creme	2 cookies	110	3	0	T	🌢
Sunshine, Hydrox	3 cookies	150	7	1	T	🌢
Sunshine, Vienna fingers	2 cookies	130	5	0	T	🌢
Sunshine, Vienna fingers, reduced fat	2 cookies	130	5	0	T	🌢

Cookies, Shortbread

	Portion	Calories	Total Fat	Dietary Fiber	Trans Fat	Guide
Keebler, Sandies, pecan	1 cookie	80	5	0	T	🌢
Nabisco, Lorna Doone	4 cookies	140	7	0	T	🌢
Nabisco, Sandies	1 cookie	80	5	0	T	🌢
Nabisco, Sandies, pecan, reduced fat	1 cookie	80	3	0	T	🌢
Pepperidge Farm	2 cookies	140	7	0	T	🌢
Rippin' Good	4 cookies	140	6	0	T	🌢

Cookies, Sugar

	Portion	Calories	Total Fat	Dietary Fiber	Trans Fat	Guide
Keebler, Cookie Stix, rainbow sugar	5 cookies	150	6	0	T	🌢
Pepperidge Farm	3 cookies	140	6	0	T	🌢
Rippin' Good	3 cookies	150	6	0	T	🌢

Cookies, Wafer

	Portion	Calories	Total Fat	Dietary Fiber	Trans Fat	Guide
Keebler, golden vanilla	8 cookies	150	7	0	T	🌢
Keebler, golden vanilla, reduced fat	8 cookies	130	4	0	T	🌢
Nabisco, Famous Chocolate	5 cookies	140	4	1	T	🌢
Nabisco, Nilla Wafers	8 wafers	140	5	0	T	🌢
Nabisco, Nilla Wafers, chocolate, reduced fat	8 wafers	110	2	0	T	🌢
Nabisco, Nilla Wafers, reduced fat	8 wafers	120	2	0	T	🌢
Sunshine, cream filled sugar	3 wafers	130	6	0	T	🌢
Sunshine, peanut butter sugar	4 wafers	170	9	1	T	🌢
Sunshine, vanilla	7 cookies	150	7	0	T	🌢

Crackers, Animal Cracker

	Portion	Calories	Total Fat	Dietary Fiber	Trans Fat	Guide
Austin, zoo animal	15 crackers	120	2	0	T	🌢
Austin, zoo animal, chocolate	13 crackers	100	2	0	T	🌢
Barnum's	12 crackers	140	4	1	T	🌢
Keebler, animal, chocolatey chip	7 cookies	130	5	0	T	🌢
Keebler, animal, sprinkled	6 cookies	150	5	0	T	🌢

Crackers, Cheese

	Portion	Calories	Total Fat	Dietary Fiber	Trans Fat	Guide
Austin, cheese on cheese	6 crackers	200	11	0	T	🌢
Austin, cheese peanut butter	6 crackers	200	11	1	T	🌢
Austin, cream cheese & chives	6 crackers	190	10	0	T	🌢
Chee-tos, cheesy cheese sandwich	1 pkg.	210	11	1	T	🌢
Doritos, nacho cheesier sandwich	1 pkg.	240	14	1	T	🌢

☺ = Eat as much as you want • ✂ = Cut Back

FOOD LISTS

	Portion	Calories	Total Fat	Dietary Fiber	Trans Fat	Guide
Frito Lay, peter pan cheese peanut butter sandwich	1 pkg.	210	10	1	T	🌢
Keebler, Munch'ems, cheddar	41 crackers	130	5	1	T	🌢
Kraft, Handi-Snacks, cheez'n breadsticks	1 unit	120	6	0	T	🌢
Kraft, Handi-Snacks, cheez'n crackers	1 unit	110	7	0	T	🌢
Kraft, Handi-Snacks, cheez'n pretzels	1 unit	100	5	0	T	🌢
Kraft, Handi-Snacks, nacho stix'n cheez	1 unit	110	6	0	T	🌢
Little Debbie, cheese on cheese	4 crackers	140	8	0	T	🌢
Little Debbie, cheese w/peanut butter	4 crackers	140	8	0	T	🌢
Little Debbie, crispy w/cream cheese & chives	4 crackers	140	7	0	T	🌢
Nabisco, Better Cheddars	22 crackers	150	8	0	T	🌢
Nabisco, Cheese Nips	29 crackers	150	6	0	T	🌢
Nabisco, Cheese Nips, reduced fat	31 crackers	130	4	0	T	🌢
Pepperidge Farm, Goldfish, cheddar cheese	55 pieces	140	6	0	T	🌢
Pepperidge Farm, Goldfish, parmesan cheese	60 pieces	140	5	1	T	🌢
Pepperidge Farm, Goldfish, reduced sodium cheddar	60 pieces	150	6	0	T	🌢
Pepperidge Farm, Snack Sticks, three cheese	8 sticks	140	6	0	T	🌢
Sargento, Mootown Snacks, cheeze & cheddar sticks	1 unit	100	6	0	T	🌢
Sargento, Mootown Snacks, cheeze & pretzels	1 unit	90	4	0	T	🌢
Sargento, Mootown Snacks, cheeze & sticks	1 unit	110	6	0	T	🌢
SnackWell's, Zesty Cheese, reduced fat	32 crackers	120	2	1	T	🌢
Sunshine, Cheez-it	27 crackers	160	8	0	T	🌢
Sunshine, Cheez-it, head & tails	37 crackers	140	6	1	T	🌢
Sunshine, Cheez-it, hot & spicy	26 crackers	160	8	1	T	🌢
Sunshine, Cheez-it, nacho	28 crackers	150	7	0	T	🌢
Sunshine, Cheez-it, reduced fat	29 crackers	140	5	0	T	🌢
Sunshine, Cheez-it, white cheddar	26 crackers	150	7	0	T	🌢
Sunshine, Krispy, mild cheddar	5 crackers	60	2	0	T	🌢

Crackers, Crisps

	Portion	Calories	Total Fat	Dietary Fiber	Trans Fat	Guide
Chatham Village, cinnamon & raisin bread crisps	3 crisps	70	3	0		🌢
Chatham Village, garlic & butter bread crisps	3 crisps	70	3	0		🌢
Nabisco, Air Crisps, cheese nips	32 crackers	130	4	0	T	🌢
Nabisco, Air Crisps, pretzel	23 crisps	110	0	0		✂
Nabisco, Air Crisps, ritz	24 crackers	140	5	0	T	🌢
Nabisco, Air Crisps, ritz, sour cream & onion	23 crackers	140	5	0	T	🌢
Nabisco, Air Crisps, wheat thins	23 pieces	140	5	1	T	🌢
Nabisco, Flavor Crisps, chicken in a basket	12 crackers	160	9	0	T	🌢
Nabisco, Flavor Crisps, sociables	7 crackers	80	4	0	T	🌢
Nabisco, Flavor Crisps, vegetable thins	14 crackers	160	9	1	T	🌢
Nabisco, Potato Air Crisps, barbecue	22 crisps	120	4	1	T	🌢
Nabisco, Potato Air Crisps, original	22 crisps	120	4	1	T	🌢
Nabisco, Sweet Crispers, caramel	18 crisps	140	3	0	T	🌢
Nabisco, Sweet Crispers, chocolate	18 crisps	130	3	1	T	🌢
Nabisco, Sweet Crispers, cinnamon	18 crisps	130	3	0	T	🌢
Nabisco, Sweet Crispers, honey	18 crisps	130	3	0	T	🌢
Nabisco, Triscuit, thin crisps, French onion	14 crackers	130	5	3	T	🌢

🌢 = Avoid • 💧 = Add for flavor

	Portion	Calories	Total Fat	Dietary Fiber	Trans Fat	Guide
Seasoned rye krisp	2 crackers	60	2	3	T	🌢

Crackers, Graham

	Portion	Calories	Total Fat	Dietary Fiber	Trans Fat	Guide
Keebler, Grahams, chocolate	8 crackers	130	4	0	T	🌢
Keebler, Grahams, cinnamon crisp	8 crackers	130	3	1	T	🌢
Keebler, Grahams, cinnamon crisp, low fat	8 crackers	110	2	0	T	🌢
Keebler, Grahams, honey	8 crackers	140	5	0	T	🌢
Keebler, Grahams, honey, low fat	9 crackers	120	2	1	T	🌢
Keebler, Snackin' Grahams, cinnamon, bite size	21 crackers	130	3	1	T	🌢
Keebler, Snackin' Grahams, honey, bite size	23 crackers	130	4	0	T	🌢
Nabisco, Grahams	4 crackers	120	3	1	T	🌢
Nabisco, Honey Maid, chocolate	8 crackers	120	3	1	T	🌢
Nabisco, Honey Maid, cinnamon	8 crackers	120	3	0	T	🌢
Nabisco, Honey Maid, cinnamon, low fat	8 crackers	110	2	0	T	🌢
Nabisco, Honey Maid, honey grahams	8 crackers	120	3	1	T	🌢
Nabisco, Honey Maid, honey grahams, low fat	8 crackers	110	2	0	T	🌢
Nabisco, Honey Maid, oatmeal crunch	8 crackers	120	3	1	T	🌢
Nabisco, Teddy Grahams, chocolate	24 pieces	140	5	1	T	🌢
Nabisco, Teddy Grahams, cinnamon	24 pieces	140	5	1	T	🌢
Nabisco, Teddy Grahams, dizzy grizzlies, chocolate frost	8 cookies	150	5	0	T	🌢
Nabisco, Teddy Grahams, dizzy grizzlies, vanilla frost	8 cookies	150	6	0	T	🌢
Nabisco, Teddy Grahams, honey	24 pieces	140	4	0	T	🌢
SnackWell's, cinnamon, fat free	20 pieces	120	0	1		✂

Crackers, Melba

	Portion	Calories	Total Fat	Dietary Fiber	Trans Fat	Guide
Devonsheer, garlic rounds	5 pieces	60	2	1		✂
Devonsheer, plain rounds	5 pieces	50	0	1		✂
Devonsheer, plain toast	3 pieces	50	0	1		✂
Devonsheer, sesame rounds	5 pieces	50	3	1		✂
Devonsheer, wheat toast	3 pieces	50	0	1		✂

Crackers, Other

	Portion	Calories	Total Fat	Dietary Fiber	Trans Fat	Guide
Austin, toasty peanut butter	4 crackers	140	7	0	T	🌢
Keebler, Club, original	4 crackers	70	3	0	T	🌢
Keebler, Club, reduced sodium	4 crackers	70	3	0	T	🌢
Keebler, Munch'ems, mesquite BBQ	41 crackers	140	5	1	T	🌢
Keebler, Toasteds, buttercrisp	5 crackers	80	4	0	T	🌢
Keebler, Toasteds, medley	5 crackers	80	4	0	T	🌢
Keebler, Townhouse	5 crackers	80	5	0	T	🌢
Little Debbie, toasty w/peanut butter	4 crackers	140	7	0	T	🌢
Nabisco, Premium, soup & oyster	23 crackers	60	2	0	T	🌢
Nabisco, Ritz	5 crackers	80	4	0	T	🌢
Nabisco, Ritz, bits sandwiches	14 sandwiches	150	8	1	T	🌢
Nabisco, Ritz, low sodium	5 crackers	80	4	0	T	🌢
Nabisco, Ritz, reduced fat	5 crackers	70	2	0	T	🌢
Nabisco, Uneeda Biscuit	2 crackers	60	2	0	T	🌢

☺ = Eat as much as you want • ✂ = Cut Back

	Portion	Calories	Total Fat	Dietary Fiber	Trans Fat	Guide
Nabisco, Waverly	5 crackers	70	4	0	T	🌢
Pepperidge Farm, Goldfish, original	55 pieces	140	6	0	T	🌢
Pepperidge Farm, Goldfish, pizza	55 pieces	140	6	1	T	🌢
Pepperidge Farm, Goldfish, pretzel	43 pieces	120	3	0	T	🌢
Pepperidge Farm, Quartet	4 crackers	70	3	0	T	🌢
Pepperidge Farm, Snack Sticks, pretzel	12 sticks	120	0	1		✂
Pepperidge Farm, Snack Sticks, sesame	8 sticks	130	5	1	T	🌢
Pepperidge Farm, butter flavored thins	4 crackers	70	3	0	T	🌢
Pepperidge Farm, three cracker assortment	4 crackers	70	3	1	T	🌢
Sargento, Mootown Snacks, chocolate chip & creme	1 unit	140	7	0	T	🌢
Sargento, Mootown Snacks, s'mores	1 unit	110	5	0	T	🌢
SnackWell's, classic golden, reduced fat	6 crackers	60	1	0	T	🌢
SnackWell's, cracked pepper	5 crackers	60	2	0	T	🌢
SnackWell's, ranch	38 crackers	130	3	0	T	🌢
SnackWell's, salsa	38 crackers	130	3	0	T	🌢
Sunshine, Hi-Ho	4 crackers	70	4	0	T	🌢

Crackers, Saltine

	Portion	Calories	Total Fat	Dietary Fiber	Trans Fat	Guide
Keebler, Zesta, original	5 crackers	60	2	0	T	🌢
Nabisco, Premium Saltine, fat free	5 crackers	60	0	0		✂
Nabisco, Premium Saltine, low sodium	5 crackers	60	2	0	T	🌢
Nabisco, Premium Saltine, multi grain	5 crackers	60	2	0	T	🌢
Nabisco, Premium Saltine, original	5 crackers	60	2	0	T	🌢
Nabisco, Premium Saltine, unsalted tops	5 crackers	60	2	0	T	🌢
Sunshine, Krispy, fat free	5 crackers	50	0	0		✂
Sunshine, Krispy, original	5 crackers	60	2	0	T	🌢
Sunshine, Krispy, unsalted tops	5 crackers	60	2	0	T	🌢

Crackers, Snack Mix

	Portion	Calories	Total Fat	Dietary Fiber	Trans Fat	Guide
Nabisco, Doo Dads, original	1/2 cup	150	7	2	T	🌢
Nabisco, Ritz, cheddar	1/2 cup	150	7	1	T	🌢
Nabisco, Ritz, traditional	1/2 cup	150	7	1	T	🌢
Pepperidge Farm, w/Goldfish	1/2 cup	150	7	2	T	🌢
Sunshine, Cheez-it, party mix	1/2 cup	140	5	1	T	🌢
Sunshine, Cheez-it, party mix, nacho	1/2 cup	130	5	1	T	🌢
Sunshine, Cheez-it, party mix, reduced fat	1/2 cup	130	3	1	T	🌢

Crackers, Vegetable

	Portion	Calories	Total Fat	Dietary Fiber	Trans Fat	Guide
Health Valley, onion, fat free	6 crackers	50	0	2		✂
Health Valley, vegetable, fat free	6 crackers	50	0	2		✂
SnackWell's, French onion, reduced fat	32 crackers	120	2	0	T	🌢

Crackers, Wheat/Grain

	Portion	Calories	Total Fat	Dietary Fiber	Trans Fat	Guide
Health Valley, whole wheat, fat free	6 crackers	50	0	2		✂
Keebler, Wheatables, garden vegetable	25 crackers	140	7	3	T	🌢
Keebler, Wheatables, ranch	29 crackers	130	4	1	T	🌢
Keebler, Wheatables, savory original	29 crackers	130	4	1	T	🌢
Keebler, Wheatables, white cheddar	27 crackers	130	4	0	T	🌢

🌢 = Avoid • 🌢 = Add for flavor

	Portion	Calories	Total Fat	Dietary Fiber	Trans Fat	Guide
Nabisco, Harvest Crisps, 5-grain	7 crackers	130	4	1	T	🍶
Nabisco, Harvest Crisps, Italian herb	13 crackers	130	4	1	T	🍶
Nabisco, Harvest Crisps, garden vegetable	15 crackers	130	4	1	T	🍶
Nabisco, Ritz, whole wheat	5 crackers	70	3	0	T	🍶
Nabisco, Triscuit, garden herb	6 wafers	130	5	3	T	🍶
Nabisco, Triscuit, low sodium	7 wafers	140	5	4	T	🍶
Nabisco, Triscuit, original	7 wafers	140	5	4	T	🍶
Nabisco, Triscuit, reduced fat	8 wafers	130	3	4	T	🍶
Nabisco, Wheat Thins	16 crackers	140	6	2	T	🍶
Nabisco, Wheat Thins, low sodium	16 crackers	140	6	2	T	🍶
Nabisco, Wheat Thins, multi-grain	17 crackers	130	4	2	T	🍶
Nabisco, Wheat Thins, reduced fat	18 crackers	120	4	2	T	🍶
Nabisco, Wheatsworth	5 crackers	80	4	1	T	🍶
Pepperidge Farm, Hearty wheat	3 crackers	80	4	1	T	🍶
SnackWell's, wheat	5 crackers	70	2	0	T	🍶

Diet/Supplement/Sport Bars

	Portion	Calories	Total Fat	Dietary Fiber	Trans Fat	Guide
Boost, chocolate crunch	1 bar	190	6	1		🍶
Boost, strawberries & cream	1 bar	190	6	1		🍶
Diet Fat Burner, chocolate coconut	1 bar	130	3	0		🍶
Ensure, chocolate fudge brownie bar	1 bar	130	3	2	T	🍶
Ensure, honey graham crunch bar	1 bar	130	3	2	T	🍶
PowerBar, chocolate	1 bar	230	2	3		✂
PowerBar, harvest, strawberry	1 bar	240	4	4		🍶
PowerBar, oatmeal raisin	1 bar	230	3	3		🍶
PowerBar, peanut butter	1 bar	230	3	3		🍶
Slim-Fast, Dutch chocolate	1 bar	140	5	2	T	🍶
Slim-Fast, Ultra, chewy caramel	1 bar	110	4	2	T	🍶
Slim-Fast, Ultra, peanut butter	1 bar	120	4	2	T	🍶
Slim-Fast, Ultra, peanut caramel	1 bar	120	4	1	T	🍶

Fruit Snacks

	Portion	Calories	Total Fat	Dietary Fiber	Trans Fat	Guide
Banana chips	1/3 cup	140	7	1		🍶
Betty Crocker, Bugs Bunny, snacks made w/fruit	1 pouch	80	0	0		✂
Betty Crocker, Fruit Gushers	1 pouch	90	1	0		✂
Betty Crocker, Fruit Roll Ups, hot colors	2 rolls	110	1	0	T	🍶
Betty Crocker, Fruit Roll Ups, peel'n build	2 rolls	110	1	0	T	🍶
Betty Crocker, Fruit Roll Ups, strawberry	2 rolls	110	1	0	T	🍶
Betty Crocker, Fruit String Thing, strawberry	1 pouch	80	1	0	T	🍶
Betty Crocker, Fruit by the Foot, strawberry	1 roll	80	2	0		✂
Branch's, Chiquita fruit snacks	1 pouch	90	0	0		✂
Branch's, Fruity O's, fruit snacks	1 pouch	90	0	0		✂
Chiquita, banana flavors	1 pouch	90	0	0		✂
Farley's, Dinosaurs	1 pouch	80	0	0		✂
Farley's, Mega Monster Roll	1 pouch	110	3	2	T	🍶
Farley's, Rugrats, fruit roll	1 pouch	70	2	1	T	🍶
Farley's, Zoo Animals	1 pouch	80	0	0		✂
Trix, snacks made w/real fruit	1 pouch	80	0	0		✂
Yogurt raisins	3 tbsp.	170	5	1	T	🍶

☺ = Eat as much as you want • ✂ = Cut Back

	Portion	Calories	Total Fat	Dietary Fiber	Trans Fat	Guide
Nuts & Seeds, Nuts						
Almond	3 tbsp.	190	16	4		🌢
Almond, roasted	28 g.	160	15	4		🌢
Almond, sliced	57 g.	359	29	7		🌢
Almond, slivered	57 g.	359	29	7		🌢
Barcelona Nuts, mixed nuts	¹/₄ cup	210	17	2		🌢
Beer nuts, classic peanut	1 oz.	170	14	2		🌢
Blue Diamond, almonds	3 tbsp.	180	16	2		🌢
Brazil nut	¹/₄ cup	200	20	2		🌢
Cashew, whole, raw	28 g.	160	13	1		🌢
Corn Nuts, barbecue flavor	¹/₃ cup	130	4	2	T	🌢
Corn Nuts, original flavor	¹/₃ cup	130	4	2	T	🌢
Corn Nuts, roasted salted	¹/₃ cup	130	4	2		🌢
MacFarms of Hawaii, milk chocolate macadamia nuts	¹/₄ cup	210	16	2		🌢
Mauna Loa, macadamia	1 oz.	220	22	2		🌢
Pecan, halves	¹/₃ cup	230	23	2		🌢
Pine nut	¹/₄ cup	190	15	4		🌢
Pistachio	1 oz.	170	14	3		🌢
Planters, P.B. Crisps	12 pieces	150	8	1	T	🌢
Planters, cashews, honey roasted	2 oz.	310	24	3		🌢
Planters, cashews, salted	2 oz.	340	29	3		🌢
Planters, mixed nuts	1 oz.	170	15	3		🌢
Planters, nut topping	2 tbsp.	100	9	1		🌢
Planters, nuts, deluxe mixed	1 oz.	170	16	2		🌢
Planters, nuts, mixed	1 oz.	170	15	2		🌢
Planters, nuts, mixed lightly salted	1 oz.	170	15	3		🌢
Planters, peanuts, cocktail	1 oz.	170	14	2		🌢
Planters, peanuts, cocktail lightly sltd	1 oz.	170	15	2		🌢
Planters, peanuts, dry roasted	1 oz.	160	13	2		🌢
Planters, peanuts, dry roasted unsalted	1 oz.	160	14	2		🌢
Planters, peanuts, honey roasted	1 oz.	150	12	2		🌢
Planters, peanuts, honey roasted, reduced fat	¹/₃ cup	130	7	2		🌢
Planters, peanuts, redskin Spanish	1 oz.	170	14	2		🌢
Planters, peanuts, salted	1 oz.	170	15	2		🌢
Walnuts	¹/₄ cup	210	20	3		🌢
Nuts & Seeds, Nuts, Peanut Butter						
Crazy Richard's, chunky	2 tbsp.	190	16	2		🌢
Crazy Richard's, creamy	2 tbsp.	190	16	2		🌢
Jif, creamy	2 tbsp.	190	16	2	T	🌢
Jif, creamy, reduced fat	2 tbsp.	190	12	2	T	🌢
Jif, crunchy, extra	2 tbsp.	190	16	2	T	🌢
Milky Way, chocolate & hazel nut spread	2 tbsp.	170	10	0	T	🌢
Nutella, hazel nut spread w/skim milk & cocoa	2 tbsp.	160	9	0	T	🌢
Peter Pan, creamy	2 tbsp.	190	16	2	T	🌢
Peter Pan, creamy, low sodium	2 tbsp.	200	18	2	T	🌢
Peter Pan, creamy, plus 8	2 tbsp.	190	16	2	T	🌢
Peter Pan, creamy, reduced fat	2 tbsp.	180	11	2	T	🌢

🌢 = *Avoid* • 💧 = *Add for flavor*

	Portion	Calories	Total Fat	Dietary Fiber	Trans Fat	Guide
Peter Pan, crunchy	2 tbsp.	190	16	2	T	🌢
Peter Pan, crunchy, reduced fat	2 tbsp.	190	12	2	T	🌢
Reese's, creamy	2 tbsp.	200	16	2	T	🌢
Skippy, creamy	2 tbsp.	190	16	2	T	🌢
Skippy, creamy, reduced fat	2 tbsp.	190	12	2	T	🌢
Skippy, creamy, roasted honey nut	2 tbsp.	190	17	2	T	🌢
Skippy, super chunk	2 tbsp.	190	17	2	T	🌢
Skippy, super chunk, reduced fat	2 tbsp.	190	12	2	T	🌢
Skippy, super chunk, roasted honey nut	2 tbsp.	190	17	2	T	🌢
Smucker's, Goober Grape, stripes	3 tbsp.	230	13	2		🌢
Smucker's, creamy	2 tbsp.	200	16	2		🌢
Smucker's, creamy, reduced fat	2 tbsp.	200	12	2		🌢

Nuts & Seeds, Seeds

	Portion	Calories	Total Fat	Dietary Fiber	Trans Fat	Guide
Flax seed, golden	28 g.	140	10	6		🌢
Planters, sunflower kernels	1/4 cup	200	17	4		🌢
Poppy seed	1/4 cup	180	15	2		🌢
Pumpkin seed, roasted in shell	1 oz.	148	12	2		🌢
Sunflower seed, BBQ flavor	1/4 cup	190	15	2	T	🌢
Sunflower seed, raw, hulled	1/4 cup	210	20	5		🌢

Popcorn, Candied

	Portion	Calories	Total Fat	Dietary Fiber	Trans Fat	Guide
Cracker Jack	1 box	150	3	1		🌢
Cracker Jack, fat free, original	3/4 cup	110	0	0		✂
Crunch'n Munch, almond supreme	1/2 cup	140	4	1	T	🌢
Crunch'n Munch, buttery toffee w/peanuts	2/3 cup	140	4	0	T	🌢
Crunch'n Munch, toffee, fat free	3/4 cup	110	0	0		✂
Planters, Fiddle Faddle	3/4 cup	140	6	1		🌢
Planters, Fiddle Faddle, fat free	1 cup	110	0	1		✂

Popcorn, Kernels

	Portion	Calories	Total Fat	Dietary Fiber	Trans Fat	Guide
Orville Redenbacher's, hot air	2 tbsp.	90	2	5		☺
Orville Redenbacher's, original	2 tbsp.	90	2	5		☺
Popping kernels, white	1/4 cup dry	110	1	5		☺
Popping kernels, yellow	2 tbsp.	110	1	5		☺

Popcorn, Microwave

	Portion	Calories	Total Fat	Dietary Fiber	Trans Fat	Guide
Betty Crocker, Pop-Secret, 94% fat free butter	3 tbsp.	120	2	4	T	🌢
Betty Crocker, Pop-Secret, 95% fat free	3 tbsp.	110	2	4	T	🌢
Betty Crocker, Pop-Secret, butter	3 tbsp.	180	12	3	T	🌢
Betty Crocker, Pop-Secret, butter light	1/4 cup	160	7	5	T	🌢
Betty Crocker, Pop-Secret, homestyle	3 tbsp.	170	12	3	T	🌢
Betty Crocker, Pop-Secret, jumbo pop butter	3 tbsp.	170	11	3	T	🌢
Betty Crocker, Pop-Secret, jumbo pop, movie theater butter	3 tbsp.	170	11	3	T	🌢
Betty Crocker, Pop-Secret, movie theater butter	3 tbsp.	180	13	3	T	🌢
Betty Crocker, Pop-Secret, movie theater butter, light	3 tbsp.	140	6	3	T	🌢
Healthy Choice, butter	3 tbsp.	120	3	5	T	🌢

☺ = Eat as much as you want • ✂ = Cut Back

	Portion	Calories	Total Fat	Dietary Fiber	Trans Fat	Guide
Jolly Time, Blast O Butter	2 tbsp.	150	11	10	T	💣
Jolly Time, Healthy Pop, butter 94% fat free	2 tbsp.	90	2	9	T	💣
Jolly Time, light	2 tbsp.	120	5	7	T	💣
Orville Redenbacher's, Double Feature, jumbo w/real butter	2 tbsp.	180	14	3	T	💣
Orville Redenbacher's, Reden-budders, movie theater butter	2 tbsp.	170	13	4	T	💣
Orville Redenbacher's, Reden-budders, movie theater butter, light	2 tbsp.	110	5	5	T	💣
Orville Redenbacher's, Reden-budders, white cheddar	2 tbsp.	170	13	3	T	💣
Orville Redenbacher's, Smart Pop, low fat butter	2 tbsp.	90	2	5	T	💣
Orville Redenbacher's, butter	2 tbsp.	170	12	4	T	💣
Orville Redenbacher's, butter light	2 tbsp.	120	6	5	T	💣
Orville Redenbacher's, butter unsalted	2 tbsp.	180	12	4	T	💣
Orville Redenbacher's, natural	2 tbsp.	160	11	4	T	💣
Orville Redenbacher's, natural light	2 tbsp.	120	5	5	T	💣
Weight Watchers, Smart Snackers	1 pkg.	100	1	7		☺

Popcorn, Ready to Eat

	Portion	Calories	Total Fat	Dietary Fiber	Trans Fat	Guide
Smartfood, white cheddar cheese	1 3/4 cups	160	10	1		💣
Smartfood, white cheddar, reduced fat	3 cups	140	6	3	T	💣
Utz, butter	2 cups	170	12	3		💣
Utz, cheese	2 cups	150	9	3	T	💣
Utz, white cheddar	2 cups	150	8	3	T	💣
Weight Watchers, Smart Snackers, butter flavored	1 pkg.	90	3	3	T	💣

Popcorn, Stove-top

	Portion	Calories	Total Fat	Dietary Fiber	Trans Fat	Guide
Jiffy Pop, butter	3 cups	140	7	3	T	💣
Jiffy Pop, natural	3 cups	140	7	3	T	💣

Rice/Corn Cakes

	Portion	Calories	Total Fat	Dietary Fiber	Trans Fat	Guide
Hain, mini, honey nut, fat free	6 cakes	60	0	0		✂
Hain, mini, peanut butter crunch	5 cakes	50	1	0		✂
Hain, mini, strawberry cheesecake	5 cakes	60	0	0		✂
Hain, mini, white cheddar, low fat	6 cakes	50	1	0		✂
Lundberg, brown rice	1 cake	70	0	0		✂
Orville Redenbacher's, caramel	1 cake	40	0	0	T	💣
Orville Redenbacher's, milk chocolate	1 cake	40	1	0		💣
Orville Redenbacher's, mini, butter popcorn	6 cakes	60	1	2	T	💣
Orville Redenbacher's, mini, caramel	6 cakes	60	0	1	T	💣
Orville Redenbacher's, mini, chocolate peanut butter crunch	6 cakes	60	1	1		✂
Orville Redenbacher's, mini, nacho	6 cakes	55	1	1	T	💣
Orville Redenbacher's, mini, peanut caramel crunch	6 cakes	60	1	1	T	💣
Orville Redenbacher's, mini, sour cream & onion	6 cakes	60	1	1		✂
Orville Redenbacher's, popcorn, low fat	1 cake	40	1	0		✂

💣 = Avoid • 🧈 = Add for flavor

	Portion	Calories	Total Fat	Dietary Fiber	Trans Fat	Guide
Quaker, apple cinnamon	1 cake	50	0	0		✂
Quaker, banana nut	1 cake	50	0	0		✂
Quaker, butter popped corn	1 cake	35	0	0		✂
Quaker, caramel chocolate chip	1 cake	60	1	0		✂
Quaker, caramel corn	1 cake	50	0	0		✂
Quaker, chocolate crunch	1 cake	60	1	0		✂
Quaker, mini, caramel corn	5 cakes	50	0	0		✂
Quaker, mini, white cheddar	6 cakes	50	0	0		✂
Quaker, monterey jack	1 cake	40	0	0		✂
Quaker, peanut butter	1 cake	60	1	0	T	💧
Quaker, salt free	1 cake	35	0	0		✂
Quaker, white cheddar	1 cake	40	0	0		✂

Snack Bars

	Portion	Calories	Total Fat	Dietary Fiber	Trans Fat	Guide
Golden Grahams Treats	1 bar	90	2	0	T	💧
Golden Grahams Treats, S'mores chocolate chunk	1 bar	90	3	0	T	💧
Golden Grahams Treats, chocolate chunk	1 bar	90	3	0	T	💧
Golden Grahams Treats, honey graham	1 bar	90	2	0	T	💧
Golden Grahams Treats, marshmallow graham w/mini marshmallows	1 bar	90	2	0	T	💧
Kellogg's, Rice Krispy treats	1 pkg.	90	2	0	T	💧
Kellogg's, Rice Krispy treats, chocolate chip	1 pkg.	90	3	0	T	💧
Nabisco, Chips Ahoy!	1 bar	150	5	0	T	💧
Nabisco, Oreo	1 bar	150	6	0	T	💧
Quaker, Cap'n Crunch's crunch berries treat	1 bar	90	2	0	T	💧
Quaker, Cap'n Crunch's peanut butter crunch treat	1 bar	90	3	0	T	💧
SnackWell's, banana	1 bar	130	2	0	T	💧
SnackWell's, chocolate cherry brownie bars	1 bar	130	2	1	T	💧
Tastykake, snack bars	1 bar	250	10	1	T	💧
Tastykake, snack bars, chocolate chip	1 bar	250	12	1	T	💧
Tastykake, snack bars, oatmeal raisin	1 bar	250	9	2	T	💧

Snack Bars, Fruit

	Portion	Calories	Total Fat	Dietary Fiber	Trans Fat	Guide
Health Valley, apple bakes, fat free	1 bar	70	0	3		✂
Health Valley, apple, fat free	1 bar	140	0	3		✂
Health Valley, date, fat free	1 bar	140	0	3		✂
Health Valley, raisin, fat free	1 bar	140	0	3		✂

Snack Bars, Granola

	Portion	Calories	Total Fat	Dietary Fiber	Trans Fat	Guide
Kudos, chocolate chip	1 bar	120	5	1	T	💧
Kudos, milk chocolate	1 bar	90	3	1	T	💧
Kudos, w/M & M's	1 bar	90	3	1	T	💧
Kudos, w/Snickers chunks	1 bar	100	4	0	T	💧
Nature Valley, crunchy granola, oats'n honey	2 bars	180	6	2		💧
Nature Valley, crunchy granola, peanut butter	2 bars	200	6	2		💧
Quaker, chewy granola bars, chocolate chip	1 bar	120	4	1	T	💧
Quaker, chewy granola bars, cookies and cream	1 bar	110	3	1	T	💧
Quaker, chewy granola bars, oatmeal cookie	1 bar	110	2	1	T	💧

☺ = *Eat as much as you want* • ✂ = *Cut Back*

	Portion	Calories	Total Fat	Dietary Fiber	Trans Fat	Guide
Quaker, chewy granola bars, peanut butter & chocolate	1 bar	120	3	1	T	💣
Quaker, chewy granola bars, s'mores	1 bar	110	2	1	T	💣
Quaker, fruit and yogurt chip	1 bar	110	2	0	T	💣
SnackWell's, fudge dipped, caramel	1 bar	120	3	1	T	💣
SnackWell's, fudge dipped, oatmeal raisin	1 bar	110	3	1	T	💣
SnackWell's, fudge dipped, original	1 bar	120	3	1	T	💣

■ SOUPS

Canned, Bean

	Portion	Calories	Total Fat	Dietary Fiber	Trans Fat	Guide
Campbell's, Chunky, hearty bean 'n' ham	1 cup	190	2	10		☺
Campbell's, Home Cookin', salsa bean	1 cup	160	1	7		☺
Campbell's, Home Cookin', savory lentil	1 cup	130	1	5		☺
Campbell's, bean w/bacon	1 cup	360	10	14		💣
Dominique's, US Senate bean	1 cup	170	2	9		☺
Goya, black bean	1 cup	210	3	10		☺
Health Valley, bean & carrots, fat free	1 cup	90	0	14		☺
Healthy Choice	1 cup	150	1	5		☺
Healthy Choice, bean & ham	1 cup	160	2	5		☺
Progresso	1 cup	140	2	7		☺
Progresso, 99% fat free	1 cup	130	2	6		☺
Progresso, hearty black bean	1 cup	170	2	10		☺

Canned, Beef

	Portion	Calories	Total Fat	Dietary Fiber	Trans Fat	Guide
Campbell's, Chunky, beef pasta	1 cup	150	3	2		💣
Campbell's, Chunky, pepper steak	1 cup	140	3	3		💣
Campbell's, Chunky, sirloin burger w/country vegetables	1 cup	180	7	4	T	💣
Campbell's, beef noodle	1 cup	140	6	2		💣
Campbell's, vegetable beef	1 cup	160	4	4		💣
Healthy Choice, beef & potato	1 cup	110	1	5		☺
Healthy Choice, vegetable beef	1 cup	100	1	2		✂

Canned, Broth

	Portion	Calories	Total Fat	Dietary Fiber	Trans Fat	Guide
Campbell's, beef	1 cup	30	1	0		✂
Campbell's, beef, consomme	1 cup	50	1	0		✂
Campbell's, chicken	1 cup	60	4	0		💣
College Inn, chicken, no fat	1 cup	10	0	0		👌
Health Valley, beef flavored broth	1 cup	20	0	0		✂
Health Valley, beef, fat free	1 cup	20	0	0		✂
Health Valley, chicken, fat free	1 cup	60	0	0		✂
Progresso, chicken	1 cup	20	2	0		✂
Swanson, beef	1 cup	20	1	0		✂
Swanson, vegetable	1 cup	20	1	0		✂
Weight Watchers, Smart Options, chicken flavor broth mix	1 pkt.	10	0	0		👌

💣 = Avoid • 👌 = Add for flavor

	Portion	Calories	Total Fat	Dietary Fiber	Trans Fat	Guide
Canned, Chicken						
Campbell's, Chunky, chicken broccoli cheese w/potato	1 cup	200	12	1		🌢
Campbell's, Chunky, chicken corn chowder	1 cup	250	15	3		🌢
Campbell's, Chunky, chicken mushroom chowder	1 cup	210	12	1		🌢
Campbell's, Chunky, hearty chicken w/vegetables	1 cup	90	2	2		✂
Campbell's, Chunky, spicy chicken & vegetables	1 cup	90	1	3		☺
Campbell's, Healthy Request, chicken rice	1 cup	120	6	0		🌢
Campbell's, Healthy Request, chicken vegetable	1 cup	160	4	2		🌢
Campbell's, Home Cookin', chicken vegetable	1 cup	130	4	3		🌢
Campbell's, chicken gumbo	1 cup	120	4	2		🌢
Campbell's, chicken vegetable	1 cup	160	4	4		🌢
Campbell's, chicken wonton	1 cup	90	2	2		✂
Healthy Choice, chicken alfredo	1 cup	120	2	0		✂
Healthy Choice, chicken corn chowder	1 cup	180	3	2		🌢
Healthy Choice, chicken pasta	1 cup	110	2	4		☺
Healthy Choice, chicken w/rice	1 cup	100	2	2		✂
Healthy Choice, hearty chicken	1 cup	130	3	3		🌢
Healthy Choice, zesty gumbo w/chicken & sausage	1 cup	90	2	3		☺
Progresso, chicken & wild rice	1 cup	100	2	1		✂
Progresso, chicken barley	1 cup	110	2	3		☺
Progresso, chicken rice, 99% fat free	1 cup	110	2	2		✂
Progresso, rotisserie seasoned chicken	1 cup	100	2	2		✂
Progresso, spicy chicken & penne	1 cup	110	2	1		✂
Canned, Chicken Noodle						
Campbell's	1 cup	140	4	2		🌢
Campbell's, Chunky, classic	1 cup	130	3	2		🌢
Campbell's, Healthy Request	1 cup	140	4	0		🌢
Campbell's, chicken & stars	1 cup	140	4	2		🌢
Campbell's, creamy chicken noodle	1 cup	260	14	4		🌢
Campbell's, double noodle in chicken broth	1 cup	200	6	4		🌢
Healthy Choice, old fashioned	1 cup	150	3	1		🌢
Progresso	1 cup	90	2	0		✂
Progresso, 99% fat free	1 cup	90	2	1		✂
Canned, Clam Chowder						
Campbell's, Home Cookin', New England	1 cup	120	3	1	T	🌢
Campbell's, New England	1 cup	200	6	2	T	🌢
Chowda, New England, frozen	1 cup	280	17	1		🌢
Healthy Choice, New England	1 cup	120	1	3		☺
Progresso	1 cup	190	10	1		🌢
Progresso, Manhattan	1 cup	110	2	3		☺
Progresso, New England, 99% fat free	1 cup	130	2	2		✂
Sea Watch, Manhattan	1 cup	90	3	2		🌢
Sea Watch, New England	1 cup	120	5	1		🌢

☺ = Eat as much as you want • ✂ = Cut Back

	Portion	Calories	Total Fat	Dietary Fiber	Trans Fat	Guide
Snow's, New England	1 cup	160	4	0	T	💣

Canned, Cream

	Portion	Calories	Total Fat	Dietary Fiber	Trans Fat	Guide
Campbell's, 98% fat free, cream of broccoli	1 cup	160	6	2	T	💣
Campbell's, 98% fat free, cream of celery	1 cup	140	6	2	T	💣
Campbell's, 98% fat free, cream of chicken	1 cup	160	6	0		💣
Campbell's, 98% fat free, cream of mushroom	1 cup	140	6	0	T	💣
Campbell's, Healthy Request, cream of celery	1 cup	140	4	2	T	💣
Campbell's, Healthy Request, cream of chicken	1 cup	140	4	0	T	💣
Campbell's, Healthy Request, cream of mushroom	1 cup	140	6	0	T	💣
Campbell's, Home Cookin', cream of mushroom	1 cup	80	2	1	T	💣
Campbell's, cream of asparagus	1 cup	220	14	2	T	💣
Campbell's, cream of broccoli	1 cup	200	12	2	T	💣
Campbell's, cream of celery	1 cup	220	14	2	T	💣
Campbell's, cream of chicken w/herbs	1 cup	160	8	2		💣
Campbell's, cream of mushroom	1 cup	220	14	2	T	💣
Campbell's, cream of potato	1 cup	180	6	2	T	💣
Campbell's, cream of shrimp	1 cup	200	14	2	T	💣

Canned, Kosher

	Portion	Calories	Total Fat	Dietary Fiber	Trans Fat	Guide
Goodman's, Quick & Hearty, chicken style	1 container	120	2	2	T	💣
Goodman's, Quick & Hearty, instant beef	1 container	120	2	1	T	💣
Manischewitz, chicken noodle	1 pkg.	140	2	0	T	💣
Manischewitz, chicken rice instant	1 pkg.	130	1	1	T	💣
Manischewitz, hearty lentil	1 pkg.	140	1	2		✂
Mrs. Manischewitz, chicken couscous	1 cup	180	2	1		✂
Mrs. Manischewitz, lentil pilaf	1 cup	140	1	2		✂
Mrs. Manischewitz, pasta marinara	1 cup	200	2	1		✂
Mrs. Manischewitz, vegetarian chili	1 cup	150	2	4		☺
Rokeach, barley & bean	1 cup	240	4	12		☺
Rokeach, vegetable	1 cup	60	0	3		☺
Tradition Instant Noodle, chicken	1 container	310	13	1		💣
Tradition Instant Noodle, tomato beef	1 container	310	14	1		💣

Canned, Minestrone

	Portion	Calories	Total Fat	Dietary Fiber	Trans Fat	Guide
Campbell's	1 cup	200	4	8		💣
Health Valley, Italian minestrone	1 cup	90	0	8		☺
Health Valley, fat free, real Italian	1 cup	80	0	11		☺
Healthy Choice	1 cup	110	1	5		☺
Progresso, parmesan	1 cup	100	3	3		💣
Progresso, season pasta, Italian herb shells	1 cup	120	2	4		☺

Canned, Potato

	Portion	Calories	Total Fat	Dietary Fiber	Trans Fat	Guide
Campbell's, Chunky, potato ham chowder, old fashioned	1 cup	220	14	3		💣
Campbell's, Home Cookin', creamy potato w/roasted garlic	1 cup	180	9	2	T	💣

💣 = Avoid • 💧 = Add for flavor

	Portion	Calories	Total Fat	Dietary Fiber	Trans Fat	Guide
Healthy Choice, baked potato	1 cup	140	2	4		☺
Progresso, 99% fat free, white cheddar potato	1 cup	140	3	2		🝡
Progresso, potato, ham & cheese	1 cup	170	7	1		🝡

Canned, Seafood

Phillips, vegetable crab, frozen	1 cup	80	2	2		✂
Sea Watch, lobster bisque	1 cup	200	15	0	T	🝡
Sea Watch, vegetable crab	1 cup	90	2	2		✂

Canned, Split Pea

Campbell's, w/ham & bacon	1 cup	360	8	10		🝡
Health Valley, split pea & carrots, fat free	1 cup	110	0	4		☺
Healthy Choice, & ham	1 cup	160	2	3		☺
Progresso, 99% fat free	1 cup	170	2	5		☺
Progresso, green	1 cup	170	3	5		✂

Canned, Tomato

Campbell's	1 cup	160	0	4		☺
Campbell's, Healthy Request	1 cup	180	4	2	T	🝡
Campbell's, Italian w/basil & oregano	1 cup	200	2	4		✂
Campbell's, tomato rice, old fashioned	1 cup	240	4	2	T	🝡
Healthy Choice, tomato garden	1 cup	100	2	5		☺
Progresso, basil	1 cup	100	2	1		✂
Progresso, hearty	1 cup	100	2	1		✂
Progresso, vegetable	1 cup	90	2	4		☺

Canned, Turkey

Campbell's, turkey noodle	1 cup	160	6	2		🝡
Healthy Choice, turkey w/white & wild rice	1 cup	90	2	2		✂
Progresso, turkey noodle	1 cup	90	2	0		✂
Progresso, turkey rice w/vegetables	1 cup	110	2	1		✂

Canned, Vegetable

Campbell's, Chunky, tomato ravioli w/vegetables	1 cup	150	3	3	T	🝡
Campbell's, French onion	1 cup	140	6	2		🝡
Campbell's, Healthy Request, hearty pasta & vegetables	1 cup	180	2	4	T	🝡
Campbell's, Healthy Request, vegetable	1 cup	180	2	4		☺
Campbell's, golden mushroom	1 cup	160	6	2	T	🝡
Campbell's, pepperpot	1 cup	200	10	2		🝡
Health Valley, 14 garden vegetable, fat free	1 cup	80	0	4		☺
Health Valley, 5 bean vegetable, fat free	1 cup	140	0	13		☺
Health Valley, barley vegetable, fat free	1 cup	90	0	4		☺
Health Valley, carotene super broccoli, fat free	1 cup	140	0	14		☺
Health Valley, country corn & vegetable, fat free	1 cup	70	0	7		☺
Health Valley, garden vegetable, fat free	1 cup	80	0	4		☺
Health Valley, healthy pasta, fat free	1 cup	100	0	4		☺

☺ = Eat as much as you want • ✂ = Cut Back

	Portion	Calories	Total Fat	Dietary Fiber	Trans Fat	Guide
Health Valley, tomato vegetable, fat free	1 cup	80	0	5		☺
Health Valley, vegetable barley, fat free	1 cup	90	0	4		☺
Healthy Choice, broccoli & cheddar	1 cup	110	2	2		✄
Healthy Choice, garden vegetable	1 cup	120	1	3		☺
Progresso, 99% fat free, tomato garden	1 cup	100	2	2		✄
Progresso, season pasta, peppercorn penne vegetable	1 cup	100	1	2		✄

Dry Mix

	Portion	Calories	Total Fat	Dietary Fiber	Trans Fat	Guide
Campbell's, onion	1 tbsp.	20	0	0		✄
Lipton, Soup Secrets, chicken noodle	3 tbsp.	80	2	0		✄
Lipton, Soup Secrets, extra noodle	3 tbsp.	90	2	0		✄
Lipton, noodle	2 tbsp.	60	2	0		✄
Nissin, Top Ramen, Oriental	$1/2$ block	190	7	1	T	☌
Nissin, Top Ramen, beef	$1/2$ block	190	7	1	T	☌
Nissin, Top Ramen, cajun chicken	$1/2$ block	180	7	1	T	☌
Nissin, Top Ramen, chicken	$1/2$ block	180	7	0	T	☌
Nissin, Top Ramen, chicken mushroom	$1/2$ block	190	7	1	T	☌
Nissin, Top Ramen, chicken vegetable	$1/2$ block	190	7	1	T	☌
Nissin, Top Ramen, creamy chicken	$1/2$ block	190	7	1	T	☌
Nissin, Top Ramen, picante beef	$1/2$ block	180	7	1	T	☌
Nissin, Top Ramen, shrimp	$1/2$ block	190	7	1	T	☌
Nissin, Top Ramen, smoked ham	$1/2$ block	180	7	0	T	☌
Westbrae Natural, brown rice ramen	$1/2$ block	140	1	2		✄
Wyler's, Soup Starter, beef vegetable	$1/8$ container	90	1	2	T	☌
Wyler's, Soup Starter, chicken noodle	$1/8$ container	80	1	1	T	☌
Wyler's, Soup Starter, hearty beef stew	$1/7$ container	80	0	2		✄
Wyler's, Soup Starter, hearty chicken vegetable	$1/7$ container	70	0	2		✄

Dry Mix, Bouillon

	Portion	Calories	Total Fat	Dietary Fiber	Trans Fat	Guide
Herbox, beef	1 pkt.	5	0	0	T	☖
Herbox, chicken	1 cube	5	0	0		☖
Wyler's, beef	1 cube	5	0	0	T	☖
Wyler's, chicken	1 cube	5	0	0	T	☖

Soup Cup, Bean

	Portion	Calories	Total Fat	Dietary Fiber	Trans Fat	Guide
Fantastic Foods, country lentil	1 pkg.	230	1	12		☺
Fantastic Foods, couscous w/lentils	1 pkg.	230	1	7		☺
Knorr, black bean soup	1 pkg.	190	1	10		☺
Knorr, hearty lentil	1 pkg.	200	1	5		☺
Nile Spice, black bean	1 pkg.	170	2	11		☺
Nile Spice, couscous lentil curry	1 pkg.	200	2	4		☺
Taste Adventure, curry lentil, Indian style	$2/3$ cup dry	210	1	19		☺

Soup Cup, Beef

	Portion	Calories	Total Fat	Dietary Fiber	Trans Fat	Guide
Campbell's, microwaveable, vegetable beef	1 container	140	1	5		☺
Maruchan Ramen, beef	$1/2$ block	190	8	1	T	☌
Nissin, Cup Noodles, beef	1 container	300	14	2	T	☌

☌ = Avoid • ☖ = Add for flavor

	Portion	Calories	Total Fat	Dietary Fiber	Trans Fat	Guide

Soup Cup, Chicken

	Portion	Calories	Total Fat	Dietary Fiber	Trans Fat	Guide
Campbell's, microwaveable, chicken noodle	1 container	130	4	2		🌢
Knorr, chicken noodle	1 pkg.	120	2	1		✂
Knorr, chicken vegetable	1 pkg.	120	2	1		✂
Lipton, Cup-A-Soup, cream of chicken	1 env.	70	2	0		✂
Lipton, Cup-A-Soup, hearty chicken	1 env.	60	1	0		✂
Maruchan Ramen, chicken	1/2 block	190	8	1	T	🌢
Maruchan Ramen, chicken mushroom	1/2 block	190	7	1	T	🌢
Nile Spice, chicken vegetable	1 pkg.	110	2	2		✂
Nissin, Cup Noodles, chicken	1 container	300	14	2	T	🌢
Nissin, Cup Noodles, chicken mushroom	1 container	300	14	2	T	🌢
Nissin, Cup Noodles, chicken vegetable	1 container	300	14	2	T	🌢
Nissin, Cup Noodles, creamy chicken	1 container	300	13	2	T	🌢
Nissin, Cup Noodles, spicy chicken	1 container	300	14	3	T	🌢

Soup Cup, Minestrone

	Portion	Calories	Total Fat	Dietary Fiber	Trans Fat	Guide
Fantastic Foods, minestrone	1 pkg.	150	1	4		☺
Nile Spice, couscous minestrone	1 pkg.	180	2	2		✂

Soup Cup, Oriental

	Portion	Calories	Total Fat	Dietary Fiber	Trans Fat	Guide
Maruchan Ramen, Oriental	1/2 block	190	8	1	T	🌢

Soup Cup, Shrimp

	Portion	Calories	Total Fat	Dietary Fiber	Trans Fat	Guide
Maruchan Ramen, shrimp	1/2 block	190	8	2	T	🌢
Nissin, Cup Noodles, w/shrimp	1 container	300	14	2	T	🌢

Soup Cup, Split Pea

	Portion	Calories	Total Fat	Dietary Fiber	Trans Fat	Guide
Fantastic Foods	1 pkg.	190	1	8		☺
Knorr	1 pkg.	150	1	4		☺
Taste Adventure	3/4 cup dry	220	1	16		☺

Soup Cup, Vegetable

	Portion	Calories	Total Fat	Dietary Fiber	Trans Fat	Guide
Fantastic Foods, corn & potato	1 pkg.	170	2	3		☺
Knorr, corn chowder	1 pkg.	140	3	2		🌢
Knorr, potato leek	1 pkg.	130	3	1		🌢
Knorr, vegetarian vegetable	1 pkg.	160	1	3		☺
Lipton, Cup-A-Soup, spring vegetable	1 env.	45	1	0		✂
Lipton, Cup-A-Soup, tomato	1 env.	90	1	0		✂
Nissin, Cup Noodles, French onion	1 container	300	12	2	T	🌢

■ SWEETNERS

Artificial

	Portion	Calories	Total Fat	Dietary Fiber	Trans Fat	Guide
Equal	1 pkt.	0	0	0		👍
Equal	1 tsp.	0	0	0		👍
Sugar Twin	1 pkt.	0	0	0		👍
Sweet'n Low	1/10 tsp.	0	0	0		👍

☺ = Eat as much as you want • ✂ = Cut Back

	Portion	Calories	Total Fat	Dietary Fiber	Trans Fat	Guide
Honey						
Sue Bee	1 tbsp.	60	0	0		✂
Sue Bee, clover spun	1 tbsp.	60	0	0		✂
Wild Flower, wild	1 tbsp.	60	0	0		✂
Jams & Jellies						
Chivers, orange marmalade, old English	1 tbsp.	50	0	0		✂
Knott's Berry Farm, boysenberry preserves	1 tbsp.	50	0	0		✂
Knott's Berry Farm, strawberry preserves	1 tbsp.	50	0	0		✂
Kraft, Sunberry Farms, grape jelly	1 tbsp.	50	0	0		✂
Kraft, Sunberry Farms, strawberry preserves	1 tbsp.	50	0	0		✂
Musselman's, apple butter	1 tbsp.	30	0	0		✂
Polaner, orange, sweet marmalade	1 tbsp.	60	0	0		✂
Polaner, preserves, chunky apricot	1 tbsp.	50	0	0		✂
Polaner, preserves, red raspberry	1 tbsp.	50	0	0		✂
Polaner, preserves, strawberry	1 tbsp.	50	0	0		✂
Polaner All Fruit, Pourable, raspberry	$^1/_4$ cup	120	0	0		✂
Polaner All Fruit, Spreadable, apricot	1 tbsp.	40	0	0		✂
Polaner All Fruit, Spreadable, black cherry	1 tbsp.	40	0	0		✂
Polaner All Fruit, Spreadable, blueberry	1 tbsp.	40	0	0		✂
Polaner All Fruit, Spreadable, grape	1 tbsp.	40	0	0		✂
Polaner All Fruit, Spreadable, peach	1 tbsp.	40	0	0		✂
Polaner All Fruit, Spreadable, pineapple	1 tbsp.	40	0	0		✂
Polaner All Fruit, Spreadable, raspberry	1 tbsp.	40	0	0		✂
Polaner All Fruit, Spreadable, raspberry, seedless	1 tbsp.	40	0	0		✂
Polaner All Fruit, spreadable, strawberry	1 tbsp.	40	0	0		✂
Reese, jellied mint sauce w/mint leaves	1 tbsp.	50	0	0		✂
Smucker's, strawberry preserves	1 tbsp.	50	0	0		✂
Welch's, Squeezable, grape, Concord jelly	1 tbsp.	50	0	0		✂
Welch's, Squeezable, strawberry spread	1 tbsp.	50	0	0		✂
Welch's, grape, Concord jelly	1 tbsp.	50	0	0		✂
White House, apple butter	1 tbsp.	35	0	0		✂
Molasses						
Grandma's Molasses	1 tbsp.	50	0	0		✂
Sugar						
Brown sugar, dark	1 tsp.	15	0	0		✂
Brown sugar, light	1 tsp.	16	0	0		✂
Domino, brown, dark	1 tsp.	15	0	0		✂
Domino, brown, dark, old fashion	1 tbsp.	15	0	0		✂
Domino, brown, golden light	1 tbsp.	15	0	0		✂
Domino, brown, light	1 tsp.	15	0	0		✂
Domino, brown, light, granulated	1 tbsp.	10	0	0		✂
Domino, confectioners 10-X	$^1/_4$ cup	120	0	0		✂
Domino, confectioners 10-X, chocolate	$^1/_4$ cup	110	0	0		✂
Domino, confectioners 10-X, lemon	$^1/_4$ cup	110	0	0		✂

	Portion	Calories	Total Fat	Dietary Fiber	Trans Fat	Guide
Domino, confectioners 10-X, strawberry	1/4 cup	110	0	0		✂
Domino, dots, cubes	1 cube	10	0	0		✂
Domino, granulated, pure sugar, packs	1 pack	15	0	0		✂
Domino, instant dissolving sugar	1 tsp.	15	0	0		✂
Estee, Fructose natural sweetener	1 pkt.	10	0	0		✂
Granulated	1 tsp.	15	0	0		✂
Hain, natural turbinado sugar	1 tsp.	15	0	0		✂
Powdered	1/4 cup	120	0	0		✂
Sugar Twin, spoonable	1 tsp.	0	0	0		✂
Sugar Twin, spoonable, brown sugar replacement	1 tsp.	0	0	0		✂
Sweet 10	10 drops	0	0	0		✂

■ VEGETABLES & BEANS

Beans, Canned

	Portion	Calories	Total Fat	Dietary Fiber	Trans Fat	Guide
B & M, barbecue	1/2 cup	170	1	6		☺
B & M, brick-oven baked	1/2 cup	180	2	7		☺
Bush's Best, baked beans	1/2 cup	110	1	8		☺
Bush's Best, baked beans w/bacon & brown sugar	1/2 cup	150	1	7		☺
Bush's Best, baked beans w/onions	1/2 cup	150	2	6		☺
Bush's Best, baked beans, bold & spicy	1/2 cup	120	1	5		☺
Bush's Best, baked beans, deluxe vegetarian	1/2 cup	130	0	6		☺
Bush's Best, baked beans, homestyle	1/2 cup	150	2	8		☺
Bush's Best, baked beans, original	1/2 cup	150	1	7		☺
Campbell's, baked beans, New England style	1/2 cup	180	3	6	T	💣
Campbell's, baked beans, brown sugar & bacon flavored	1/2 cup	170	3	7	T	💣
Campbell's, baked brown sugar & bacon	1/2 cup	170	3	6		💣
Campbell's, pork & beans	1/2 cup	130	2	6		☺
Cannellini, white kidney beans	1/2 cup	100	1	5		☺
Chili beans, Mexican style	1/2 cup	110	1	6		☺
Fava	1/2 cup	110	0	5		☺
Garbanzo beans	1/2 cup	110	1	7		☺
Goya, black beans	1/2 cup	90	1	6		☺
Goya, chick peas	1/2 cup	100	2	7		☺
Goya, pink beans	1/2 cup	80	1	7		☺
Goya, pinto beans	1/2 cup	80	1	8		☺
Goya, red & black beans	1/2 cup	160	0	3		☺
Goya, red kidney beans	1/2 cup	90	1	8		☺
Goya, small red beans	1/2 cup	90	1	6		☺
Great Northern beans	1/2 cup	110	0	7		☺
Green Giant, Mexican	1/2 cup	110	1	6		☺
Green Giant, barbecue	1/2 cup	130	1	7		☺
Green Giant, honey bacon	1/2 cup	160	1	6		☺
Hanover, baked beans, brown sugar & bacon	1/2 cup	130	1	7		☺
Hanover, baked beans, hickory flavored	1/2 cup	150	0	6		☺
Hanover, baked beans, honey mustard	1/2 cup	170	1	6		☺

☺ = Eat as much as you want • ✂ = Cut Back

	Portion	Calories	Total Fat	Dietary Fiber	Trans Fat	Guide
Hanover, baked beans, vegetarian	1/2 cup	150	5	6		💣
Hanover, beans & rice	1/2 cup	200	1	7		☺
Hanover, pork & beans in tomato sauce	1/2 cup	120	2	7		☺
Hunt's, vegetarian	1/2 cup	140	1	5		☺
Kidney beans, dark red	1/2 cup	110	0	6		☺
Kidney beans, redskin	1/2 cup	110	0	6		☺
Old El Paso, refried beans w/green chiles	1/2 cup	100	1	6		☺
Old El Paso, refried beans, vegetarian	1/2 cup	100	1	6		☺
Old El Paso, refried beans, black	1/2 cup	110	2	6		☺
Ortega, refried beans, fat free	1/2 cup	120	0	9		☺
Pink	1/2 cup	80	1	7		☺
Pinto	1/2 cup	100	0	5		☺
Taco Bell, refried beans, fat free	1/2 cup	110	0	6		☺
Three bean salad	1/3 cup	100	1	3		☺
Van Camp's, Beanee Weenee	7.5 oz.	230	9	7		💣 ☺
Wax	1/2 cup	25	0	2		

Beans, Dry

	Portion	Calories	Total Fat	Dietary Fiber	Trans Fat	Guide
Adzuki	1/4 cup	160	1	6		☺
Baby lima	1/4 cup dry	70	0	15		☺
Black beans	1/4 cup dry	70	0	15		☺
Blackeye peas	1/4 cup dry	90	0	10		☺
Cranberry	1/2 cup	136	1	5		☺
Fava	1/4 cup	120	1	9		☺
Flageolet	1/4 cup	174	1	13		☺
Great Northern	1/4 cup dry	70	0	13		☺
Green split peas	1/4 cup dry	110	0	11		☺
Hurst's, HamBeens, 15 bean soup	3 tbsp.	120	1	9	T	💣
Hurst's, HamBeens, cajun 15 bean soup	3 tbsp.	120	1	9		☺
Hurst's, HamBeens, pinto beans w/ham flavor	3 tbsp.	120	1	6	T	💣
Large lima	1/4 cup dry	70	0	12		☺
Lentils	1/4 cup dry	70	0	9		☺
Lentils, French green	1/4 cup	160	1	14		☺
Lentils, brown	1/4 cup	168	1	13		☺
Lentils, orange	1/4 cup	160	1	9		☺
Mung	1/4 cup	160	1	9		☺
Navy beans	1/4 cup dry	80	0	12		☺
Pinto beans	1/4 cup dry	60	0	14		☺
Red kidney beans	1/4 cup dry	70	0	14		☺
Soy	85 grams	150	8	5		💣

Beans, Tofu

	Portion	Calories	Total Fat	Dietary Fiber	Trans Fat	Guide
Frieda's, soft tofu	3 oz.	45	3	0		💣
Mori-nu, silken style, extra firm	3 oz.	45	2	0		✂
Mori-nu, silken style, extra firm lite	3 oz.	35	1	0		✂
Mori-nu, silken style, firm	3 oz.	50	3	0		💣
Nasoya, tofu	1/5 block	90	5	0		💣

💣 = Avoid • ✂ = Add for flavor

	Portion	Calories	Total Fat	Dietary Fiber	Trans Fat	Guide
Vegetables, Canned						
Allens, collard greens, sunshine chopped	1/2 cup	30	1	3		☺
Artichoke hearts	1/2 cup	30	0	1		☺
Chun King, chow mein vegetables	2/3 cup	15	0	1		☺
Corn, cream style	1/2 cup	90	1	2		☺
Del Monte, carrots, fresh cut, sliced	1/2 cup	35	0	3		☺
Del Monte, corn, fresh cut, fiesta	1/2 cup	50	1	2		☺
Del Monte, corn, whole kernel sweet	1/2 cup	70	1	3		☺
Del Monte, peas & carrots	1/2 cup	60	0	2		☺
Del Monte, tomato, chunky chili style	1/2 cup	30	0	2		☺
Del Monte, tomato, chunky pasta style	1/2 cup	45	0	2		☺
Del Monte, tomato, stewed cajun recipe	1/2 cup	35	0	2		☺
French's, onions, french fried real	2 tbsp.	45	4	0	T	🍂
Goya, jalapeño	2 peppers	10	0	0		☺
Goya, peas, green pigeon	1/2 cup	70	0	4		☺
Goya, peppers, pickled hot	1 tsp.	0	0	0		☺
Goya, peppers, serrano	4 peppers	15	0	1		☺
Green Beans, cut & French style	1/2 cup	20	0	2		☺
Green Giant, Mexicorn	1/3 cup	60	0	1		☺
Green Giant, asparagus spears	4.5 oz.	20	0	1		☺
Green Giant, corn, green bean & carrots	1/2 cup	40	0	2		☺
Green Giant, corn, niblets	1/3 cup	70	0	2		☺
Green Giant, mushrooms, sliced	1/2 cup	30	0	2		☺
Green Giant, peas, sweet w/tiny pearl onions	1/2 cup	60	0	4		☺
Hanover, three bean salad	1/3 cup	100	1	3		☺
Hunt's, tomato, Italian style	2 tomatoes	20	0	0		☺
Hunt's, tomato, crushed	1/2 cup	30	0	1		☺
Hunt's, tomato, diced	1/2 cup	25	0	1		☺
Hunt's, tomato, paste	2 tbsp.	25	0	0		☺
Hunt's, tomato, puree	1/4 cup	25	0	0		☺
Hunt's, tomato, stewed	1/2 cup	30	0	0		☺
Kame, corn, baby cocktail	1/2 cup	20	0	2		☺
Kame, ginger, sliced	20 pieces	17	0	0		☺
Kame, mushrooms, straw	1/2 cup	20	0	0		☺
La Choy, bean sprouts	1 cup	10	0	1		☺
La Choy, fancy mixed Chinese	2/3 cup	10	0	0		☺
Lavictora, jalapeño peppers, marinated	1.5 pieces	10	0	0		☺
Lesueur, asparagus spears, tender green	4.5 oz.	20	0	1		☺
Lesueur, carrots, whole	1/2 cup	35	0	3		☺
Lima beans	1/2 cup	80	0	4		☺
Mitchell's, corn, Shoepeg white	1/2 cup	100	1	2		☺
Old El Paso, green chiles, chopped	2 tbsp.	5	0	1		☺
Old El Paso, green chiles, peeled	2 tbsp.	5	0	1		☺
Old El Paso, jalapeño slices	2 tbsp.	10	0	1		☺
Old El Paso, tamales	3 tamales	330	19	5		🍂
Onions, whole	1/2 cup	40	0	1		☺
Ortega, jalapeño, sliced	1/4 cup	10	0	0		☺
Peas, sweet	1/2 cup	60	0	4		☺
Potato, Irish	1/2 cup	60	0	1		☺

☺ = Eat as much as you want • ✂ = Cut Back

	Portion	Calories	Total Fat	Dietary Fiber	Trans Fat	Guide
Potato, sweet, whole	1/2 cup	100	0	1		☺
Progresso, artichoke hearts	1 piece	15	0	1		☺
Progresso, tomato, crushed	1/4 cup	20	0	1		☺
Read, Potato, German salad	1/2 cup	120	3	2		🌢
Sliced beets	4 slices	20	0	0		☺
Spinach, whole leaf	1/2 cup	30	0	2		☺
Sun of Italy, hot giardiniera	1/4 cup	5	0	0		☺
Sun of Italy, mushrooms, marinated	1/4 cup	10	0	0		☺
Sun of Italy, peppers, cherry, hot, ground	1 tbsp.	5	0	0		☺
Sun of Italy, peppers, roasted	1/2 cup	25	0	0		☺
Trappey's, okra, cut	1/2 cup	25	0	3		☺
Tyling, stir fry mixed Chinese vegetables	2/3 cup	15	0	2		☺
Vlasic, pepper, hot rings	12 pepper rings	5	0	0		☺
Vlasic, pepper, mild rings	12 pepper rings	5	0	0		☺
Vlasic, pepperoncini, salad peppers	2 peppers	5	0	0		☺
Vlasic, peppers, Mexican, hot tiny	9 peppers	10	0	0		☺
Whole beets	1/2 cup	40	0	2		☺
Zucchini	1/2 cup	30	0	1		☺

Vegetables, Dry Mix, Potato

	Portion	Calories	Total Fat	Dietary Fiber	Trans Fat	Guide
Betty Crocker, 4 cheese mashed	1/2 cup prepard	90	1	1	T	🌢
Betty Crocker, Potato Buds	1/3 cup mix	80	0	1		☺
Betty Crocker, au gratin	1/2 cup prepard	100	1	1	T	🌢
Betty Crocker, butter & herb mashed	1/2 cup prepard	100	2	1	T	🌢
Betty Crocker, cheddar & bacon	1/2 cup prepard	100	2	1	T	🌢
Betty Crocker, hash brown, real	1/2 cup prepard	130	0	2		☺
Betty Crocker, ranch	1/2 cup prepard	100	1	1	T	🌢
Betty Crocker, roasted garlic mashed	1/2 cup prepard	90	2	1	T	🌢
Betty Crocker, scalloped	1/2 cup prepard	100	1	1	T	🌢
Betty Crocker, sour cream & chives	1/2 cup prepard	100	2	1	T	🌢
Betty Crocker, sour cream & chives mashed	1/3 cup	90	1	1	T	🌢
Betty Crocker, three cheese, real	1/2 cup prepard	110	2	1	T	🌢
Fantastic Foods, Stuffed-Mashed, cheddar cheese	1/4 cup	100	2	2		✂
Fantastic Foods, Stuffed-Mashed, sour cream & chives	1/4 cup	100	2	2		✂
Hungry Jack, au gratin	1/2 cup	110	1	1	T	🌢
Hungry Jack, mashed	1/2 cup prepard	80	0	1	T	🌢
Idaho Spuds	1/3 cup flakes	80	0	1		☺
Pillsbury, Idaho mashed	1/2 cup prepard	90	0	2		☺
Pillsbury, Idaho spuds	1/2 cup prepard	80	0	1		☺
Washington, instant mashed	1/3 pkg. mix	85	0	1		☺

Vegetables, Fresh

	Portion	Calories	Total Fat	Dietary Fiber	Trans Fat	Guide
Alfalfa, sprouts	1 cup	30	1	2		☺
Artichoke	3.5 oz.	40	2	2		✂
Arugula	1 oz.	7	0	1		☺
Asparagus	1 cup	29	0	1		☺

🌢 = Avoid • 👌 = Add for flavor

	Portion	Calories	Total Fat	Dietary Fiber	Trans Fat	Guide
Bamboo shoots	1/2 cup	21	0	1		☺
Beans, green, snap or string, cooked	1 cup	31	0	1		☺
Beets	1 cup	54	1	1		☺
Bok choy, baby	1 cup	24	0	1		☺
Broccoli	1 cup	40	0	2		☺
Brussels sprouts	1/2 cup	19	0	2		☺
Cabbage, Chinese	1 cup	16	0	1		☺
Cabbage, green	1 cup	24	0	1		☺
Cabbage, red	1 cup	22	0	1		☺
Cabbage, savoy	1 cup	17	1	1		☺
Carrot	1 med.	35	0	2		☺
Carrot, baby	1 cup	45	0	2		☺
Cauliflower	1 cup	28	0	1		☺
Celery	1 cup	21	0	1		☺
Chile, hot	1 med.	18	0	1		☺
Chives	1 tbsp.	1	0	1		☺
Cilantro	1/4 cup	6	0	1		☺
Corn	1/2 cup	89	1	2		☺
Corn	1 med. ear	80	1	3		☺
Cress, garden	1/2 cup	8	0	1		☺
Cucumber	1 med.	38	0	2		☺
Eggplant	1/2 cup	25	0	1		☺
Endive	1 cup	9	0	1		☺
Escarole	1 cup	9	0	1		☺
Fennel	3.5 oz.	28	0	1		☺
Garlic	1 clove	4	0	1		☺
Ginger, crystalized	3 pieces	100	0	1		✄
Ginger root, sliced	1/4 cup	17	0	1		☺
Green chard	1 cup	26	0	1		☺
Greens, collard	1 cup	88	1	1		☺
Greens, dandelion	1 cup	26	0	1		☺
Greens, kale	1 cup	31	1	1		☺
Greens, mizuna	1 cup	43	1	0		☺
Greens, mustard	1 cup	43	1	1		☺
Greens, turnip	1 cup	14	0	1		☺
Kohlrabi, sliced	1/2 cup	19	0	3		☺
Leeks, chopped	1/2 cup	32	0	1		☺
Lettuce, Boston	1 cup	8	0	1		☺
Lettuce, butterhead	1 head	21	0	2		☺
Lettuce, iceburg	1 cup	7	0	1		☺
Lettuce, leaf, green	1 cup	9	0	1		☺
Lettuce, leaf, red	1 cup	10	0	1		☺
Lettuce, romaine	1 cup	12	0	1		☺
Lettuce, romaine, red	1 cup	12	0	1		☺
Mushrooms	5 med.	20	0	1		☺
Mushrooms, enoki	1 cup	20	0	1		☺
Mushrooms, jumbo	1 cup	20	0	1		☺
Mushrooms, portobello	1 cup	20	0	1		☺
Mushrooms, portobello, dried	3.6 g.	11	0	1		☺

☺ = Eat as much as you want • ✄ = Cut Back

	Portion	Calories	Total Fat	Dietary Fiber	Trans Fat	Guide
Mushrooms, shiitake	1 cup	20	0	1		☺
Okra, sliced	1/2 cup	19	0	1		☺
Onion	1 med.	60	0	3		☺
Onion, green, chopped	1 cup	60	0	1		☺
Onion, pearl	1 cup	61	0	1		☺
Parsley, Italian, chopped	1 cup	26	0	1		☺
Parsley, chopped	1 cup	26	0	1		☺
Parsnip, diced	1 cup	102	1	3		☺
Peas, green, shelled	1/2 cup	58	0	4		☺
Peas, snow, cooked	1 cup	64	0	2		☺
Peas, sugar snap	1/2 cup	57	0	2		☺
Pepper, bell, green	1 pepper	16	0	1		☺
Pepper, bell, red	1 pepper	23	0	1		☺
Pepper, bell, yellow	1 pepper	16	0	1		☺
Peppers, chili, green & red	1 med.	18	0	1		☺
Potato	1 med.	100	0	3		☺
Potato, red	1 med.	88	0	7		☺
Potato, sweet	1 med.	136	0	4		☺
Pumpkin, cubes	1/2 cup	15	0	1		☺
Radicchio, shredded	1/2 cup	5	0	1		☺
Radish	3 radishes	8	0	1		☺
Radish, Asian	1 med.	62	0	5		☺
Rhubarb, diced	1/2 cup	13	0	1		☺
Rutabaga, cubed	1/2 cup	25	0	2		☺
Seaweed, kelp	1 oz.	12	0	1		☺
Shallot	1 tbsp.	7	0	1		☺
Spinach	1 cup	14	0	1		☺
Squash, butternut	1/2 cup	32	0	1		☺
Squash, chayote	1 cup	22	0	1		☺
Squash, summer	1/2 med.	20	0	1		☺
Squash, yellow	1 cup	26	0	1		☺
Squash, zucchini	1 cup	22	0	1		☺
Tomato	1 med.	35	1	1		☺
Tomato, green	1 med.	30	0	2		☺
Tomato, roma	4–5 each	27	0	1		☺
Turnip	1 cup	29	0	1		☺
Water chestnuts, Chinese	4 med.	38	0	1		☺
Watercress	1 cup	24	0	1		☺
Yam	1 med.	136	0	4		☺

Vegetables, Frozen

	Portion	Calories	Total Fat	Dietary Fiber	Trans Fat	Guide
Beans, green, cut	2/3 cup	25	0	2		☺
Beans, green, petite	3/4 cup	25	0	3		☺
Beans, lima, baby	1/2 cup	110	0	5		☺
Birds Eye, Pasta Secrets, Italian pesto	2 1/3 cups	240	9	2	T	💣
Birds Eye, Pasta Secrets, primavera	2 1/3 cups	230	10	3	T	💣
Birds Eye, Pasta Secrets, three cheese	2 cups	230	8	2	T	💣
Birds Eye, Pasta Secrets, white cheddar	2 cups	240	10	2	T	💣
Birds Eye, Pasta Secrets, zesty garlic	2 cups	240	10	2	T	💣

💣 *= Avoid* • 👍 *= Add for flavor*

Total	Portion Dietary	Calories Trans				
Birds Eye, stir fry, Oriental	2 1/4 cups	210	4	2		💧
Birds Eye, stir fry, asparagus	2 cups	90	1	3		☺
Birds Eye, stir fry, pepper	3 oz.	25	0	2		☺
Birds Eye, stir fry, spicy Asian	2 1/4 cups	230	2	3		☺
Birds Eye, stir fry, sugar snap	1 cup	40	0	2		☺
Birds Eye, stir fry, teriyaki	2 cups	210	3	3		💧
Broccoli, florets	4 florets	25	0	2		☺
Brussels sprouts, petite	1/2 cup	40	0	4		☺
Cauliflower, florets	4 pieces	20	0	2		☺
Corn, sweet, yellow	2/3 cup	80	1	1		☺
Corn, white	2/3 cup	80	1	1		☺
Dole, peeled mini carrots	3 oz.	40	0	2		☺
Green Giant, Pasta Accents, Oriental style	2 1/2 cups	270	10	4	T	💧
Green Giant, Pasta Accents, alfredo	2 cups	210	8	4	T	💧
Green Giant, Pasta Accents, creamy cheddar	2 1/3 cups	250	8	5	T	💧
Green Giant, Pasta Accents, garlic seasoning	2 cups	260	10	3	T	💧
Green Giant, Pasta Accents, lasagna style	2 cups	260	10	4	T	💧
Green Giant, broccoli spears	3.5 oz.	25	0	2		☺
Green Giant, sugar snap peas	2/3 cup	50	0	3		☺
Mixed	2/3 cup	60	1	3		☺
Okra, cut	3/4 cup	25	0	3		☺
Peas, sugar snap	3/4 cup	30	0	3		☺
Peas, sweet	2/3 cup	70	1	4		☺
Pepper, green, diced	3/4 cup	20	0	2		☺
Spinach, creamed	1/2 cup	120	6	3	T	💧
Spinach, packed leaf	1 cup	20	0	2		☺

☺ = Eat as much as you want • ✂ = Cut Back

▰ NOTES

Journal Abbreviations Used

Am J Clin Nutr = American Journal of Clinical Nutrition

Am J Epidemiology = American Journal of Epidemiology

Am J Hypertension = American Journal of Hypertension

Archives Internal Med = Archives of Internal Medicine

Bol Assoc Med P R = Asociacion Medica de Puerto Rico

Br Med J = British Medical Journal

Cancer Epidemiol Biomarkers Prev = Cancer Epidemiology Biomarkers and Prevention

Cancer Res = Cancer Research

Contemp Nutr = Contemporary Nutrition

Diabetes Res Clin Pract = Diabetes Research and Clinical Practice

Eur J Clin Nutr = European Journal of Clinical Nutrition

Hum Nutr Clin Nutr = Human Nutrition Clinical Nutrition

Int Clin Nutr.= International Journal of Clinical Nutrition

Int J Cancer = International Journal of Cancer

J Am Diec Assoc = Journal of the American Dietetic Association

J Natl Cancer Inst = Journal of the National Cancer Institute

JAMA = Journal of the American Medical Association

N Eng J Med = New England Journal of Medicine

Nutr Cancer = Nutrition and Cancer

Chapter One—Counting Your Way to Health

1. Centers for Disease Control and Prevention, "Update: Review of overweight among children, adolescents and adults—United States, 1988-1994." *Morbidity and Mortality Weekly* Report 46 (9): 199-201 (March 7, 1997).

2. Centers for Disease Control and Prevention, "Prevalence of Overweight among adolescents—United States, 1988–1991." *Morbidity and Mortality Weekly* Report 43 (44): 818–20 (November 11, 1994).

3. Marelen Cimons, "As obesity standard drops, dieters' spirits may follow," *Los Angeles Times*, 5 June, 1998, A16.

4. M. Fumento, *The Fat of the Land* (New York: Penguin Putnam, 1997), xi.

Chapter Two—The 20/30 Rationale

1. See, for example: J. Polivy, "Psychological consequences of food restriction," *J Am Diet Assoc*: 96 (6): 589–592 (June 1996).

2. Steve Blair, American Heart Association's Annual Epidemiology meeting, 20 March, 1994.

3. C. Bouchard, "Is weight fluctuation a risk factor?" *New England J Med*, 1887-1889 (27 June, 1991). L. Lissner, et al, "Variability of body weight and health outcomes in the Framingham population," 1839–1843.

4. Jing Ma, Meir J Stampfer et al. "Methylenetetrahydrofolate Reductase Polymorphism, Dietary Interactions, and Risk of Colorectal Cancer," *Cancer Res*, (March 1997) 1098-1101.

5. R. L. Gebhard et al, "The role of gallbladder emptying in gallstone formation during diet-induced rapid weight loss," *Hepatology* 24 (3): 544–548 (September 1996).

6. A. Stafleu et al, "Nutritional knowledge and attitudes towards high-fat foods and low-fat alternatives in three generations of women," *Eur J Clin Nutr* 50 (1): 33-41 (January 1996).

7. V. Ganji and N. Betts, "Fat, Cholesterol, Fiber and Sodium Intakes of US Population: Evaluation of Diets Reported in 1987-88 Nationwide Food Consumption Survey," *Eur J Clin Nutr* 49 (12): 915-20 (December 1995).

8. M. B. Katan, "High-Oil Compared with Low-Fat, High-Carbohydrate Diets in the Prevention of Ischemic Heart Disease," *Am J Clin Nutr* 66 (Suppl 4): S974-S979 (October 1997). M. F. Oliver, "It is More Important to Increase the Intake of Unsaturated Fats Than to Decrease the Intake of Saturated Fats: Evidence from Clinical Trials Relating to Ischemic Heart Disease," *Am J Clin Nutr* 66 (Suppl 4): S980-S986 (October 1997). D. P. Rose, "Dietary Fatty Acids and Cancer," *Am J Clin Nutr* 66 (Suppl 4): S998-S1003 (October 1997). A. Ascherio and W. C. Willett, "Health effects of trans fatty acids." *Am J Clin Nutr* 66 (Suppl 4): S1006-S1010 (Oct. 1997). S. Shapiro, "Do Trans Fatty Acids Increase the Risk of Coronary Artery Disease? A Critique of the Epidemiologic Evidence," *Am J Clin Nutr* 66 (Suppl 4): S1011-S1017 (Oct. 1997). S. L. Connor and W. E. Conner, "Are Fish Oils Beneficial in the Prevention and Treatment of Coronary Artery Disease?" *Am J Clin Nutr* 66 (Suppl 4): S1020-S1031 (October 1997). B. Haber, "The Mediterranean Diet: a View from History." *Am J Clin Nutr* 66 (Suppl 4): S1053-S1057 (October 1997). See also D. C. Hatton, et al. "Improved Quality of Life in Patients with Generalized Cardiovascular Metabolic Disease on a Prepared Diet." *Am J Clin Nutr* 64 (6): 935-43 (December1996), which showed that giving busy people prepared low-fat, high-fiber food helps prevent heart attacks and strokes.

9. T. R. Kirk, S. Burkill, and M. Cursiter. "Dietary Fat Reduction Achieved by Increasing Consumption of a Starchy Food— an intervention study," *Eur J Clin Nutr* 51 (7): 455-61 (July 1997).

10. ibid.

Chapter Three—Preventing Disease the 20/30 Way

1. See, for example: A. Tannenbaum, "Genesis and Growth of Tumors: Ill Effects of a High-Fat Diet," *Cancer Res* 2: 468-75 (1942).

2. K. Yeung et al, "Comparisons of Diet and Biochemical Characteristics of Stool and Urine Between Chinese Populations with Low and High Colorectal Cancer Rates," *J Natl Cancer Inst* 82: 46-50 (1991).

3. See, for example, P. J. Goodwin and N. F. Boyd. "Critical Appraisal of the Evidence that Dietary Fat Intake is Related to Breast Cancer Risk in Humans," *J Natl Cancer Inst* 79 (3): 473-485 (September 1987).

A. Schztzkin et al, "The Dietary Fat-Breast Cancer Hypothesis is Alive." *JAMA* 261 (22): 3284-87 (1989).

4. G. Howe et al, "Dietary Factors and Risk of Breast Cancer: Combined Analysis of 12 Case-Control Studies," *J Natl Cancer Inst* 82: 561-9 (1990).

5. A. Whittemore et al, "Diet, Physical Activity, and C cancer Among Chinese in North America and China." *J Natl Cancer Inst* 82: 915-26 (1990). For more on the link between fat and colon cancer, see J. H. Weisburger, "Dietary Fat and the Risk of Chronic Disease: Mechanistic Iinsights from Experimental Studies," *J Am Diet Assoc* 97 (7 Suppl): S16-23 (July 1997).

6. C.L. Bird et al, "Obesity, Weight Gain, Large Weight Changes, and Adenomatous Polyps of the Left Colon and Rectum," *Am J Epidemiology* 147 (7): 670-80 (April 1, 1998).

7. D. Y. Kim, K. H. Chung and J. H. Lee, "Stimulatory Effects of High-Fat Diets on Colon Cell Proliferation Depend on the Type of Dietary Fat and Site of the Cancer," *Nutr Cancer* 30 (2): 118-123 (1988).

8. R. J. Calvert et al, "Reduction of Colonic Carcinogenesis by Wheat Bran Independent of Fecal Bile Acid Concentration," *J Natl Cancer Inst* 79 (4): 875-880 (October 1987).

9. D. A. Snowdon, Letter, *JAMA* 254 (3): 356-7 (1985).

10. See, for example, P. Greenward and E. Lanza, "Dietary Fiber and Colon Cancer," *Bol Assoc Med* P R 78 (7): 311-313 (1986). See also J. Slavin, D. Jacobs, and L. Marquart, "Whole-Grain Consumption and Chronic Disease: Protective Mechanisms," *Nutr Cancer* 27 (1): 14-21 (1997), which looks at the role whole grains play in combating cancer.

11. D. P. Rose. "Dietary fiber and breast cancer." *Nutr Cancer* 13:1-8, 1990.

12. R. E. Hughes, "Hypothesis: A New Look at Dietary Fiber," *Hum Nutr Clin Nutr* 40C: 81-86 (1986).

13. "Study Shows Link Between Diet and Breast Cancer," Tel Aviv University Report October 12,1986.

14. P. Greenward and E. Lanza, "Dietary Fiber and Colon Cancer." *Bol Assoc Med* P R 78 (7): 311-313 (1986).

15. G. A. Colditz et al, "Increased Green and Yellow Vegetable Intake and Lowered Cancer Deaths in an Elderly Population," *Am J Clin Nutr* 41 (1): 32-6 (1985).

16. C. LaVecchia et al, "Dietary Factors in the Risk of Bladder Cancer," *Nutr Cancer* 12: 93-101 (1989).

17. C. LaVecchia et al, "Dietary Factors and The Risk of Breast Cancer," *Nutr Cancer* 10: 205-14 (1987).

18. See, for example, K. M. Egan et al, "Risk Factors for Breast Cancer in Women with a Breast Cancer Family History," *Cancer Epidemiology Biomarkers Prev* 7 (5): 359-364 (May 1998).

19. R. Verreault et al, "A Case-Control Study of Diet and Invasive Cervical Cancer," *Intl J Cancer* 43: 1050-54 (1989).

20. F. Barbone et al, "Diet and Endometrial Cancer," Abstract. *Am J Epidemiology* 132: 783 (1990).

21. R. Zeigler et al, "Carotenoid Intake, Vegetables, and the Risk of Lung Cancer Among White Men in New Jersey," *Am J Epidemiology* 123 (6): 1080-93 (1986).

22. R. Ziegler et al, "Diet and the Risk of Vulvar Cancer," *Am J Epidemiology* 132: 778 (1990).

23. See, for example, R. Kearny, "Promotion and Prevention of Tumor Growth: Effects of Endotoxin, Inflammation and Dietary Lipids," *Int Clin Nutr* 7 (4): 157-68 (1987).

24. Roberto Marchioli, MD and Rosa Maria Marfisi et al, "Meta-Analysis, Clinical Trials, and Transferability of Research Results Into Practice: The Case of Cholesterol-Lowering Interventions in the Secondary Prevention of Coronary Heart Disease," *Archives Internal Med* 156 (11): 1158-1169 (June 1996).

25. M. A. Denke. "Role of Beef and Beef Tallow, an Anriched Source of Stearic Acid, in a Cholesterol-Lowering Diet," *Am J Clin Nutr* 60 (6 Suppl): S1044-1049 (December 1994). R. M. Dougherty, M. A. Allman and J. M. Iacono, "Total and Low-Density–Lipoprotein Cholesterol Lipoprotein fractions and Fecal Fatty Acid Excretion of Men Consuming Diets Containing High Concentrations of Stearic Acid," *Am J Clin Nutr* 60 (6 Suppl): S1043 (December 1994).

26. J. P. Midgley et al, "Effect of Reduced Dietary Sodium on Blood Pressure: a Meta-Analysis of Randomized Controlled Trials," *JAMA* 275 (20): 1590-1597 (May 22, 1996).

27. M. H. Alderman et al, "Low Urinary Sodium is Associated with Greater Risk of Myocardial Infarction Among Treated Hypertensive Men," *Hypertension* 25 (6): 1144-1152 (June 1995). M. H. Alderman et al, "Dietary Sodium Intake and Mortality: The National Health and Nutrition Examination Survey." *Lancet*: 351 (9105): 781-785 (March 13, 1998).

28. U. Appel et al, "A Clinical Trail of the Effects of Dietary Patterns on Blood Pressure," *N Eng J Med* 326: 1117-1124 (April 17, 1997). T.A. Kotchen et al, "Nutrition and Hypertension Prevention," *Hypertension* 18 (Suppl 1): 115-120 (September 1991). Hsui-Yueh Su et al, "Effective Weight Loss and Blood Pressure in Insulin Resistance in Normaltensive and Hypertensive Obese Individuals," *Am J Hypertension* 8 (11): 1067-1071 (November 1995).

29. P. Schlamowitz et al, "Treatment of Mild to Moderate Hypertension with Dietary Fibre," Letter. *Lancet* 2: 622-23 (1987).

30. A. Wright et al, "Dietary Fibre and Blood Pressure," *Br Med J* 2: 1541-42 (1979).

31. J. Barone et al, "Dietary Fat and Natural-Killer Cell Activity," *Am J Clin Nutr* 50: 861-67 (1989).

32. D. S. Kelley et al, "Energy Restriction Decreases Number of Circulating Natural Killer Cells and Serum Levels of Immunoglobulins in Overweight Women," *Eur J Clin Nutr* 48 (1): 9-18 (January 1994).

33. D. H. Han et al, "Insulin Resistance of Muscle Glucose Transport in Rats Fed a High-Fat Diet: a Reevaluation," *Diabetes* 46 (11): 1761-7 (November 1997). N. D. Oakes et al, "Mechanisms of Liver and Muscle Insulin Resistance Induced by Chronic High-Fat Feeding," *Diabetes* 46 (11): 1768-74 (November 1997). R. G. Moses et al, "The Recurrence of Gestational Diabetes: Could Dietary Differences in Fat Intake be an Explanation?" *Diabetes Care* 20 (11): 1647-50 (November 1997).

34. M. Toeller et al, "Protein Intake and Urinary Albumin Excretion Rates in the EURODIAB IDDM Complications Study," *Diabetologia* 40 (10): 1219-26 (October 1997).

35. E. M. Berry, "Dietary Fatty Acids in the Management of Diabetes Mellitus," *Am J Clin Nutr* 66 (4 Suppl): 991S-997S (October 1997).

36. E. M. Berry. "Dietary Fatty Acids in the Management of Diabetes Mellitus," *Am J Clin Nutr* 66 (4 Suppl): 991S-997S (October 1997).

37. N. Okauchi et al, "Is Caloric Restriction Effective in Preventing Diabetes Mellitus in the Otsuka Long Evans Tokushima Fatty Rat, a Mode of Spontaneous Non-Insulin–Dependent Diabetes Mellitus?" *Diabetes Res Clin Pract* 27 (2): 97-106 (February 1995).

Chapter Four—Phytochemicals, The "Medicines" In Foods

1. Paul Knekt, Ritva Jarvinen et al, "Dietary Flavonoids and the Risk of Lung Cancer and Other Malignant Neoplasms," *Am J Epidemiology* 146 (3): 223-230 (August 1997). Lee-Chen Yong, Charles C. Brown et al, "Intake of Vitamins E, C, and A and Risk of Lung Cancer. The NHANES I Epidemiologic Followup Study," *Am J Epidemiology* 146 (3): 231-243 (August 1997). Marc T. Goodman, Lynne R. Wilkens et al, "Association of Soy and Fiber Consumption with the Risk of Endometrial Cancer," *Am J Epidemiology* 146 (4): 294-304 (August 1997).

Chapter Five—Playing For Better Health

1. S. B. Racette et al, "Exercise Enhances Dietary Compliance During Moderate Energy Restriction in Obese Women," *Amer J Clin Nutr*, 62 (2): 345-349 (August 1995).

2. S. J. Whiting, D. J. Anderson, and S. J. Weeks, "Calciuric Effects of Protein and Potassium Bicarbonate but Not of Sodium Chloride or Phosphate can be Detected Acutely in Adult Women and Men," *Am J Clin Nutr* 65 (5):1465-1472 (May 1997).

3. A. Sebastian, "Improved Mineral Balance and Skeletal Metabolism in Post-Menopausal Women Treated with Potassium Bicarbonate," *N Eng J Med* 330: 1776-1781 (June 23, 1994).

4. I. Thune, "Physical Activity and the Risk of Breast Cancer," *N Eng J Med* 336: 1269-75 (May 1, 1997).

5. A. Hakim et al, "Effects of Walking on Mortality Among Nonsmoking Retired Men," *N Eng J Med* 338 (2): 94-99 (January 1998).

The source for the BMI chart is the National Center for Health Statistics.

INDEX

A

aerobic exercise, 50-52, 54, 61
African Berbere Spice Blend, 98
antioxidants, 42
artichokes
  Artichoke Dip, 143
  Spaghetti Squash Soup with
    Artichokes, 109
asparagus
  Chinese Asparagus Salad, 114
  Cream of Asparagus Soup, 107
  Quinoa with Asparagus and
    Mushrooms, 131

B

bananas
  Banana-Pineapple Ice, 148
  Banana "Rice" Pudding, 149
Barbecue Beans and Barley, 131
barley
  Barbecue Beans and Barley, 131
  Barley-Bean Salad, 118
  Barley Biryani, 137
  Fastest Beans and Barley, 133
  Mango Salad with Barley and
    Beans, 112
  Mushroom-Barley Soup, 102
  Split Pea-Barley Pot, 108
  Sweet Potato and Barley Chili, 121
beans, 71-72
  Barbecue Beans and Barley, 131
  Barley-Bean Salad, 118
  Bean-Eggplant-Tomato Casserole, 217
  Bean-Pepper Salsa, 140
  chilis, 120-121
  Creole Beans 'n' Greens, 132
  Fastest Beans and Barley, 133
  Kasha-Bean "Meatballs," 142
  Mango Salad with Barley
    and Beans, 112
  Smoked Salmon-Butter
    Bean Salad, 115
  Three-Bean Curry, 124
bioflavonoids, 44
blood pressure, 20/30 Plan and, 34-36.
    See also cardiovascular disease
body fat, measuring, 51. See also Body
    Mass Index; obesity; weight loss
Body Mass Index (BMI), 2-3, 61-62
bouillon, 95
brain, stroke and, 33-34
breakfast cereals, 24, 69

Broccoli Stalk Slaw, 110
bulgur
  Spring Tabbouleh, 113
  Sweet and Zingy Bulgur Salad, 116

C

cancer, 20/30 Plan and, 26-30
carbohydrates, sugar and, 18-20.
    See also refined grains; whole grains
cardiovascular disease
  exercise and, 50-52
  20/30 Plan and, 30-33
Caribbean Caviar, 144
Caribbean Lentil Salad, 115
Caribbean Lentil Soup, 105
Cassoulet, 134
Catfish Gumbo, 126
chick peas
  Chick Pea Soup, 103
  Quick Curried Chick Peas, 124
chicken, 33
chilis, 120-121
Chinese Asparagus Salad, 114
cholesterol
  cancer and, 27
  exercise and, 52
  fat consumption and, 14
  HDL vs. LDL, 32-33
Clam Chowder, 106
Clementine Sorbet, 147
couscous, 122-123
Cream of Asparagus Soup, 107
Creamy Fruit Sorbet, 150
Creole Beans 'n' Greens, 132
Cuban Hash, 126
Cuban Sweet Potato Salad, 117
curries, 124-125
  Curried Lentils and Mushrooms, 123
  Curried Quinoa, 138

D

desserts, 145-150
Dessert Spice Blend, 99
diabetes
  blood sugar levels and, 68
  20/30 Plan and, 38-40
dieting, effects of, 10-11.
    See also weight loss
dining out, 80-81
doom & gloom, 88-89
Double Mushroom-Grain Soup, 101

E

emotional state, exercise and, 52
entrees, 120-135
estrogen, cancer and, 28-29.
    See also phytoestrogens
exercise, 48-62
    aerobic, 50-52, 54, 61
    flexibility and, 52-53, 56-57
    options, 60
    programs, 57-60
    strength and, 52-53, 54-56

F

Falafel Bites, 141
Fall Mulligatawny Soup, 105
Farmer's Paella, 132
fast foods, 80
Fastest Beans and Barley, 133
fat. See body fat
fat-free foods, 7, 77
fats
    blood pressure and, 35-36
    cancer and, 26-28
    consumption of, 3-4, 14-17
    fatty foods, 78
    good vs. bad, 11-14
    partially hydrogenated oils, 79
    reducing intake of, 64-65
Festive Wild Rice Salad, 113
fiber
    benefits of, 17-21
    blood pressure and, 36
    cancer and, 28-29
    consumption of, 4-5, 21-23
    increasing intake of, 65-66
    low-fiber foods, 78-79
fish, health benefits of, 34
flavor boosting tips, 64
flexibility, exercise and, 52-53, 56-57
Florentine Pea Soup, 104
foods, choosing, 76-81
fortified foods, 77
free radicals, 42
fruit
    desserts, 145-150
    peeling vs. not, 94-95
Fruity Nuggets, 147

G

Gallo Pinto, 128
Garam Masala Spice Blend, 98
Golden Soup, 108
grains. See refined grains; whole grains
gram counter keychain, 6-7
Greek Pilaf, 139

H

Harissa Sauce, 99
heart disease. See cardiovascular disease
high-protein diets, 11
Hot and Sour Mushroom Soup, 101
hypertension. See blood pressure

I

immune system, 20/30 Plan and, 37
impotence, 20/30 Plan and, 36
injury, avoiding and treating, 58
Irish Spring Soup, 100
isoflavones, 45

K

Kamut Waldorf Salad, 119
Kasha-Bean "Meatballs," 142
key chain counter, 6-7

L

labels, reading, 76-78
Lebanese Split Peas with Spinach
    and Lemon, 134
lentils
    Caribbean Lentil Salad, 115
    Caribbean Lentil Soup, 105
    Curried Lentils and Mushrooms, 123
    Lentil-Amaranth CanapÈs, 143
    Lentil Chili, 121
    Lentil Sprouts Salad, 117
    Lentil-Sweet Potato Dal, 104
    Summer Harira, 100
"light" foods, 77
liquids, flavored, 95-96

M

Malaysian Salad, 112
mangoes
    Mango-Melon Mist, 145
    Mango Salad with Barley
    and Beans, 112
    Sweet Potato-Mango Soup, 109
mayonnaise, 96
menu planning, 7-8
metabolism, exercise and, 49-50
Mexican Slaw, 110
Minestrone, 106
Minty Orange and Quinoa Salad, 114
Moroccan Fruit Pudding, 146
Moroccan Seafood Stew, 125
Mulligatawny Soup, 105
mushrooms
    Curried Lentils and Mushrooms, 123
    Double Mushroom-Grain Soup, 101

Hot and Sour Mushroom Soup, 101
Mushroom-Barley Soup, 102
Mushrooms with Grains, 138
Mushroom Pâté, 140

N

natural foods, 77-78
New England Clam Chowder, 106
Nineteen-Meals Rule, 8, 80

O

obesity
    diabetes and, 38-39
    diet and, 2-5
    exercise and, 61
    See also weight loss
omega fatty acids, 14
Orange and Quinoa Salad, 114
organic foods, 77-78

P

Paella, 132
partially hydrogenated oils, 79
Pâté, 140
peaches, baked, 145
pears, mulled, 146
peas. See split peas
phytochemicals, 42-46
phytoestrogens, 45
Picadillo, 126
Pineapple "Upside-Down Cake"
    Pudding, 148
Porotos Granados, 127
portion size, 77
potatoes
    Potato "Egg" Salad, 111
    Potato Goulash, 130
protein
    diabetes and, 38
    false promises of, 53
psychological state, exercise and, 52
pumpkin
    Pumpkin Soup, 103
    Wild Rice-Pumpkin Soup, 102

Q

quinoa
    Curried Quinoa, 138
    Malaysian Salad, 112
    Minty Orange and Quinoa
        Salad, 114
    Quinoa with Asparagus and
        Mushrooms, 131
    Quinoa Pilaf with Cherries, 136

R

recipes, 94-150
refined grains, 18-20, 67-68
restaurant eating, 80-81

S

salad dressings, 96
salads, 110-119
Salmon Mousse, 141
Salsa, 140
salt, blood pressure and, 35
Seafood Stew, 125
Sicilian Minestrone, 106
side dishes, 136-139
Smoked Salmon-Butter Bean Salad, 115
snacks, 140-144
soups, 100-109
Southwestern Salad, 118
spaghetti squash. See squash
Spanish "Rice," 130
Speedy Chick Pea Soup, 103
spice blends, 97-99
Spiced Fruit Compote, 150
split peas
    Florentine Pea Soup, 104
    Golden Soup, 108
    Lebanese Split Peas with Spinach
        and Lemon, 134
    Split Pea-Barley Pot, 108
Spring Couscous, 123
Spring Tabbouleh, 113
Spring Tonic Soup, 107
squash
    Porotos Granados, 127
    Spaghetti Squash Soup with
        Artichokes, 109
    Spaghetti Squash, Thai Style, 133
    Zippy Zucchini, 136
Stir-fry du Jour, 135
strength, exercise and, 52-53, 54-56
stroke, 33-34
sugar
    carbohydrates and, 18-20
    sugary foods, 78
Summer Harira, 100
Sushi Salad Supreme, 116
sweet potatoes
    Cuban Sweet Potato Salad, 117
    Lentil-Sweet Potato Dal, 104
    Sweet Potato and Barley Chili, 121
    Sweet Potato Curry with Bananas
        and Okra, 128
    Sweet Potato-Mango Soup, 109
Sweet and Sour Tofu, 129
Sweet and Zingy Bulgur Salad, 116

T

Tabbouleh, 113
Three-Bean Curry, 124
time saving tips, 72-73
tofu
    Potato "Egg" Salad, 111
    Sweet and Sour Tofu, 129
    Tofu Dressing, 119
    Tofu "Fried Rice," 129
triglycerides, 33
Two-Corn Green Chili, 120
Two-Grain Tropical Treat, 149
two-step secret to success, 84-92

V

vegetables
    cooking times for, 96-97
    peeling vs. not, 94-95

W

Waldorf Salad, 119
water consumption, benefits of, 55
weight loss
    exercise and, 49-50, 61-62
    guidelines for, 5-6
    20/30 formula for, 23-24
whole grains, 66-71
wild rice
    Wild Rice-Pumpkin Soup, 102
    Wild Rice Salad, 113
    Wild Rice with Snow Peas
        and Raspberries, 137
wrong reasons, 89-91

Y

Yogurt Dipping Sauce, 142
yo-yo dieting, 10

Z

Zippy Zucchini, 136
"Zone, The," 11